HANDBOOK

for Health Care Research

Second Edition

ROBERT L. CHATBURN, RRT-NPS, FAARC

Research Manager, Respiratory Institute
Cleveland Clinic
Cleveland, Ohio

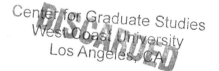

JONES AND BARTLETT PUBLISHERS
Sudbury, Massachusetts
BOSTON   TORONTO   LONDON   SINGAPORE

World Headquarters

Jones and Bartlett Publishers
40 Tall Pine Drive
Sudbury, MA 01776
978-443-5000
info@jbpub.com
www.jbpub.com

Jones and Bartlett Publishers
Canada
6339 Ormindale Way
Mississauga, Ontario L5V 1J2
Canada

Jones and Bartlett Publishers
International
Barb House, Barb Mews
London W6 7PA
United Kingdom

Jones and Bartlett's books and products are available through most bookstores and online booksellers. To contact Jones and Bartlett Publishers directly, call 800-832-0034, fax 978-443-8000, or visit our website www.jbpub.com.

Substantial discounts on bulk quantities of Jones and Bartlett's publications are available to corporations, professional associations, and other qualified organizations. For details and specific discount information, contact the special sales department at Jones and Bartlett via the above contact information or send an email to specialsales@jbpub.com.

The author, editor, and publisher have made every effort to provide accurate information. However, they are not responsible for errors, omissions, or for any outcomes related to the use of the contents of this book and take no responsibility for the use of the products and procedures described. Treatments and side effects described in this book may not be applicable to all people; likewise, some people may require a dose or experience a side effect that is not described herein. Drugs and medical devices are discussed that may have limited availability controlled by the Food and Drug Administration (FDA) for use only in a research study or clinical trial. Research, clinical practice, and government regulations often change the accepted standard in this field. When consideration is being given to use of any drug in the clinical setting, the health care provider or reader is responsible for determining FDA status of the drug, reading the package insert, and reviewing prescribing information for the most up-to-date recommendations on dose, precautions, and contraindications, and determining the appropriate usage for the product. This is especially important in the case of drugs that are new or seldom used.

Production Credits

Publisher: David Cella
Acquisitions Editor: Kristine Jones
Associate Editor: Maro Gartside
Production Manager: Julie Champagne Bolduc
Associate Production Editor: Jessica Steele Newfell
Marketing Manager: Grace Richards
Manufacturing and Inventory Control Supervisor: Amy Bacus
Composition: Spearhead Global, Inc.
Cover Design: Kristin E. Parker
Cover Image: © Loongar/Dreamstime.com
Printing and Binding: Malloy, Inc.
Cover Printing: Malloy, Inc.

Library of Congress Cataloging-in-Publication Data
Chatburn, Robert L.
  Handbook for health care research / Robert L. Chatburn. — 2nd ed.
      p. ; cm.
    Includes bibliographical references and index.
    ISBN 978-0-7637-7805-7 (pbk. : alk. paper)
1. Medicine—Research—Handbooks, manuals, etc.   I. Title.
    [DNLM: 1. Health Services Research—methods—Handbooks. 2. Research Design—Handbooks.
  W 49 C492h 2010]
  R850.C43 2010
  610.73072—dc22
                                     2009031526
6048

Printed in the United States of America
14 13 12 11 10   10 9 8 7 6 5 4 3 2

Dedication

Allied health professionals are rarely given formal training in research methodology. And even when they are, it is never more than a cursory overview. The real learning happens in apprenticeship. One must have a good mentor who can pass on the benefit of his knowledge and experience. I have been blessed with four of the best mentors a person could have.

The first is Marvin Lough, MBA, RRT, FAARC. Marv gave me my first job in the profession and helped me create a dedicated research position. He taught me that it is not what a person holds in memory that counts, but rather what he knows how to find. He has exemplified to me, in every way, what it means to be a professional, a leader, and a gentleman.

The second is Frank P. Primiano Jr., PhD. Frank has the most disciplined, logical and penetrating mind that I have ever encountered. He taught me the basic skills of a scientist. He taught me that brilliance lies in paying attention to the details and the supreme importance of defining and understanding the words you use. But most importantly, he taught me "If you explain something so that even a fool *can understand it…then only a fool* will *understand it."*

The third is Terry Volsko, MHHS, RRT, FAARC. I have never met anyone with a greater hunger for knowledge or a stronger will to succeed. She has been a brilliant and tireless colleague, an insightful critic, and a compassionate friend.

Fourth is James K. Stoller, MD, MSc, FAARC. Jamie taught me that scholarship without leadership is hollow. He convinced me that authority can be wielded with both humor and compassion to coax extraordinary results from talented people.

Brief Contents

Contents

Preface

Learning to conduct research is like learning to ride a bicycle: reading a book is not much help. You need to learn by doing, with someone holding you up the first few times. Yet, the student of health sciences research must be familiar with basic concepts that can be studied by reading. The trick is for an author to select the right topics and present them in a way that is both relevant and interesting.

Handbook for Health Care Research, Second Edition, is the result of my research experience in the field of respiratory care over the last 30 years. I have selected topics and statistical procedures that are common to medical research in general as well as to allied health care in particular. It is by no means an exhaustive treatise on any particular aspect of medical research. Rather, it is a practical guide to supplement specialized statistics textbooks, although it can function as a stand-alone text for a short course in research for a two- or four-year respiratory care or other allied health program. In fact, this book grew out of the notes I used for seven years to teach research at Cuyahoga Community College.

On one level, the book is geared for the student or health care professional who wants to become involved with research. Basic concepts are presented along with real-world examples. Naturally, because I am a respiratory therapist, the examples focus on respiratory care. However, the concepts are applicable to any area of medical research. I have tried to keep the theory and mathematics at the most elementary level. I assume that the reader will have basic computer skills and will have access to software that will handle the math. For that reason, unlike many books on the topic, this book gives no probability tables for calculating things like the critical values of the *t*-statistic. Computers have made hand calculations all but obsolete. What the student really needs to know is which procedure to use, when to use it, and why to use it.

For the experienced researcher, the book is organized for easy look-up of basic research procedures and definitions. When you are in the middle of a project, you do not want to have to dig through pages and pages of theory when you simply want to be reminded of which test to use or how to format the data for computer entry.

Not every health care professional will be directly involved with research. However, everyone will be involved with the results of research. Most will be involved with some sort of continuous quality improvement project, which will inevitably require familiarity with research techniques. Therefore, this book, if nothing else, is an excellent tool to help you become an "educated consumer" of research. After all, how can you appreciate the information in professional journals if you do not even know what a *p* value is? Researchers who publish in journals are trying to sell you their ideas. If you do not understand the procedures they use to generate their ideas and the language they use to sell them, you could end up "buying a lemon."

New to the Second Edition

For the *Second Edition* of *Handbook for Health Care Research*, the tables and figures have been fully updated and revised. Chapter 6, "Reviewing the Literature," has been rewritten to reflect the latest Internet resources. Appendix I is brand-new, and it provides valuable insight for improving your scientific writing skills. Chapter 15, "The Abstract," has been revised, and a new model paper is presented in Appendices V and VI.

Features of Handbook for Health Care Research

Several features in this book are unique. For example, the descriptions of statistical tests are standardized in a practical format. For each procedure, a hypothetical (or sometimes real-world) study problem is introduced, the hypothesis is stated, the data are given in the format that they are entered into the computer, and then a detailed report from an actual statistical program is given.

Another unique feature is Chapter 15, which focuses on writing the stand-alone abstract. The new researcher's first experience with publishing research will usually be in the form of an abstract rather than a full-text article. For this reason, I have placed particular emphasis on how to write an abstract that will pass peer review. There are model abstracts that have been published in *Respiratory Care*, along with examples of abstracts that show what *not* to do. I review each example in detail and explain the mistakes made. These detailed examples are intended to give the reader a mentor, someone looking over his or her shoulder and providing help and encouragement. In fact, this text is written in a conversational style throughout. This helps to illustrate the relevance of each new concept that might otherwise seem dull and intangible.

Finally, Appendix I is an unique tutorial for improving your science writing, authored by Matti Mero, an experienced copyeditor for *Respiratory Care*. As a copyeditor for a major medical journal, Matti has seen every kind of mistake. His suggestions will help you avoid them and make the experience of peer review much easier once you submit your manuscript for publication.

Also included in the appendices is a model manuscript that was published in *Respiratory Care*. I include the comments of the peer reviewers along with the authors' responses. One of the biggest obstacles for new researchers is that they have a hard time accepting critical comments about a manuscript they have submitted for publication. Many, maybe even most, are so discouraged that they do not make the suggested revisions, and their work goes to waste. My hope is that by reading actual reviewers' comments and the authors' responses, you will understand that (1) every researcher, no matter how experienced, will be criticized, and (2) the criticism leads to a better product if you follow through. I always tell my students that the first thing they have to learn is to put their egos on the shelf.

I hope *Handbook for Health Care Research, Second Edition*, becomes your practical go-to guide.

Acknowledgments

Much thanks to David J. Pierson, MD, for writing Chapter 16, "The Case Report." David first wrote this chapter for my book *Fundamentals of Respiratory Care Research*—now long out of print—and then the chapter reappeared in the *First Edition* of this book. Fortunately, David's advice is timeless.

Mathew "Matti" Mero, MA, is the author of the new Appendix I, "Basic Science Writing." Matti is a copyeditor for *Respiratory Care* and has a unique perspective honed from many years of rooting out mistakes and rounding the rough edges of countless authors (me among them). What he writes is pure gold, and you are not likely to find anything like it in other books. I am indebted to Matti for catching many a "slip of the pen" over the many years that I have been submitting manuscripts to *Respiratory Care*.

Charles G. Durbin, Jr., MD, FAARC, of the University of Virginia Health System, Charlottesville, contributed to Chapter 6, "Reviewing the Literature," based on a paper he published in *Respiratory Care* in October 2009, pages 1366–1371. Charlie has been a friend and colleague for many years.

About the Author

Robert L. Chatburn, RRT-NPS, FAARC, is an Adjunct Associate Professor in the Department of Medicine at the Lerner College of Medicine of Case Western Reserve University and a Fellow of the American Association for Respiratory Care. Mr. Chatburn is currently the Clinical Research Manager of the Respiratory Institute at the Cleveland Clinic. Previously, he was the Technical Director of respiratory care at University Hospitals for 20 years. He is the author of nine textbooks and over 240 publications in medical journals. He is an Associate Editor of *Respiratory Care* and is recognized internationally as a research scientist and authority on mechanical ventilation and pediatric respiratory care.

Mr. Chatburn was born and raised in the Cleveland area. He received an AS degree from Cuyahoga Community College and a BS degree from Youngstown State University. He began his career at Rainbow Babies & Children's Hospital in 1977. In 1979 he was promoted to research coordinator. In 1986 he took the position of Technical Director of pediatric respiratory care and in 1995 annexed the adult division as well. In 1997 he became Adjunct Assistant Professor of pediatrics at Case Western Reserve University and was promoted to Adjunct Associate Professor in 1998. In 2006 Mr. Chatburn became Clinical Research Manager of the Respiratory Institute at the Cleveland Clinic. Mr. Chatburn was among the first 13 people awarded fellowship in the American Association for Respiratory Care in 1998 and was the recipient of the 2007 Forrest M. Bird Lifetime Scientific Achievement Award.

Contributing Authors

Charles G. Durbin, Jr., MD, FAARC
Professor of Anesthesiology and Surgery
University of Virginia

Matthew Mero, MA
Respiratory Care

David J. Pierson, MD
Medical Director, Respiratory Care
Harborview Medical Center
Professor of Medicine
University of Washington

Section I

Introduction

CHAPTER 1

Why Study Research?

The ability to read and critically evaluate published research reports is required of all health care professionals, who must be able to assess such things as the usefulness of new equipment, the effectiveness of present and proposed treatment modalities, the quality of services provided, and the adequacy of teaching materials available. Without this skill, no meaningful evaluation of current practices can be made and no research can be planned.

The pursuit of scientific knowledge in any field must ultimately rest on the testing and retesting of new ideas and their practical application. Growing numbers of clinicians, educators, and administrators are conducting their own investigations and critically examining research done by others in their particular field of interest. Even if you never conduct a study, you still must be familiar with the basic concepts of research in order to practice as a professional whose understanding grows from continuing education. The word *research* is here used in a generic sense to mean a systematic method of inquiry.

The main purpose of the *Second Edition* of *Handbook for Health Care Research* is to help you become an educated consumer of medical research. If you want to actually perform research, the best thing you can do is find a mentor, someone who has experience conducting scientific studies and publishing the results. A mentor can help you turn the ideas in this book into practical realities.

Table 1.1 describes the five basic phases of research. Health care workers are usually involved with the second phase, the application of research results in the clinical setting. Within the research continuum, however, infinite opportunities exist to become involved in seeking the answers to questions relating to the practice of health care.

The following discussion outlines several areas of health care where we may apply the principles of scientific analysis to provide a sound basis for patient care. These include health care education, professional accountability, and administration of services.

Health Care Education

Colleges are responsible for graduating practitioners who are knowledgeable and current in the practice of their profession. Educators must stay up to date with new ideas and technology in medicine that affect the diagnosis and treatment of disease.

Table 1.1

The Five Phases of Research

1. *Basic Research.* Seeks new knowledge and furthers research in an area of knowledge rather than attempting to solve an immediate problem.
2. *Applied Research.* Seeks to identify relationships among facts to solve an immediate practical problem.
3. *Clinical Investigations.* Seek to evaluate systematically the application of research findings in the clinical setting, usually in a relatively small patient population.
4. *Clinical Trials.* Seek to determine the effectiveness and safety of clinical treatments in samples of patients drawn from larger populations.
5. *Demonstration and Education Research.* Seek to examine the efficacy of treatments designed to promote health or prevent disease in defined populations.

Critical Evaluation of Published Reports

Keeping abreast of new product and treatment developments is essential for educators. In deciding whether to present a particular piece of equipment or treatment modality to students, instructors must first discern whether the claims for its use and potential benefits rest on a solid scientific foundation. To do so, they must be able to read and critically evaluate reports and tests of function and reliability. A critical reading of scientific journals will provide the basis for decisions concerning classroom demonstrations, guides, and the planning process. Educators may wish to conduct their own investigations as well.

The results of published reports should never be accepted uncritically. Consider this example: the use of intermittent mandatory ventilation (IMV) was claimed to decrease the time required to wean a patient from mechanical ventilation. Yet recent studies have shown that the average length of time a patient spends on the ventilator and in the hospital actually *increased* by the use of IMV.

How much credence should we give to each study's results? Is one or the other limited by its design? Does a non-uniformity of patient populations exist? Were the types of IMV systems used the same in each study? What criteria were used for judging a patient's readiness for removal from mechanical ventilation? Health care educators must ask these types of questions of all studies before passing the results on to their students; they must do more than simply take a study's conclusions at face value.

Continuing Education

To ensure that health care practitioners keep informed of recent developments in their fields, hospital department managers must establish and maintain continuing education programs. Inservice programs provide opportunities to explore and discuss new trends, ideas, and research that occur in the field. Allied health professionals are taking an increasing role in patient education as well as in clinical practice. As they keep current on data relating to, for example, the relationship of cigarette smoking to heart disease or cancer, they can increase a patient's awareness of the appropriateness of particular treatment modalities.

Research on health care practices leads to the reeducation of practitioners and the updating of department procedure manuals. It also leads to the development of new guidelines that improve clinical competence. This occurs as state-of-the-art data on equipment, care modalities, physical diagnosis, and monitoring procedures are made available and their validity tested.

Professional Accountability

Health care professionals are accountable not only to their patients, departments, and hospital administrators but also to government agencies, third-party payers, and the public at large. Our nation's entire health care system is under increasing pressure to justify the cost of services it provides. Government agencies and third-party payers want to know that services provided are both necessary and beneficial.

In times of economic austerity, funding of health care agencies, such as the Food and Drug Administration (FDA) and the Centers for Disease Control and Prevention (CDC), often is reduced. The functioning of these agencies—as well as Medicare, Medicaid, and Blue Cross/ Blue Shield—affects health care both directly and indirectly. Investment in health care for the elderly and poor by the government is under close scrutiny to make sure that funds are going to pay for justifiable services. Understandably, with an increased federal role in paying the bills, there is increased pressure to ensure the quality and quantity of care and that it is cost efficient.

The high cost of health care must be supported by scientific research. Regulations governing medical services and reimbursement are based on the current state of knowledge. Relevant questions about a service pertain to its necessity for the treatment of an established medical problem and whether it is of demonstrable benefit to a patient. The task of medical officials is to ensure that the appropriate regulatory body has this information at its disposal. The task of health care researchers is to make certain that the information is based on reliable scientific data.

Administration of Health Care Services

Health care department managers and hospital administrators alike look to the results of carefully completed studies to help solve problems relating to areas of concern such as cost containment, productivity assessment, departmental organization, and employee stress management. Managers are responsible for staffing their departments with qualified personnel, providing services that are delivered in a professional and timely manner, and making certain that infection control, safety, and preventative maintenance programs are ongoing and productive. How can managers best evaluate these services and programs? Which method of providing infection control, for instance, should a manager choose? Knowing that equipment can be a major source of nosocomial infection, the manager needs a reliable method to assess the possible change in infection rate affected by a program of disinfection or sterilization. The manager will also consider the cost effectiveness of different methods. He or she will ask the same type of questions in evaluating patient and employee safety programs as well as organization, delivery, and evaluation of patient care.

Evaluation of the quality of departmental programs and services is difficult. Empirical observation must not be the basis for acceptance or rejection. The costs of trial and error are too prohibitive for this type of decision-making.

Continuous Quality Improvement

Continuous quality improvement implies the identification of gaps between the current state and the future state as well as a correction process for eliminating the gaps. This correction process is accomplished through the careful and rigid manipulation of variables and the measurement of any effects; in other words, using the scientific method. Only in this way can the physician, patient, patient's family, hospital, and government administrator be assured of the quality of cost-effective services.

Evaluating New Equipment and Methods

Validating Manufacturers' Claims

To meet the changing needs of health care, medical equipment manufacturers introduce to the market new diagnostic and support instruments. Because of the relatively short product life cycle in the market of technical equipment, new products are introduced frequently. But *new* does not necessarily mean *better*. At times, the development of new technology outpaces the need for that technology. When this happens, product marketers have not done their job in accurately assessing demand. Medical professionals must take the lead in ensuring that they are not left in the position of trying to invent ways to use new equipment. New equipment should ideally satisfy a well-established need. Although manufacturers often engage in extensive testing and market research, the final burden of proof as to a product's ultimate function and benefit falls to the end users.

For example, unlike drugs, *modes of mechanical ventilation* are introduced on the market without having the burden of proving that they are effective at improving patient outcomes. What makes this particular example so frustrating is that many of these modes are called by the same name, but the drugs perform very differently on different brands of ventilators. The end users must question whether a new mode makes a difference in any measurable sort of way. Does it make a difference in terms of patient safety, comfort, or duration of mechanical ventilation? Are the potential benefits worth the added expense of this new ventilator feature? These types of critical questions must be asked and systematically addressed when any new piece of equipment is made available in a field. Rather than accept on faith that a new technology will do exactly what its manufacturer claims, health care practitioners should validate claims and conduct comparison tests with existing equipment.

Questions

Definitions

Define the following terms:

1. Basic research
2. Applied research
3. Quality assurance

True or False

1. The most important reason for studying research methodology is to gain the ability to read and critically evaluate studies published in medical journals.
2. The best thing you can do if you want to really learn how to do research is to find a mentor.

Multiple Choice

1. In which of the following area(s) may the principles of scientific analysis to improve patient care be applied?
   a. Education
   b. Continuous quality improvement
   c. Evaluation of new equipment
   d. All of the above

CHAPTER 2

Ethics and Research

T he health care industry today is confronted with a multitude of laws, regulatory constraints, and standards that govern the conduct of the industry itself and the individuals who work in it. Conducting health care in this environment requires constant attention to a multitude of details. Conducting health care research demands additional attention to a special set of regulatory and ethical considerations.

Research involving human subjects—which we refer to as *clinical* research—invokes legal, ethical, and sociologic concerns related to the safety and protection of the subject's basic human rights.* Research involving animals requires responsible attention to several important concerns as well. Regardless of the type of study subjects, those engaged in medical research must be reminded that the importance of their work should never overshadow but, rather, complement society's health care goals. Complex procedures must strictly adhere to legal guidelines so that subjects are not exploited. Innovative and controversial research must be ethically conducted and honestly reported.

The current and future prospects for productive and informative research in health care are as high now as they have ever been. In pursuing these prospects, the health care researcher must be concerned not only with the proper methodologies and logistics of running the actual study, but with legal and ethical issues that are no less important. Structuring research that is within the bounds of ethically and scientifically rigorous standards is an important and complex task, with a multitude of subtleties. The research investigator must achieve scientific rigor while at the same time maintaining the highest ethical standards.

A complete discussion of all the ethical and legal implications of clinical research is beyond the scope of this text. The goal of this chapter is, first of all, to familiarize you with the institutional approval process researchers need to navigate to begin research involving human subjects. Second, this chapter is designed to heighten your awareness with respect to several legal and ethical concerns that investigators will undoubtedly encounter as they design and conduct their research endeavors in our modern environment.

Note: Classes on Protection of Human Subjects and Responsible Conduct of Research are required and mandated by federal regulations for anyone participating in human subject clinical studies funded by the Public Health Service. Free training is available online from the National Institutes of Health.

Institutional Review and Human Subjects' Rights

When human beings are used in scientific research, great care must be taken to ensure that their rights are protected. Institutional review boards have been established to ensure that proposed studies do not violate patient rights.

Functions of the Institutional Review Board

The health care researcher cannot and should not begin an investigation involving human subjects without formal approval from the appropriate hospital's institutional review board (IRB), also known by such names as the Institutional Review Committee, Human Subjects Review Committee, Human Investigation Committee, or Research Surveillance Committee. These committees, boards, and other groups are formally designated by an institution to review biomedical research involving human subjects. They meet at certain specified intervals to review, recommend, and approve study proposals.

The main functions of an IRB are to protect the rights, well-being, and privacy of individuals, as well as to protect the interests of the hospital or center in which the research is conducted. Specific IRB procedures will vary from institution to institution. In each case, health care workers must review those guidelines applicable in their own institution.

IRBs are typically established, operated, and function in conformance with regulations set forth by the U.S. Department of Health and Human Services (DHHS), established to protect the rights of human subjects that apply to all institutions receiving federal funds. The DHHS issues regulations that must be followed for biomedical and behavioral human research to receive such funds.

Consideration of risks, potential benefits, and informed consent typically occupies the majority of the IRB's time. Generally, before an IRB will approve a research protocol, the following conditions must be met:

1. The risks to the (research) subject are so outweighed by the sum of the benefits to the subject and the importance of the knowledge to be gained as to warrant a decision to allow the subject to accept these risks.
2. Legally effective informed consent will be obtained by adequate and appropriate methods.
3. The rights and welfare of any such subjects will be adequately protected.

Review of research involving human subjects must always occur before the initiation of research and may be required at specified intervals during the lifetime of the research activity. If an application for external funding is being considered, the researcher should thoroughly review the study proposal before submission to the funding agency. It is common for an IRB to ask an investigator to modify a research plan to comply with Food and Drug Administration (FDA) and DHHS regulations as well as ethical norms. However, the IRB is not a police force. There is a presumption of trust that the approved research protocol will indeed be followed consistently. Nevertheless, investigators have been known to deviate from the agreements reached with an IRB.

Composition of the Institutional Review Board

To provide input representing a wide variety of concerns, the IRB committee is typically composed of members with diverse backgrounds. An IRB characteristically includes representatives of administration, staff, and legal areas of both the institution and the community. This diversity encourages that proposed research be reviewed for acceptability not only in terms of scientific standards but in terms of community acceptance, relevant law, professional standards, and institutional regulations as well.

As well as a diverse background, committee members exhibit a high standard of personal and professional excellence. IRB members should exhibit sufficient maturity, experience, and competence to ensure that the board will be able to discharge its responsibilities and that its determinations will be accorded respect by investigators and the community served by the institution. The quality of an IRB decision is thus a direct reflection of the degree of maturity, experience, and competence of its members.

Approval of the Institutional Review Board

The investigator must formally apply for IRB approval before beginning a study. A thorough IRB application typically includes the components listed in **Table 2.1**. First, a formal research protocol must be established. This description of the study's intended purpose and procedures is then followed by human subjects information, which should describe sources of potential subjects and the anticipated number required. Also included should be a description of the consent procedures and a description of potential risks and benefits as they relate both to the subjects and to society.

An integral part of the study protocol, and a necessary component for IRB review, is the patient or subject consent form, discussed in greater detail later in this chapter. To prepare this form properly, a number of issues (Table 2.1) must be thoroughly addressed. The content of each of these areas of concern must then be prepared with the consent form for the information of the potential study subject.

Table 2.1

Typical Components of an IRB Proposal

1. A complete description of the study's intended purpose and procedures to be followed.
2. A description of potential risks the subject may incur from participation in the study.
3. A description of potential benefits, either direct or indirect, the subject may incur from participation in the study.
4. A description of how data will be handled such that the subject's identity remains anonymous.
5. A statement that the subject may withdraw from the study at any time without a prejudicial effect on his or her continuing clinical care.
6. The name and number of the investigator, should any questions arise regarding the subject's participation in the study.
7. Copy of the complete informed consent form.
8. A list of available alternate procedures and therapies.
9. A statement of the subject's rights, if any, to treatment or compensation in the event of a research-related injury.

Informed Consent

Informed consent is the voluntary permission given by a person allowing him- or herself to be included in a research study after being informed of the study's purpose, method of treatment, risks, and benefits.

A key principle of ethical conduct in research is that participation in studies must be voluntary. In turn, voluntary consent is predicated on communicating all the information the potential subject needs to be self-determining. The consent form represents the culmination of much effort devoted to protect the rights of research subjects through the process of fully informing them before their involvement in clinical research.

Background

The Nuremburg Trials after World War II revealed the atrocities committed by Nazi physicians in the name of research. As a result of these revelations, voluntary informed consent became a central focus of biomedical ethics. The doctrine of informed consent is designed to uphold the ethical principle of *respect for persons*. As such, this doctrine is now grounded in a body of medicolegal decisions that cite a failure to obtain adequate informed consent as either *battery* or *negligence*.

Having received critical commentary for many years, the protection of human subjects' rights has received formal legislative attention. In legitimizing this emphasis, the World Medical Association adopted the Declaration of Helsinki in 1964. This declaration recommended that informed consent be obtained. Before this, potential volunteers were protected only by the assumed responsibility of the individual investigator to explain fully the nature of the research. Abuses of this responsibility led to the development and implementation of the informed consent requirement.

Role Today

Today, informed consent is a crucial feature of virtually all clinical trials. No research involving human subjects should be initiated without the informed and voluntary consent of those subjects. Competent patients must be offered the opportunity to accept or reject a medical intervention proposed as part of their participation in a research study. Likewise, incompetent patients must be offered the same opportunity through the mediation of a legal guardian or surrogate.

For consent to be *informed*, the potential subject must be given information regarding all the possible pros and cons of the proposed medical intervention. We always move toward maximizing the patients' best interests while enhancing their participation in decision-making. The consent form will clearly summarize the IRB application. It must contain all the elements listed in Table 2.1 so that a patient's rights will be protected should he or she elect to participate in the research study.

Revocation of Consent

A subject may withdraw from a research activity at any time during the course of the study, within the limits of the research. Any request for withdrawal should be honored promptly. As spelled out in the consent form, revocation of consent and participation in the research study should never result in a subject being penalized or made to forfeit benefits to which he or she is otherwise entitled. However, the subject's commitment to participate in a research study is seen by some to represent a moral obligation. In this context, research can be viewed as a joint venture between investigator and subject. The subject has made a promise to participate and to bear the inconvenience of testing in return for the benefit he or she hopes to derive.

Nevertheless, should a subject wish to withdraw from participation in research, the investigator must fully inform the subject of the potential dangers in doing so. Alternatives to the current mode of therapy must be described so the pros and cons of withdrawal from the study can be properly evaluated. In all instances, the implications of withdrawal from therapy must be made clear to the subject, and arrangements must be made for a smooth, uneventful transition to standard clinical care.

Ethical Issues

Basic Principles

Professional ethics in health care ethics is a subset of the category of medical ethics, which in turn is a division of the much broader philosophy of ethics. Although the law sets a minimum level of expected behavior, ethics generally requires more than the minimum, and often aims toward the ideal. Every clinical researcher, regardless of the study, has relevant ethical responsibilities to which he or she is held accountable. The following discussion will address ethical decisions in the field of clinical research as they concern health care investigations.

Three fundamental ethical principles relevant to clinical research are *respect for persons*, *justice*, and *beneficence*. Respect for persons is interpreted to mean that those conducting clinical research will endeavor to treat potential subjects as autonomous, self-determining individuals. Furthermore, those subjects not capable of making considered judgments (incompetent), those either immature or incapacitated, are entitled to protection. The principle of justice requires that all persons be treated fairly and equally. Finally, beneficence can best be understood as a commitment to do no harm and to maximize the potential benefits while minimizing potential harms. Incumbent in this definition is the understanding that no person will be asked to accept risks of injury in the interest of producing societal benefits.

Research studies that violate these standards have been documented and serve as a basis for the contemporary balance between human experimentation and legal regulation of medical research. For example, in 1932 male prisoners with syphilis were recruited without consent and misinformed as to their treatment.[1] When penicillin became available for the treatment of syphilis, these men were not informed. In another study (the Jewish Chronic Disease Hospital Study), patients with various chronic debilitating diseases were injected with live cancer cells.

Consent was said to have been negotiated, but was never documented due to the investigator's contention that informing the patients of the procedure would frighten them unnecessarily. These and other abuses have combined to tighten both legal regulations and ethical guidelines for clinical research.

Ethical concepts differ substantially from legal concepts. Ethical concepts have evolved into the various professional standards and principles that guide the practice of medicine. Professional standards do not carry the weight of law; only statutes and common law have any legal authority in this country. However, many statutes and many court decisions have been, and will continue to be, extensively based on the moral and ethical convictions of the health care professions. Health care ethics may be considered a subset of the larger field of medical ethics. No longer is the physician the absolute ruler and his or her ancillary helpers mere followers who cannot be expected to exercise any moral judgment of their own. Furthermore, medical care is no longer delivered solely by physicians and nurses. The contemporary health care industry employs a variety of professional health care practitioners, each with a high and noble ethical code of conduct no less meaningful than the Hippocratic Oath. For example, the field of respiratory care operates under an ethical code represented by the American Association for Respiratory Care (AARC) Statement of Ethics and Professional Conduct (**Table 2.2**). The issues of health care ethics are becoming more numerous and complex with nearly every major medical advance that is implemented. A partial list of the pressing issues of the early twenty-

Table 2.2

American Association for Respiratory Care Statement of Ethics and Professional Conduct

In the conduct of professional activities the Respiratory Therapist shall be bound by the following ethical and professional principles. Respiratory Therapists shall:
- Demonstrate behavior that reflects integrity, supports objectivity, and fosters trust in the profession and its professionals. Actively maintain and continually improve their professional competence, and represent it accurately.
- Perform only those procedures or functions in which they are individually competent and which are within the scope of accepted and responsible practice.
- Respect and protect the legal and personal rights of patients they care for, including the right to informed consent and refusal of treatment.
- Divulge no confidential information regarding any patient or family unless disclosure is required for responsible performance of duty, or required by law.
- Provide care without discrimination on any basis, with respect for the rights and dignity of all individuals.
- Promote disease prevention and wellness.
- Refuse to participate in illegal or unethical acts, and refuse to conceal illegal, unethical, or incompetent acts of others.
- Follow sound scientific procedures and ethical principles in research.
- Comply with state or federal laws, which govern and relate to their practice.
- Avoid any form of conduct that creates a conflict of interest, and shall follow the principles of ethical business behavior.
- Promote health care delivery through improvement of the access, efficacy, and cost of patient care.
- Refrain from indiscriminate and unnecessary use of resources.

Source: American Association for Respiratory Care. (1994). AARC Statement of Ethics and Professional Conduct. Accessed July 13, 2009. Available at: http://www.aarc.org/resources/position_statements/ethics.html.

first century includes death with dignity, euthanasia, discontinuation of life-support systems, organ transplantation, genetic engineering, behavior modification, use of animal experimentation, and a further subset of issues that come under the general heading of human experimentation for health care research. In addition to the basic ethical principles of respect for persons, justice, and beneficence, what other issues can the health care researcher expect to confront? Several issues discussed below deserve consideration.

Objective Patient Care

Under the auspices of a physician, the health care practitioner contractually undertakes to give a patient the best possible treatment. Indeed, at the core of modern medical ethics is the Hippocratic promise to do one's best for every patient and to do no harm. Does the very act of enrolling a patient in a randomized clinical trial violate this obligation? Does this subject fully understand the implications of potentially falling into the placebo group? Does a subject fully understand that randomization to the control group may mean that treatment may be very different from what he or she is accustomed to (e.g., in terms of frequency or intensity)? Some critics believe that if a clinician or investigator has reason to believe that the experimental treatment is better than the control treatment, he or she must recommend the experimental option. For example, suppose a new aerosolized drug seems to be highly effective and superior to the standard treatment of patients with acute respiratory distress syndrome. A controlled clinical trial is undertaken, with 50 patients randomized to receive conventional therapy. Another 50 patients are randomized to the treatment group and receive a new drug in addition to conventional therapy. Now suppose that 15 patients in the experimental group die, as opposed to 30 patients in the control group. Is the clinical investigator guilty of unethical behavior? Is he or she guilty of a crime, a sin of omission?

Unfortunately, there are no clear-cut answers. As is made clear in the Nuremberg codes, the degree of risk to be taken should never exceed that determined by the humanitarian importance of the problem to be solved by the experiment. In other words, there should always be a favorable balance between harm and benefit. The fundamental ethical principle is that of beneficence. Furthermore, justice and respect for persons are served when a study's potential harms and benefits are clearly and properly presented to the subject for his or her informed consent.

Reporting Research Results

Scientific investigations are based to a very high degree on trust. We trust that each investigator will conduct his or her research in accordance with the protocol approved by the appropriate IRB. And we trust that all research findings will be reported accurately and without intentional bias. Abandoning trust would lead to overwhelming suspicion and make scientific investigation impossible. Without trust in the honesty and integrity of published findings, how would progress in science and medicine be possible?

Fortunately, fraud in science is rare, due to the skepticism of the scientific community. No experiment is accepted until it has been independently repeated. Research results, no matter how sensational, are quickly forgotten if they cannot be obtained from other investigators duplicating the study methodology.

Questions

Definitions

Define the following terms:

- IRB
- Informed consent

True or False

1. The IRB is intended to protect the rights of patients involved in research studies.
2. The IRB is composed of the people who designed the research study.

Multiple Choice

1. Typical components of an IRB proposal include:
   a. Description of study purpose
   b. Potential risks and benefits
   c. Informed consent form
   d. Description of investigator's previous experience
   e. All of the above
   f. Only a, b, and c
2. Three fundamental ethical principles relevant to clinical research are:
   a. Respect for persons
   b. Cost containment
   c. Justice
   d. Beneficence
   e. Only a, b, and d
   f. Only a, c, and d
3. At the core of modern medical ethics is the Hippocratic Oath, which obligates caregivers to:
   a. Treat everyone fairly
   b. Do no harm
   c. Give only treatment proven by scientific methods
   d. Obtain informed consent before entering a person in a study

Reference

1. Centers for Disease Control and Prevention. (2009). U.S. Public Health Service Syphilis Study at Tuskegee. Accessed July 13, 2009. Available at: http://www.cdc.gov/tuskegee.

CHAPTER 3

Outcomes Research

O utcomes research is starting to make its mark in defining optimal health care practices. With the need for cost containment, outcomes research becomes a double-edged sword used both to cut nonessential practices and to protect those that maintain quality of care. The profession of health care has a long history of research and a commitment to basing practice on science. However, much of the published research is still focused on devices and procedures rather than the broader issues of patient outcomes and economic effects. We need to evolve our paradigms to accommodate the larger vision of disease management, which encompasses the arenas of outcomes research and evidence-based medical practice.

In this chapter, I will give a brief history of the outcomes research movement to provide some sense of context. Then, I will try to demystify the language of outcomes research and review some of its themes and methods. Finally, I will present specific examples of outcomes research found in the pages of *Respiratory Care* to illustrate some of the methods of outcomes research and stimulate future studies.

A Brief History

Florence Nightingale may have been the first outcomes researcher in medicine. She had a flair for collecting, analyzing, and presenting data. She even invented the polar-area chart, where the statistic being represented is proportional to the area of a wedge in a circular diagram. But of course, she had as much trouble finding appropriate data as we do today. Nevertheless, her most effective weapon was the presentation of solid, relevant data.

The modern outcomes movement in the United States began in the early 1980s. An increasing focus on cost containment led to interest in identifying and eliminating unnecessary procedures. Perhaps more intriguing was the recognition that there were substantial variations in medical practice, apparently based on geography or race. Indeed, some researchers claimed that "geography was destiny" because medical practices as commonplace as hysterectomy and hernia repair were performed much more frequently in some areas than in others, with no differences in the underlying rates of disease.

Given that there are variations in practice and differences in outcomes, we may logically assume that some practices produce better outcomes than others. So the stage was set to improve efficiency and quality if only the right data were available. But where to look? Consider the vast array of devices and techniques used in medicine and how few of them are supported by evidence from randomized controlled trials. This is not surprising, given that clinical trials can cost millions of dollars and last years. One might speculate that data collected for administrative or billing purposes (e.g., Medicare and Medicaid tapes collected by the Health Care Financing Administration) might contain valuable outcome data such as mortality, length of hospital stay, resource use, and costs. On the one hand, such data can be quickly analyzed, without requiring patient consent or interfering with medical care. On the other hand, this type of research is limited by the quality and completeness of the available data.

New data must be collected in a systematic fashion with a specific focus on outcomes. In 1989 Congress created the Agency for Health Care Policy and Research (AHCPR). It consisted of 11 major components, including the Center for Outcomes and Effectiveness Research, the Center for Cost and Financing Studies, and the Center for Quality Measurement and Improvement. The initial focus of the AHCPR was to create Patient Outcomes Research Teams (PORTs; five-year studies of specifically identified diseases with highly focused methods), the Pharmaceutical Outcomes Research Program, and the Minority Health Research Centers. In time, the AHCPR changed its name and its focus. According to the Agency for Healthcare Research and Quality (AHRQ), the purpose of outcomes research is to answer four basic questions:

- What works?
- What doesn't?
- When in the course of an illness (does it work or not)?
- At what cost?

These questions suggest the scope and focus of modern outcomes research.

Understanding the Jargon

Like any new discipline, the field of outcomes research suffers from a lack of consistent definitions and a unifying conceptual framework. Many seemingly unrelated terms are encountered in the literature, such as efficacy, effectiveness, quality of life, patient-centered care, evidence-based medicine, and so on. All these terms signify a paradigm shift in which the emphasis is on populations rather than individuals, on practice guidelines rather than anecdotal justifications for treatment, and on capitation rather than fee-for-service payments. I have found it helpful to view this new paradigm in terms of the general concept of "disease management" within which the specific activities of outcomes research and evidence-based medicine interact in a process of continuous quality improvement.

Disease management (also called outcomes management) can be defined as a systematic, population-based approach to identify patients at risk, intervene with specific programs, and measure outcomes. The basic premise of disease management is that an optimal strategy exists for reduced cost and better outcomes. Disease management emphasizes identifying populations of interest, creating comprehensive interventions, explicitly defining and measuring outcomes, and providing a strategy for continuous quality improvement.

Continuous quality improvement (CQI) is a cycle of activities focused on identifying problems or opportunities, creating and implementing plans, and using outcomes analysis to

Figure 3.1

Continuous quality improvement expressed in the traditional format of a cycle of "plan, do, check, act" and an equivalent cycle showing the interaction of plans and implementations through goals.

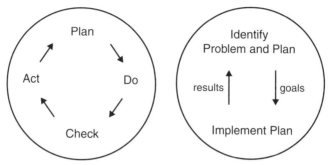

redefine problems and opportunities. CQI was started decades ago by pioneers such as Walter A. Shewert, W. Edwards Deming, and Joseph M. Juran and is currently embraced by The Joint Commission (TJC). The "plan, do, check, act" cycle endorsed by TJC can be viewed as simply creating plans and implementing them. The plan leads to implementation through the creation of specific goals. Implementation leads to more plans through the analysis of results (**Figure 3.1**).

Outcomes research can be defined as the scientific study of the results of diverse therapies used for particular diseases, conditions, or illnesses. The specific goals of this type of research are to create treatment guidelines, document treatment effectiveness, and to study the effect of reimbursement policies on outcomes.

Evidence-based medicine is an approach to practice and teaching that integrates pathophysi-ological rationale, caregiver experience, and patient preferences with valid and current clinical research evidence. To implement evidence-based medicine, the practitioner must be able to define the patient problem, search for and critically appraise data from the literature, and then decide whether, and how, to use this information in practice.

If we view disease management as a universe of activities, then outcomes research (e.g., epidemiological studies, clinical trials, quality of life surveys, efficacy and effectiveness studies, and cost analyses) and evidence-based medicine (e.g., creation and use of practice guidelines and care paths) can be seen as subset activities linked by the general structure of continuous quality improvement (**Figure 3.2**).

Outcomes Research: Focus and Methods

Outcomes research can be distinguished from traditional clinical research more by its focus than by the methods it employs. This difference in focus is highlighted in **Table 3.1**. Appropriate outcomes can be roughly grouped into three categories: clinical, economic, and humanistic (**Table 3.2**).

Outcomes research uses a variety of techniques (**Table 3.3**). *Qualitative research* often produces large amounts of textual data in the form of transcripts and observational field notes.

Figure 3.2

Disease management expressed as a continuous quality improvement cycle showing the interaction of plans (created by outcomes research) and implementations (evidence-based medicine tools) through goals (desired outcomes) and measured results (actual outcomes).

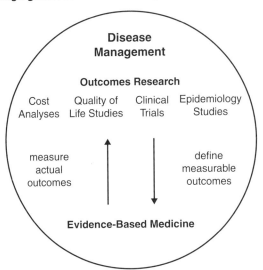

Table 3.1

Differences Between Traditional Clinical Research and Outcomes Research

Traditional Clinical Research	Outcomes Research
Disease-centered	Patient- and community-centered
Drugs and devices	Processes and delivery of care
Experimental	Observational
Methods from "hard sciences" (e.g., physics, biochemistry)	Methods from "social sciences" (e.g., economics, epidemiology)
Efficacy	Effectiveness
Mechanisms of disease	Consequences of disease on patients
Effects of biochemical and physiologic factors	Effects of socioeconomic factors

Rather than trying to identify a statistically representative set of observations, qualitative research uses analytical categories to describe and explain social phenomena. Qualitative research generates hypotheses (although not necessarily hypothesis tests) and attempts to identify the relevance of findings to specific groups of people.

Quantitative research uses both experimental and nonexperimental designs. The classic experimental design of the randomized controlled trial can be applied to outcomes research if

Table 3.2

Various Types of Outcome Measures Used in Outcomes Research

Category	Type	Example
Clinical	Clinical events	Myocardial infarct
	Physiologic measures	Pulmonary function indices
	Mortality	Asthma deaths
Economic	Direct medical costs	Hospital and outpatient visits
	Indirect costs	Work loss, restricted activity days
Humanistic	Symptoms	Dyspnea scores
	Quality of life	SF-36 Questionnaire, St. George's
	Functional status	Respiratory Questionnaire
	Patient satisfaction	Activities of daily living

Table 3.3

Methods Used in Outcomes Research

Qualitative Methods (formal hypothesis testing not necessarily required)

Generate hypotheses
Describe complex phenomena
Identify relevance of findings to specific patient groups

Quantitative Methods

Experimental
  • Randomized controlled trials
Nonexperimental
  • Data synthesis
  • Meta-analysis
  • Decision analysis
  • Economic analysis
Observational studies
  • Cohort
  • Case control
  • Survey

it is set up to evaluate effectiveness (as opposed to efficacy; see definitions below). Nonexperimental designs can focus on either data synthesis or observational study designs.

In keeping with the population-based theme of outcomes research, methods are needed to synthesize data from numerous studies as opposed to interpreting the results of a single study. One such method is called *meta-analysis*. Meta-analysis is a method of combining the results of several independent studies (usually drawn from the published literature) to improve the reliability of general conclusions that may be used to evaluate therapeutic effectiveness and plan new studies. The method consists of four steps:

1. A thorough literature review
2. Calculation of an effect size for each study
3. Determination of a composite effect size from the weighted combination of individual effect sizes
4. Calculation of a failsafe number (number of unpublished results) to assess the certainty of the composite size

Decision analysis is used to determine optimal strategies when there are several alternative actions and an uncertain or risk-filled pattern of future events. This technique is a derivative of operations research and game theory. It involves identifying all available choices and the potential outcomes of each. Usually a model is created in the form of a decision tree. The tree is used to represent the strategies available to the clinician and the likelihood that each outcome will occur if a particular strategy is chosen. The relative value of each outcome can also be described.

Several basic types of economic evaluations are applied to health issues. *Cost identification* is simply the description of the costs of providing an intervention. It is the first step in all the other types of analyses, but it is often the only one reported in a study. *Cost of illness* analysis estimates the total cost of a disease or disability to society. *Cost minimization* is applied when two or more interventions are being compared on the same outcomes and the outcomes seem to yield similar effectiveness. Then the question is simply which is least expensive. An example would be the question of whether to repair or replace a mechanical ventilator. When the same outcomes are measured but the effectiveness differs, then they are compared on the basis of cost per outcome (e.g., dollars per life saved or dollars per additional year of life) using *cost effectiveness* analysis. If both outcomes and effectiveness differ, then a *cost-benefit analysis* first attempts to express both outcomes and benefits in terms of dollars. Then the interventions are evaluated in terms of the overall economic tradeoffs among them. In this way the cost of, for example, a smoking prevention program can be compared with that of lung reduction surgery, and both can be compared with other programs, such as highway development or job training. *Cost utility* analysis is similar to cost effectiveness except that the effectiveness is expressed as a "utility" that is the product of a clinical outcome, such as years of life saved, and a subjective weighing of the quality of life to be had during those years. Utility is often expressed as quality-adjusted life years (QALYs). For example, quality of life is often measured on a linear scale where 0 indicates death (or indifference to death) and 1.0 represents perfect health. Suppose a patient is discharged to a chronic ventilator weaning facility for six months and dies on the ventilator. If the patient rates the utility of life on the ventilator as 0.2, the patient has experienced $0.5 \times 0.2 = 0.1$ QALYs. If the assumptions are correct, this means that six months on a ventilator in a weaning facility is approximately equal in value to the patient as one month (0.1 year) in perfect health. Economic analyses can seem overly complicated.

Quality of life (QOL) measures have been important in research since the 1970s. Uses of QOL data include distinguishing patients or groups, evaluating therapeutic interventions, and predicting patient outcomes. However, there are many QOL instruments and much theory, but there is no unified measurement approach. And there is little agreement on definitions and interpretations. Some authors argue that because QOL is a uniquely personal perspective, patient-specific measures should be used.

Another issue that seems confusing is the difference between efficacy studies and effectiveness studies. An example of the type of question answered by an *efficacy* study is as follows: "Does the intervention work in a tertiary care setting with carefully selected patients under tightly controlled conditions?" This type of study generally requires a priori hypotheses, randomization of subjects to predefined treatments, homogeneous patient populations at high risk for the outcome, experienced investigators following a specific protocol, a comparative intervention (e.g., a placebo), and intensive follow-up. Conclusions from this type of study prompt relatively high levels of confidence. However, because the design is so restrictive, the results may not be generalizable to a broad range of patients in usual practice settings. Thus, efficacy studies may not be appropriate for cost-effectiveness analyses.

In contrast, *effectiveness* studies are designed to answer questions such as: "Does the intervention work in clinical practice settings with unselected patients, typical care providers, and usual procedures?" Many effectiveness studies have been conducted as observational (often retrospective) studies in which observed groups were not randomly assigned and neither patients nor providers knew they were being studied. The weakness of this study design is that selection bias may be a problem (i.e., the groups may not have the same prevalence of confounding variables, which are unforeseen and unaccounted-for variables that threaten the reliability and validity of an experiment), so adjustment for factors such as severity of illness and case mix becomes important. Prospective effectiveness trials have been reported. They differ from typical clinical trials in that they enroll heterogeneous participants, impose few protocol-driven interventions, and report outcome measures relevant to the delivery system.

The Outcome of Outcomes Research

Not everyone believes that outcomes research is good. Some authors voice both practical and philosophical arguments against the outcomes movement. They claim the outcomes movement exaggerates its usefulness by understating several difficulties. For example, how much time and money will be required to determine the effectiveness of many commonly used (and continuously evolving) medical procedures? How will physicians use outcomes data when making multiple consecutive decisions in the rush of daily patient care? And how will compliance with practice guidelines be enforced?

Some data suggest that clinical practice guidelines have been remarkably unsuccessful in influencing physician behavior. Reasons for this include the fact that some guidelines are not written for practicing physicians, the issue of physician disagreement with or distrust of guidelines written by so-called national experts, and physicians choosing to ignore guidelines because of nonclinical factors such as financial incentives or fear of malpractice litigation.

This last issue is echoed by the opinion that many physicians are opposed to the kind of micromanagement and attendant loss of clinical autonomy envisioned by the participants in the outcomes movement. Some proclaim that uncertainty and subjectivity are at the heart of the clinical encounter and this will always be the case. Also, by criticizing the uncertainty of physicians, the outcomes movement may set the unrealistic goal of creating important certainties for practitioners, and thereby it misrepresents the terms of the clinical encounter and inadvertently undermines confidence in the physician's ability to act wisely in the face of inevitable uncertainty.

Examples from Respiratory Care

Outcomes research, along with its methodologies and core curriculum, can be viewed as an important discipline for the field of respiratory care. Specific areas where outcomes research techniques could be employed include:

1. Determining the effectiveness of CQI initiatives.
2. Comparing variations in respiratory care practices in order to identify optimum strategies.
3. Developing and assessing innovations.
4. Evaluating resource utilization in areas employing respiratory care professionals compared with similar settings without them.

Indeed, the profession's scientific journal, *Respiratory Care*, has published a substantial amount of outcomes research in the last few years. A quick survey of articles in the Original Contribution category of *Respiratory Care* from 1997 through 2000 showed that about 28% of articles could be classified as outcomes research. While the majority of articles are still focused on devices and procedures, a number of those focused on problem solving and quality improvement may serve as examples. What follows is a brief description of the methodology used in a few of these studies.

Stoller, Orens, and Ahmad (1998) is an observational study that qualifies as outcomes research because it is an evaluation of clinical outcomes in a "real world" setting during variations in respiratory therapy practices.[1] The authors hypothesized that the use of a respiratory care consult service would decrease over-ordering of respiratory care services and decrease the volume of respiratory care services delivered. Data were obtained from the departmental management information system and from the hospital's cost management software. They compared baseline data from 1991, prior to establishment of a respiratory care consult service in 1992, to clinical data from 1996. Results were reported using descriptive statistics (averages, percentages, and trend graphs) of numbers of therapies, numbers of patients treated, and costs of therapies.

Adams, Shapiro, and Marini (1998) is an example of an epidemiology study.[2] Epidemiology studies describe the distribution and size (prevalence and incidence) of disease problems in human populations. The authors developed the study question "Did cost constraints and changes in care settings and techniques affect the number of ventilator-assisted individuals (VAI), their sites of care, or methods used for ventilatory assistance?" They defined VAIs and specified inclusion and exclusion criteria. Data were generated from surveys sent to all sites providing VAI care. Results were reported using descriptive statistics (averages, medians, percentages, and bar graphs), numbers of patients treated, and diagnostic categories.

Espie et al (2008) is an example of a controlled clinical trial designed as an effectiveness study (i.e., a heterogeneous patient population treated by usual caregivers in a standard acute care environment).[3] The purpose of this study was to investigate the clinical effectiveness of protocol-driven cognitive behavior therapy (CBT) for insomnia delivered by oncology nurses. This was a randomized, controlled, two-center trial of CBT versus treatment as usual (TAU) in 150 patients who had completed therapy for cancer. The results indicated that CBT was associated with reductions in wakefulness at night compared with no change for the group with usual treatment. The authors concluded that CBT for insomnia may be both clinically effective and feasible to deliver in real world practice.

Parker and Walker (1998) provide a good example of how to assess quality of life (QOL) issues.[4] The researchers created a priori hypotheses and described the study population based on diagnosis and physiologic measures. They defined the intervention as rehabilitation classes at a specific frequency and duration along with an exercise program. Their QOL survey was abstracted from other published, validated QOL instruments. They used inferential statistics to compare charges and QOL scores. Results were reported using graphs and mean values.

Smith and Pesce (1994) is an example of cost-utility analysis, as defined previously, because the results are expressed in terms of patient utility (using a QOL score on a scale of $0 = $ death to $1.0 = $ perfect health) and quality-adjusted life-years.[5] This article provides an excellent description of a complex topic, showing how a decision tree model is constructed, how probabilities of different outcomes are estimated, how costs are attributed, and how utility is calculated. In addition, it provides an example of how sensitivity analysis is used to evaluate the effects of varying baseline values (i.e., assumptions) within the model.

Benchmarking

Most of the medical procedures we practice each day have never been and never will be supported by formal scientific research. There simply is not enough time or money to do so. However, we can still logically justify what we do. The next best thing to scientific research is *benchmarking*. A benchmark is literally a standard or point of reference in measuring quality. As it relates to industry or health care, benchmarking is the process of comparing your performance with your peers' to see who is the most successful. Benchmarking often is defined as a continuous process of measuring products, services, and practices against one's toughest competitors or renowned industry leaders, and then learning from them.

Three types of benchmarking are generally recognized: collaborative, functional, and internal. Collaborative benchmarking enables an organization to learn from the best practices within a voluntary network of health care providers. Collaborative benchmarking is often managed by a professional organization such as the University Hospitals Consortium.

Functional benchmarking compares a work function with the functional leader even when the leader is in a different industry. However, clinical functions, by their technical nature, restrict the search for benchmarking partners to health care organizations.

Internal benchmarking involves the identification of best practices within one's own organization. Internal benchmarking is both an effort to improve performance and a low-risk way to share performance data. By publishing your performance data in medical journals, others can learn what a high-performing organization is doing to achieve results.

Benchmarking depends on the disciplined collection and use of objective information. The paradigm is simple, and entails:

- Identifying critical success factors and determining key indicators
- Collecting information relevant to the key indicators

- Searching to identify extraordinary performers, as defined by the data
- Identifying the factors that drive superior performance
- Adopting or adapting those factors that fit into your processes

There are three types of benchmarking indicators: ratio, process, and outcome.

Ratio indicators establish a relationship between two measures (e.g., worked hours per unit of service). Ratio indicators are generally indicative of productivity or of a volume measurement. They provide a comparative performance point to other departments or hospitals but do not reveal information about the practices that drive the performance.

Process indicators measure a process with a beginning point and an ending point (e.g., blood gas measurement turnaround time). Process indicators lead to investigations of the practice that drives the performance.

Outcome indicators measure clinical outcomes (e.g., patient returns to the emergency department within 24 hours). Outcome indicators lead to an understanding of the practices that provide the best possible clinical outcomes.

Once the key indicators have been identified, useful information (data) about existing processes are collected. Most quality improvement tools depend on accurate data. The methods of data collection (except perhaps financial data) are not much different from the methods of formal research. Keep in mind that when one attempts to compare data from one department with that of another, the comparison is impossible unless the measures are defined in such a way apples are being compared to apples.

Once data are gathered, they are analyzed using the same procedures as those used in formal research projects. These procedures include both descriptive and inferential statistics and graphic illustrations. In benchmarking jargon, this phase is sometimes called "gap analysis" because the researcher is trying to identify any gaps or differences among benchmarking participants.

Once the gap analysis is complete and the results are known, individuals typically respond in one of three ways: denial, rationalizing, or learning.

Seldom will the results of a benchmarking project proclaim any department "best of class" across the board. More often the news is less than uplifting, perhaps even discouraging. The natural response from a manager is denial, insisting that the data cannot be correct. Unfortunately, they probably are. Facing reality is often the most difficult part of benchmarking.

The second response is rationalization. In the attempt to explain away the gaps identified in the data analysis, managers usually try to find errors in the data or methods used to collect the data. If an error can be uncovered, then they think business can continue as usual. The cry is often "We're unique!" and the implication is that just because a methodology worked in Hospital A does not mean that it will work for us, because we are different.

Learning is the third response. Learning comes from accepting reality and taking actions to change it. Corrective action begins with accepting that the benchmarking data are probably correct, asking the right questions, and realizing that lessons can be learned.

The overriding objective of benchmarking is to identify and learn about best practices. But unless we implement the best practices, we have engaged in nothing more than an intellectual exercise with little value.

Summary

Outcomes research seeks to understand the end results of particular health care interventions. End results include effects that people experience and care about, such as change in ability to function. In particular, for individuals with chronic conditions (where cure is not always possible) outcome results include quality of life as well as mortality. By linking the care people get to the outcomes they experience, outcomes research has become the key to developing better ways to monitor and improve the quality of care.

The methods of outcomes research vary significantly from those of traditional clinical research. Health care workers need to be familiar with these methods to be educated consumers of (and to participate in) future studies.

Questions

Definitions

Define the following terms:

- Disease management
- Continuous quality improvement
- Outcomes research
- Evidence-based medicine
- Benchmarking

True or False

1. Qualitative research uses classical experimental designs, whereas quantitative research relies on textual data in the form of observational field notes.
2. Outcomes research is centered on patients and communities, while traditional clinical research is disease-centered.
3. Two types of *clinical* measures used in outcomes research are patient symptoms and quality of life.
4. One of the main challenges for outcomes studies is to move from description and methods development to problem solving and quality improvement.
5. *Efficacy* studies attempt to answer the question "Does the intervention work in a tertiary care setting under controlled conditions?" while *effectiveness* studies attempt to answer the question "Does the intervention work in clinical practice settings?"

Multiple Choice

1. An economic evaluation that is applied when two or more interventions are compared on the same outcomes and the outcomes have similar effectiveness is:
   a. Cost identification
   b. Cost minimization

c. Cost effectiveness

d. Cost utility

2. An economic analysis used when the same outcomes are measured but effectiveness differs is:

a. Cost identification

b. Cost minimization

c. Cost effectiveness

d. Cost utility

3. The main value of benchmarking is:

a. It is a practical alternative when there is not enough time or money for a scientific study.

b. It is better than continuous quality improvement.

c. No patient data are needed.

d. Many hospitals can collaborate.

4. A benchmarking indicator that establishes a relationship between two measures such as worked hours per unit of service is called a:

a. Process indicator

b. Ratio indicator

c. Outcome indicator

d. All of the above

5. Common responses of managers confronted with benchmarking results include all but:

a. Arguing that the data are incorrect

b. Attempting to explain away results by asserting that their situation is unique

c. Learning from the experience of others

d. Insisting on performing a gap analysis

References

1. Stoller JK, Orens D, Ahmad M. Changing patterns of respiratory care service use in the era of respiratory care protocols: An observational study. *Respir Care.* 1998;43(8):637–642.

2. Adams AB, Shapiro R, Marini JJ. Changing prevalence of chronically ventilator-assisted individuals in Minnesota: Increases, characteristics, and the use of noninvasive ventilation. *Respir Care.* 1998; 43(8):643–649.

3. Espie CA, Fleming L, Cassidy J, Samuel L, Taylor LM, White CA, Douglas NJ, Engleman HM, Kelly HL, Paul J. Randomized controlled clinical effectiveness trial of cognitive behavior therapy compared with treatment as usual for persistent insomnia in patients with cancer. *J Clin Oncol.* 2008;26(28): 4651–4658.

4. Parker L, Walker J. Effects of a pulmonary rehabilitation program on physiologic measures, quality of life, and resource utilization in an HMO setting. *Respir Care.* 1998;43(3):177–182.

5. Smith KJ, Pesce RR. Pulmonary artery catheterization in exacerbations of COPD requiring mechanical ventilation: A cost-effectiveness analysis. *Respir Care.* 1994;39(10):961–967.

Section II

Planning the Study

CHAPTER 4

The Scientific Method

Research attempts to find answers using the *scientific method*. Science is simply organized curiosity. The scientific method is the organizational structure by which we formulate questions and answers during experiments. The key purpose of this organizational structure is to allow experiments to be repeated and thus validated by other researchers. In this way, we develop confidence in our findings. Contrary to popular belief, science does not attempt to *prove* anything. You can never prove the truth of an assumption simply because you can never test all the factors that could possibly affect it. Scientific theories are never "true," they are simply useful to various degrees, and their life spans are inversely proportional to the amount of research done on them.

The Scientific Method

The scientific method is usually thought of as a series of steps that lead from question to answer (and then usually to more questions).

Step 1: Formulate a Problem Statement

Research projects usually start out as a vague perception of some problem, either real or imagined. The first step is to refine this vague notion into a concise statement, usually only one or two sentences in length. Think in terms of (1) what you see happening and (2) why it is important. For example, if you find a coin lying on the ground, your problem statement might be "I need to identify this coin so I can decide whether or not to spend it."

Step 2: Generate a Hypothesis

A hypothesis is a short statement that describes your belief or supposition about a specific aspect of the research problem. The hypothesis is what you test with an experiment. Nobody knows where hypotheses come from; forming one is a creative act. All you can do is prepare yourself by studying all aspects of the problem thoroughly so your mind becomes a fertile

Figure 4.1

Algorithm illustrating the scientific method.

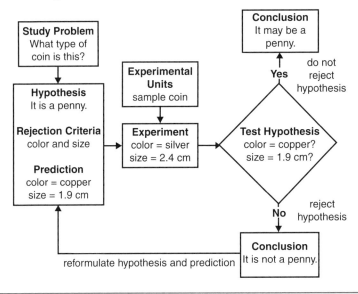

ground for hypotheses to grow. Continuing with our example, we might hypothesize that the coin is a penny (see **Figure 4.1**).

Step 3: Define Rejection Criteria

The purpose of the experiment is to provide data. We will use the data to either reject the hypothesis as false or accept it for the time being as a useful assumption. The fact that we can never prove the truth of a hypothesis leads us to focus on trying to prove it false. We prove that a hypothesis is false by comparing the experimental data with a set of criteria we have established before the experiment began. If the experimental data do not meet the criteria, we reject the hypothesis (hence the name "rejection criteria"). In order to define the rejection criteria, we need to specify what we can measure during the experiment. For example, we could measure the coin's diameter and note its color.

Step 4: Make a Prediction

Next, we make a prediction based on our hypothesis that specifies the rejection values. For example, we can say, "If the coin is a penny, it will have a diameter of 1.9 centimeters and a copper color." The rejection criteria are thus: diameter = 1.9 centimeters and color = copper.

Step 5: Perform the Experiment

The rejection criteria determine the measurements that are required in the experiment. Many factors are involved with designing experiments, some of which we will discuss in the next section. Much of experimental design is based on statistical theory, most of which is beyond the scope of this book. However, the basic idea is to determine (1) what variables to measure, (2) how the measurements should be made, and (3) what experimental units (subjects) will be used for making measurements. In our simple example we have only one experimental unit (the coin), and we need only a ruler and our eyes for making the measurements.

Step 6: Test the Hypothesis

It is the hypothesis, not the experimental subject, that is being tested (despite the fact that we say things like "the patient was tested for cystic fibrosis"). The hypothesis is tested by comparing the experimental data with the rejection criteria. If the data contradict the prediction we made, then the hypothesis is rejected. If not, the hypothesis is accepted as possibly true until further data can be obtained. For example, suppose that the diameter of the coin is 2.1 centimeters and it is silver. Obviously, we would reject the hypothesis that it is a penny. We would then create a new hypothesis (perhaps that the coin is a dime) and a new prediction (based on the diameter and color of a dime).

But suppose the diameter is indeed 1.9 centimeters and the color is copper. Does that mean it is definitely a penny? What if there is a foreign coin that just happens to have those characteristics? So, we simply acknowledge that we may be wrong, but until we have further information, we will suppose the coin is a penny. This example shows that we can do everything right in terms of following the scientific method and still end up with a wrong conclusion. It also shows the critical nature of selecting the right rejection criteria and making accurate measurements as well as how science usually produces more questions than answers.

Steps in Conducting Scientific Research

We will now expand on the basic scientific method to give an overview of the entire process of conducting a research project. Each step in the process will be explained further in later sections of this book.

Develop the Study Idea

The first step is to develop your ideas about the study problem and the specific hypotheses. Ideas come from everyday work experiences, talking with colleagues, and reading professional journals. You must also consider the feasibility of actually conducting the experiment. A great project that you do not have the resources to finish is a waste of time.

Search the Literature

An important step in the research process is a thorough search of the literature. A literature search helps you to find what is already known about your subject and provides ideas for methods you might use for experiments.

Consult an Expert

Before you begin writing the plan for your project, discuss your ideas with someone who has experience with research and statistics. Advice at this point can help you refine the study question, identify appropriate experimental methods, and develop an implementation plan.

Design the Experiment

Three basic study designs are commonly used in health care: (1) the case study, (2) the device or method evaluation, and (3) the clinical study. The case study is a description of a particular patient care episode that has exceptional teaching value. There is usually no need for statistical analysis, so the case study may be a good choice for a novice researcher.

A device or method evaluation has at least some descriptive statistics and may even involve hypothesis testing to determine the efficacy of a treatment or compare the performance of a new device with the performance of older devices. While this design is a little more complicated than the case study, it is very popular among beginning researchers because it usually does not involve the hassle of working with patients.

A clinical study is the most advanced design and usually involves sophisticated statistical procedures, medical equipment, patient care, permission to perform studies, and a variety of other logistical complications. Clinical practice is based on this type of research. However, you should not attempt this type of research until you have some experience and a good mentor.

Write the Protocol

A brief but detailed research protocol serves as a set of instructions for investigators. It also serves to communicate your plans to others, like those from whom you must obtain cooperation or permission to conduct the study.

Obtain Permission

Before conducting a study, you need permission from your immediate supervisor and from any others who will be affected (e.g., physicians, nurses, staff, lab personnel). If the study involves the potential for risk to study subjects, the research protocol will have to be approved by the institutional review board (IRB), which is sometimes called the committee for protection of human subjects. If your study involves the medical treatment of patients (or even animals) you will probably have to get a physician to act as principal investigator in order to obtain permission from the IRB. In addition, any such study requires written consent from the study subjects or their guardians. The decision to participate in a study must be voluntary and the subject must be allowed to withdraw at any time.

Collect the Data

The best-laid plans often fall apart during implementation. Many times, data collection requires more time than originally anticipated. Often the protocol must be revised as problems occur. When planning for the study, make sure you consider how data will be collected, what forms will be used to record the data, and who will be responsible for it.

Analyze the Data

Once the data collection phase is completed, the data are summarized in tables and graphs using basic descriptive statistics. If the study design requires it, formal statistical procedures are used to test hypotheses. Finally, you must interpret the findings and form your conclusions.

Publish the Findings

There is no point in doing all the work of a study if you do not communicate your findings to your colleagues. And you cannot effectively communicate them unless you write a report. Of course, as long as you are going to write anyway, you might as well use a style recommended by one of the medical journals. The manuscript can be a simple one-page abstract. You can then submit the abstract to a journal for review and possible publication. If it is published, it will be preserved as part of medical history in copies of the journal worldwide.

Questions

Definitions

Define the following terms:

- Hypothesis
- Rejection criteria

True or False

1. Experiments are designed to prove that a hypothesis is true.
2. The following is the correct series of steps for using the scientific method:
   a. Formulate the problem
   b. Generate a hypothesis
   c. Define the rejection criteria
   d. Perform the experiment
   e. Test the hypothesis

Multiple Choice

1. All of the following are steps in conducting scientific research except:
   a. Search the literature
   b. Design the experiment
   c. Analyze the data
   d. Survey patients
   e. Publish the results
2. Comparing the experimental results with the rejection criteria is a part of which step in the scientific method?
   a. Creating the problem statement
   b. Formulating the hypothesis
   c. Creating the prediction
   d. Formulating a conclusion
   e. Testing the hypothesis

CHAPTER 5

Developing the Study Idea

P eople often say that emotion and personal belief play no part in the scientific method, that only through detached objectivity can the truth be revealed. If this were in fact the case, there would be no human scientists. Without passion, there could be no hypothesis; without a hypothesis there could be no experiment; and without experimentation there would be no science. This chapter examines the factors that motivate and guide the development of a research protocol.

Sources of Research Ideas

Choosing and defining a research topic are the first steps in applying the scientific method to a clinical research problem. This process implies concern or question about some concept or observation. Indeed, the scientific method itself can be viewed as nothing more than organized curiosity. Curiosity about the details of one's everyday activity provides the impetus for finding out how or why events are related. The scientific method simply provides a standardized and efficient technique for describing these relationships in a way that can be verified by other observers. Curiosity and the creative energy it engenders are vital ingredients of a productive research effort.

In choosing a research topic, your interest may be stimulated in a number of ways. One of the most obvious ways is to read peer-reviewed medical journals to discover what other research-ers are doing. Often one investigator's results will not completely answer the questions another investigator seeks to answer. Perhaps the authors themselves suggest areas where further work needs to be done. Occasionally, the results of an article contradict those of a previous study, creat-ing the need for yet another look at the research problem. Review articles that cover the state of the art in some area of research are especially fruitful in generating ideas along these lines.

The basic concept to remember is that research breeds more research. With this idea in mind, another source of research problems can be identified. You can start with a well-established theory or concept of patient care and test whether or not it is true for a particular set of circumstances. Opportunities arise from the proliferation of technological advancements, as seen in the never-ending stream of medical advertisements. Many, or perhaps even most, new devices have never been closely compared to competing devices outside the engineering laboratories where they were developed. Medical device evaluations and comparisons provide an ideal starting point for beginning researchers.

A third major source of research topics is the realm of personal experience. Your day-to-day work experience constantly provides opportunities to ask, "Why are things done this way?" or "What would happen if … ?" Consider how many daily decisions are based on tradition or authority, without any apparent objective rationales. Often an event that causes a sense of irritation, especially if it is a recurrent event, can be turned into a legitimate research problem that may result in a solution or a better way to do things. Talking with coworkers can also be a valuable source of insight and ideas.

Trying to develop research topics from personal experience is often the most frustrating approach for a beginning researcher. The natural tendency is to choose a general problem that everyone seems to recognize but no one does anything about. The difficulty lies in trying to narrow the general idea to a specific problem statement. There are at least two reasons for this difficulty. First, a general problem, by its nature, is often spoken about in vague, undefined terms. Second, in attempting to describe the problem explicitly, the investigative task may appear to be overwhelming. One may easily become frustrated to the point of not being able to write anything.

One way to avoid this situation is to start small. Begin with a specific incident that stimulated either curiosity or irritation. Simply state what you see happening and why it is important. Write a narrative, first-person account of the incident. This will help you to begin to formulate the research problem with a feeling of involvement and prevent impulsive generalizations.

Developing a Problem Statement

Once a specific idea for a research topic has been selected, the next step is to develop a formal problem statement. This problem statement is the foundation of the actual study design. It dictates the concepts and methods used to gather data. It also determines the theoretical context in which the conclusion will be interpreted. Moving from a loose set of ideas to a formal problem statement, however, is a complex process. It involves many false starts, as original notions are discarded or modified after careful consideration.

The development process begins with an expansion of the scope of the original problem. This stage involves an *inductive* reasoning process of going from specific observations to general theories. At this point, the words and concepts used must be explicitly defined. Definitions not only help to organize one's thoughts but also make it possible to relate the topic to previous research. Explicit definitions also facilitate communication with experts whose experiences are helpful in forming a more realistic perspective of the problem.

The next step is to begin reviewing the literature, using key definitions to speed the search. Try to find analogous problems in other disciplines to create original experimental approaches. For example, many problems concerning clinical measurement (e.g., airway pressure measurement) have been solved in the context of electrical or mechanical engineering. Another aspect of expanding the problem's scope is the identification of any pertinent theories that might be useful in establishing a relationship among a problem's many elements.

For example, suppose you were originally concerned about the maximum respiratory rates that mechanical ventilators were capable of delivering. Perhaps no guidelines exist for selecting a maximum frequency for a patient, and you believe that rates as high as 100 to 150 breaths per minute may be inappropriate. Perhaps you have observed a few patients whose condition deteriorated when ventilated with high rates. In the original narrative account of the research problem, the term *gas trapping* was used. During the process of expanding the original idea, consulting with experts, and reviewing the literature, the concept of gas trapping is found to relate to other specifically defined terms, such as lung compliance, airway resistance, and functional residual capacity. Note that the definitions used here are *operational* definitions; that is, they are defined in terms of the specific operations, observations, or measurements used in gathering the data. Now the problem can be stated more explicitly, forming some general concepts that seem promising.

Your focus of attention should shift from a review of clinically oriented literature to articles dealing more specifically with pulmonary physiology. You may find that the interaction among ventilator frequency, lung compliance, and airway resistance is sometimes described using the concepts of impedance, time constant, and frequency response. A new idea is discovered: the actions of the various components of the respiratory system can be modeled using electrical analogs. Thus, you are led to review electrical engineering texts for a complete understanding of these concepts. This is an excellent example of how a study of analogous problems in related disciplines can help create a general theory by enlarging the scope of the problem.

Once a generalized theoretical framework has been established relating the various concepts that are associated with the research topic, you must narrow and refine those ideas. This is a *deductive* process of going from general theory to a specific application and experimental design. At this stage you need to formulate a specific hypothesis and describe specific experiments to test it. The experimental plan is a description of the variables that will be measured and how they will be interpreted. Using the previous example, you may decide to measure pulmonary compliance and resistance, cardiac output, and the FRC in a series of ten patients. These measurements will be used to test the hypothesis that patients with high resistance and compliance require lower ventilatory frequencies to avoid inadvertent increases in FRC and concomitant decreases in cardiac output.

A formal statement of the research problem might be: "The optimum ventilator frequency for patients with chronic obstructive pulmonary disease is less than that for patients with normal lungs." Of course, the term *optimum* must be defined in terms of measurable criteria. The problem statement, along with the supporting theoretical framework and experimental design, constitutes the research protocol.

Finally, a formal research protocol must be drafted using the specific outline required by your institutional review board. This outline will include a consent form that must be written in nontechnical lay terms.

Keep in mind that not all research topics should be developed in exactly this format. Development of the topic depends on the level of the research. There are three basic levels of research. At the first level, you are primarily interested in describing *what* occurs in a particular situation. Typically, little or no literature is available on the topic, and the research design tends to be exploratory or descriptive. The problem statement is often declarative in nature, and the research method centers on specific laboratory or patient observations and questionnaires. The data analysis is usually based on descriptive statistics. Examples of this type of research appear frequently in the "Methods and Devices" section of medical journals.

The second level of research includes a description of the *relationships* between or among variables. Usually there is some literature available on the topic, but not enough to predict the action of the variables. The problem statement may be in the form of a question, and the research method is often a descriptive survey using structured questionnaires or physiologic measurements. This method differs from that of the previous level in that some conclusion can be made about *how* variables are related. The data analysis typically involves correlation and regression statistics. Examples of this type of research can be found in the many studies comparing transcutaneous blood gas values with traditional arterial blood gas analysis or comparing arterial oxygen saturation via pulse oximetry with directly measured oximeter values.

The third level of research seeks to explain *why* variables are related in a particular manner. Usually enough literature is available on the topic to predict the action of specific variables based on a particular theoretical framework. The problem statement should be in the form of a hypothesis, and the research method involves randomized controlled experiments. Data analysis is usually in the form of statistical procedures that distinguish significant differences between estimated population parameters.

Judging the Feasibility of the Project

The process of identifying and defining a research topic, because of the personal commitment involved, can be very nearsighted. That is, after all the effort you put into developing a research topic, you may find it difficult to see that others might not be interested in supporting the project or that feasibility problems make the study's implementation questionable. Thus, before beginning the study, step back mentally and evaluate the overall worth of the project in a larger context. The major considerations are listed in **Table 5.1**.

Significance of the Problem

In the early stages of the project, you should ask questions like: What are the potential implications of the study results? Will a specific population of patients, the medical community, or society in general benefit from the proposed study? Will the results lead to practical applications or an expansion of medical knowledge? Will the findings support or challenge untested assumptions?

Examine your own personal motives. Will the research effort culminate in a published journal article? If you are interested in describing a *breakthrough* discovery in a *classic* article, the scope of your research problem should be able to be linked to a general theory so that the

Table 5.1

Factors Affecting the Feasibility of a Research Project

1. Significance or potential benefits of study results
2. Measurability of research variables
3. Duration and timing of study
4. Availability of research subjects
5. Availability of equipment and funds
6. Knowledge and experience of investigators

results will have broad application. Alternatively, problems of a more limited scale can be very relevant to departmental policy making. Every author enjoys the satisfaction of having a manuscript accepted for publication. The goal of a study, however, should never be the advancement of personal prestige. Concentrate your efforts on providing the highest quality of research. Fame will take care of itself.

Measurability of the Problem

To use the scientific method to investigate a research topic, the problem statement must involve *variables* that can be precisely *measured* and *defined*. Thus, questions concerning morals or ethics are usually not appropriate research topics. However, such questions may possibly be modified to allow research of a related aspect of the general issue. For example, the research question "Do patients have the right to die?" is too arbitrary to be an appropriate topic. Consider an alternative question: "Does a health care worker's experience reflect his or her opinion about euthanasia?" This topic may be studied by means of a survey, and the knowledge gained might be useful in developing an understanding of the general ethical issue, which in turn facilitates future decision making.

Time Constraints

A good research plan specifies the expected amount of time necessary to complete the project. This is necessary to evaluate other factors, such as patient availability and cost. In addition, it may be necessary to time the study to coincide with optimum data collection. For example, a study of postoperative cardiac patients should coincide with surgeons' schedules if there are seasonal fluctuations in the types of patients they see.

Availability of Subjects

Research subjects may be anything from ultrasonic nebulizers to rabbits to human infants. If the study will use inanimate objects, make sure you have an adequate supply of functional units. If the study involves animals, ensure that suitable facilities are available and adhere to specific guidelines to ensure their humane care. If the experimental subjects are humans, the cooperation of a physician will be needed.

  If the study will test a hypothesis, the most crucial aspect of determining subject availability is knowing how many subjects you will need. You must perform some elementary statistical calculations *before* gathering data to ensure the usefulness of the statistical conclusion *after* the data are gathered (see discussion of sample size in Chapter 10).

Cost and Equipment

In addition to planning for the proper equipment and space to conduct a study, consider the cost involved. If you intend to apply for a research grant, you must itemize expected costs. Expense categories might include:

- *Literature:* Index cards, journals, literature searches, manuscript copies, and illustration fees

- *Labor:* Reimbursement to subjects for cooperation, salary support for technicians and secretaries, laboratory tests, and consultation fees
- *Supplies and laboratory equipment:* Paper, notebooks, recorders, transducers, and amplifiers
- *Transportation:* If the results will be presented at a national convention

Experience

Although you may be able to obtain help with the various aspects of the study, you should avoid sophisticated measuring instruments or complex statistical analysis for your first study. Planning the project from beginning to end helps to avoid the demoralizing experience of having to abandon the study because of being "in over your head."

Summary

Selecting a clinical research problem is a nebulous process. William I.B. Beveridge has said, "It is not possible deliberately to create ideas or to control their creation. When a difficulty stimulates the mind, suggested solutions just automatically spring into the consciousness. The variety and quality of the suggestions are functions of how well prepared our mind is by past experience and education pertinent to the particular problem. What we can do deliberately is to prepare our minds in this way, voluntarily direct our thoughts to a certain problem, hold attention on that problem, and appraise the various suggestions thrown up by the subconscious mind."[1]

Appraising the various aspects of a given research problem is the process of identifying and defining specific variables and placing these variables into a unifying theoretical framework. This appraisal is essentially an inductive intellectual process, moving from specific observations to general theories. What follows is the deductive process of reasoning from these general theories to particular hypotheses, and the creation of experiments to test them. There can be no rigid order to the steps used in formulating a research statement. The general thought process, however, should roughly follow the flow chart illustrated in **Figure 5.1**. Experience will dictate your personal style. Remember to include operational definitions, a literature review, and an assessment of feasibility.

Questions

Definitions

Define the following terms:

- Inductive reasoning
- Deductive reasoning
- Operational definitions
- Feasibility analysis

Figure 5.1

General thought process involved in developing a formal research protocol.

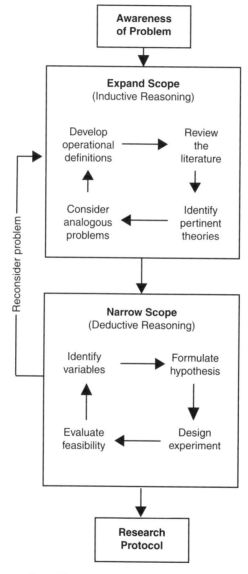

Beginning with an awareness of a problem, the scope of the topic is expanded by a recursive process of creating definitions, reviewing the literature, identifying relevant theories, and considering similar problems in other areas. A theoretical framework or conceptual model can then be created. Next, specific variables and hypotheses suggested by the model are developed, and experiments are designed to test the hypotheses. If the experiments do not seem feasible, reconsider the study problem. You may have developed a new perspective that would lead you to start over using a slightly different line of reasoning.

True or False

1. A major source of potential research ideas is medical journals.

2. The problem statement is important because it dictates the concepts and methods used to gather data.

3. The general thought process in developing a research protocol is to go from a narrow scope to an expanded scope.

Multiple Choice

1. Deciding whether the results of a study may lead to practical applications applies to which factor in the feasibility analysis?

    a. Significance of study results

    b. Measurability of research variables

    c. Duration and timing of study

    d. Availability of research subjects

    e. Availability of equipment and funds

    f. Knowledge and experience of investigators

2. Deciding to consult a statistician applies to which factor in the feasibility analysis?

    a. Significance of study results

    b. Measurability of research variables

    c. Duration and timing of study

    d. Availability of research subjects

    e. Availability of equipment and funds

    f. Knowledge and experience of investigators

3. Realizing that the sample size required will take too long to gather applies to which factor in a feasibility analysis?

    a. Significance of study results

    b. Measurability of research variables

    c. Duration and timing of study

    d. Availability of research subjects

    e. Availability of equipment and funds

    f. Knowledge and experience of investigators

4. Which factor in a feasibility analysis would prompt you to see if rabbits were available in the medical school's animal lab?

    a. Significance of study results

    b. Measurability of research variables

    c. Duration and timing of study

    d. Availability of research subjects

    e. Availability of equipment and funds

    f. Knowledge and experience of investigators

Reference

1. Beveridge WIB. (1950). *The Art of Scientific Investigation.* New York: Vintage.

CHAPTER 6

Reviewing the Literature*

Once you have identified a clinical problem, the next step is to review the available literature. A thorough investigation of others' works at this point can save time, money, and trouble. Ample research may already have been done on a particular area of interest. Also, opportunities for further research may be quickly revealed. Regardless of the techniques and sources used, literature review is a vital step in any research project.

Why conduct a review? First, the literature review enables you to discover whether related studies have already been done. If there have been six studies showing that the highest obtainable F_{IO_2} reached with a particular manual resuscitation bag is greater than 0.90, then another study is obviously not needed to reconfirm these findings. If, however, there has been only one study comparing the aerosol output of two ultrasonic nebulizers and the results are highly controversial, this could be a useful area to explore. In fact, any area in which there is a great amount of controversy would be worthy of further exploration. A single study is not conclusive. A study's original findings are considered valid only after several other investigations have replicated them.

Researchers must immerse themselves in the literature on a specific topic to become knowledgeable about previous related studies. Research on a particular subject should be conducted by those who are well versed in this area and are able to converse intelligently on all aspects of the topic. Consider the benefit of communicating with other researchers and experts in the field, and being able to "pick their brains" if a problem arises during the course of the research. You are encouraged to communicate directly with recognized experts in an area of inquiry who are on the cutting edge of knowledge. Although other studies may have been done in a certain area, you may have a completely different approach. You may find you need to reassess your plan of action. Perhaps the scope of your project should be narrowed or even refocused on another area entirely.

A further reason for performing a literature search is to learn how others designed their studies. Proper design can make the difference between a significant study and a useless one. If the intent is to replicate earlier work, this investigation will enable use of the earlier author's design, if it is a good one. By looking at several different study designs, you can judge which

---

*This chapter is based on articles by Robert Chatburn and Charles Durbin published in *Respiratory Care* (October 2009).

may be best suited to address the current problem. Perhaps an entirely different design will better serve the purpose. In fact, by noting where previous authors had difficulty, you can avoid duplicating earlier mistakes.

Conducting the Literature Search

Scope of the Review

If your investigation is of a relatively new device or procedure, a search of all available literature on the topic is not only possible but desirable if a limited number of articles about it exist.

Other areas of inquiry may have a much more extensive base in the literature. In these cases, fiscal and temporal constraints will make an exhaustive search impossible. Therefore, you will have to decide how to limit the inquiry. One way of limiting the number of citations included in a search is to look at only the past three or five years. Such a search will provide the most recent research, some of which may be replications of and thus confirmations or refutations of earlier studies. Recent articles will likely refer to a few significant earlier works that formed the basis for many subsequent studies. Reading a few of those earlier articles may give you the historical "flavor" of a particular topic. This is especially important if there is controversy surrounding the topic.

If you have difficulty in narrowing the field to a manageable size, a search of the past year will show the most popular topics. This search may also change the direction of your proposed study. The topic of interest may have been extensively and conclusively detailed by others. Conversely, you may note an obvious gap in the literature that merits further study.

The importance of performing a proper literature search at this stage cannot be overemphasized. As a first-time researcher, you will have many questions about general principles that a more experienced researcher can answer. Identifying a mentor to provide guidance throughout the process is essential if you want to complete your first project successfully. This mentor can provide assistance in obtaining funding, serve as a sounding board when difficult decisions need to be made, and identify other resource persons to assist in specific areas, such as statistical analysis.

Sources of Information

Books

You may think that textbooks would be the first place to look for information about the research problem. The problem with books is that the information they contain is usually outdated before it is even published. Consider that it takes between two and five years from the time an author starts writing to the time the book appears on store shelves. Consider further that the reference papers the book is based on take one to two years to get published, and most of the papers referenced are not new. So, at best, the information in textbooks is three to seven years old, and most of it is much older than that.

However, textbooks are usually a good place to look for basic theories and concepts that you can use as a foundation for building your own hypotheses. They are also good for learning about measurement, statistical, and even patient care techniques needed for designing your experiments. Finally, textbooks often have good lists of reference articles that can be a start in further literature searches. Pay particular attention to the names of authors who seem to be authorities on particular subjects. You will want to search for more recent articles by these authors.

Journal Articles

Most of the information you will use in formulating your research plan will come from medical journal articles. The question is how to find the right information. You must first understand that for just about any topic that has been researched, you will find conflicting results in published papers. That means you must try to read at least the abstracts of all papers published in the last three to five years on your topic, if such papers exist. Then, you must distinguish the controversial areas from those that are relatively settled. The controversial areas will provide ideas for new research, and the settled areas provide ideas for experimental designs.

Look also for recent papers that are reviews of existing knowledge. For example, you might find an article entitled "Alternative to percussion and postural drainage: A review of mucus clearing therapies." Such an article will save you a lot of work because the author has already searched the literature to find and summarize the published articles on that particular topic. Not only will the review itself be helpful, but its list of references will also be useful for further searches.

A growing number of periodicals summarize the best evidence in traditional journals. They provide structured abstracts of the best studies and expert commentaries. These new journals include *Evidence-Based Medicine*, *Evidence-Based Nursing*, and *Evidence-Based Cardiovascular Medicine*. Such journals summarize the best evidence from high-quality studies selected from all the journals of relevance to our research interests.

Databases

A database is a structured collection of facts. A list of names and phone numbers on a piece of paper is a database. A spreadsheet containing a business profit and loss statement is a database. And, of course, a project created with a software database design program like Microsoft Access is a database. The structure is called the database model (e.g., a relational model), but the specifics are beyond the scope of this book. Part of the database structure is the *index*, or mechanism for locating specific data and for enforcing rules, such as preventing duplicate entries. Data are often indexed using a *controlled vocabulary*, a carefully selected set of words and phrases such that each concept is described using only one term in the set and each term in the set describes only one concept. For example, an article about continuous positive airway pressure (CPAP) might be indexed using a hierarchical controlled vocabulary such as:

1.0. Therapeutics
1.1. Respiratory Therapy
   1.1.1. Respiration, Artificial
      1.1.1.1. Positive-Pressure Respiration
        • Continuous Positive Airway Pressure

The power of the computer has allowed us to create gigantic databases with very complex structures. Such databases allow us to define many different ways of relating the data (i.e., information or creating meaning), to find that information more quickly than any other time in history, and to display it in whatever form we can imagine. There are three basic database categories commonly used for storing medical data: bibliographic, citation, and synthesized.

Bibliographic Databases

A bibliographic, or library, database contains information on books, book chapters, reports, citations, abstracts, and either the full text of the articles indexed or links to the full text. Perhaps the most popular bibliographic database is PubMed (www.ncbi.nlm.nih.gov/sites/entrez?db=pubmed), a free service of the U.S. National Library of Medicine that includes over 18 million citations from MEDLINE and other life-science journals for biomedical articles dating back to 1948 (**Table 6.1**). PubMed includes links to full-text articles and other related resources in medicine, nursing, dentistry, veterinary medicine, health care systems, and pre-clinical sciences. It provides a Clinical Queries search filters page as well as a Special Queries page. The site also provides automatic e-mailing of search updates, the ability to save records, and filters for search results using "My NCBI." PubMed also lets you save your search results in a variety of ways.

Another free bibliographic medical database you should know about is SearchMedica (www.searchmedica.com). According to the SearchMedica Web site, "SearchMedica . . .

Table 6.1

Useful Internet Sites

PubMed: www.ncbi.nlm.nih.gov/sites/entrez?db=pubmed
SearchMedica: www.searchmedica.com
ISI Web of Knowledge: http://isiwebofknowledge.com
The Cochrane Collaboration: www.cochrane.org
UpToDate: www.uptodate.com
National Guideline Clearinghouse: www.guideline.gov
MDConsult: www.mdconsult.com
Oxford Reference: oxfordreference.com
STAT!Ref: statref.com
Safari Books Online: safaribooksonline.com
Amazon.com: www.amazon.com
EndNote software: www.endnote.com
RefWorks software: www.refworks.com
Zotero software: www.zotero.org

[delivers] only the most clinically reputable content intended for practicing medical clinicians. With guidance from our advisory board of specialty physicians and our staff editors, Search-Medica scans well-known, credible journals, systematic reviews, and evidence-based articles that are written and edited for clinicians practicing in primary care and all major specialties. Using similar expertise, SearchMedica also selects and scans patient-directed websites, online CME courses, and government databases of clinical trials and practice guidelines."[1]

Citation Databases

A citation database is specially designed so that you can track the progress of an idea or research topic by searching the published works that cite a particular author or article. The most popular citation database is probably the ISI Web of Knowledge (http://isiwebof knowledge.com). This site includes 700 million cited references from 23,000 journals covering 256 scientific disciplines. It has access to 9,000 Web sites, 110 conference proceedings, 23 million patents, and over 100 years of back files.

Synthesized Databases

Synthesized databases are pre-filtered records for particular topics. They are usually subscription based with relatively large fees. This type of database may provide the "best" evidence without extensive searches of standard bibliographic databases. The leading database in this category is the Cochrane Collaboration (www.cochrane.org). Cochrane reviews are designed to be exhaustive reviews of the literature on a given topic. The results provide a comprehensive analysis of the existing evidence and are presented in the following format:

* Objectives (of the review)
* Search strategy (e.g., databases used)
* Selection criteria (types of studies included in the reviews; e.g., randomized controlled trials)
* Data collection and analysis (e.g., emphasis on allocation concealment, adherence to intention-to-treat principle)
* Main results (e.g., number of studies included in the report, total number of patients studied, statistical meta-analyses)
* Authors' conclusions (a concise statement of the take-home message)

Another synthesized database, UpToDate (www.uptodate.com), is a subscription-based service that claims to be the largest clinical community in the world dedicated to synthesizing knowledge for clinicians and patients. It has 3,800 expert clinicians who function as authors, editors, and peer reviewers and 320,000 users who provide feedback and questions to the editorial group. They cover 7,400 topics in 13 medical specialties. The service provides graded treatment recommendations based on the best medical evidence.

There is a free synthesized database you may find useful: the National Guideline Clearinghouse (NGC; www.guideline.gov). The NGC is a comprehensive database of evidence-based clinical practice guidelines and related documents created by the Agency for Healthcare

Research and Quality (AHRQ), U.S. Department of Health and Human Services. According to the Web site, "The NGC mission is to provide physicians, nurses, and other health professionals, health care providers, health plans, integrated delivery systems, purchasers and others an accessible mechanism for obtaining objective, detailed information on clinical practice guidelines and to further their dissemination, implementation and use."[2]

Portals

Portals are Web pages that act as a starting point for using the Web or Web-based services. One example of a subscription-based service is MDConsult (www.mdconsult.com), which provides links to books, journals, patient education resources, and images. Another example is Ovid, which provides links to books, journals, evidence-based medicine databases (e.g., Cochrane Collaboration), and the Cumulative Index to Nursing and Allied Health Literature (CINAHL). Most medical libraries will have subscriptions to both of these services.

Electronic Journals and Books

Many medical journals are now available online. Of note, the *Journal of Physiology* has articles dating back to 1878.

Many electronic versions of textbooks are available on the Internet. From the PubMed homepage, select "Search Books" from the drop-down menu (instead of "Search PubMed"), enter a search term, and you will get a results page with tabs for books and figures from books. Subscription services include Oxford Reference Online (oxfordreference.com), STAT!Ref (statref.com; great source for nursing and drugs), and Safari Books Online (safaribooksonline.com; excellent source of technical reference books). Your medical library will probably have subscriptions to these services.

Google (google.com) will let you search for books, too. Just select the "More" link at the top of the page and then select "Books."

Also, do not forget Amazon.com. Books on this site are all for sale, but often you can find them (even those out of print) used for a small fraction of their original cost. If you do not want to buy the book, use Amazon for ideas before you go to the library.

General Internet Resources

There are many free search engines of which you are probably already aware. Sites like Google, Yahoo!, AltaVista, and Ask are all useful. But remember, these sites use proprietary search algorithms rather than controlled vocabularies like PubMed, so you are likely to get unexpected results. You might also consider so-called meta-search engines (such as clusty.com, dogpile.com, and surfwax.com) that transmit your search terms simultaneously to several individual search engines.

Suggestions for Conducting Searches

The first and most important suggestion I can offer is to talk to a professional librarian. These people can show you all the tricks of the trade—things you never imagined could be done. In some cases, they will even do the search for you. Some libraries offer free courses on how to use all kinds of software tools for conducting searches.

Aside from that, I suggest that you make sure you understand your topic (e.g., the basic concepts and relevant terminology) before getting started. Then, start with review articles and look at their reference lists. Use the key words from relevant articles as your search terms. Be specific. Learn about Medical Subject Headings (MeSH terms, used by the United States National Library of Medicine to index articles in Index Medicus and MEDLINE) at PubMed. Use the "Related Articles" links at PubMed and other sites to help guide your search. Finally, buy and use bibliographic software such as EndNote or RefWorks. These programs let you import the results of your reference searches into your own database for future use. If you are an author, they will also help you manage the references in your manuscripts. Programs like these will save you a lot of time and effort. A great free bibliographic software program called Zotero can be downloaded at www.zotero.org.

How to Read a Research Article

This is the *Information Age*. New knowledge is accumulating at an exponential rate. Acquiring new knowledge is essential to providing acceptable medical care throughout one's career. For most individuals, reading, whether from print or electronic media, remains the most common way of acquiring new information. Information is not enough to create knowledge. Experts have defined information literacy as consisting of several identified skills and abilities. Broad categories of these competencies are listed in **Table 6.2**.

Reading can take many forms. Casual perusal of news reports or digested summaries of published papers are daily activities in an active reader's life. This chapter develops an approach to reading and appraising a scientific research paper efficiently and critically. In accordance with the broad competencies and skills described in Table 6.2, this section will deal with

Table 6.2

Necessary Competencies of Lifelong Learning

Critical and creative thinking
Problem analysis
Ability to gather and organize information
Abstract reasoning
Interpretive and assessment skills
Insight and intuition in generating knowledge
Effective communication
Information literacy competency, which consists of the following abilities:
- To recognize the need for information
- To know how to access information
- To understand how to evaluate information
- To know how to synthesize information
- To be able to communicate information

recognizing the need for information, evaluation of new information, and to a limited degree, synthesis of this information.

It is through research that new therapies and ideas that have the potential to improve health care are developed and evaluated. Research papers are the written reports of experiments created by the clinician scientists who performed these experiments. A research paper provides the details of the experiment to allow readers decide if the findings are likely to be useful to patients in their care. Unfortunately, reading a research paper is hard work and it takes time to do well. Not all research work is of high quality, and it is helpful to decide if the quality of the study merits reading the paper. Judging the quality of a research paper is important to the potential reader for several other reasons. Since time for reading is limited and attention span is short, the first task of an efficient reader is to select quality reports. The second important task is to read the selected papers efficiently. Most casual readers prefer brief summaries of new thoughts and ideas rather than a detailed description of the scientific study that led to the advance. However, to achieve understanding at a deeper level demands accessing and reading the primary data sources. This level of involvement also leads to more pleasure as command of a field of knowledge develops in the reader. Further reading and understanding builds on past mastery, and continued study becomes second nature rather than a duty or task to be accomplished. However, there is never enough time, so proper selection and systematic reading are important skills to develop.

Selecting a Research Paper to Read

The first question a reader must answer is: "Why read this research paper at all?" As part of lifelong learning, most clinicians use several methods to keep up with current published information. Subjects of particular and continuing interest are often approached with broad electronic searches of medical information databases, such as the National Institute of Medicine's MEDLINE. A successful search strategy can be automated and deliver updated results by e-mail, identifying potentially useful papers on a routine basis. Another way to keep up is to review the table of contents of current medical journals for titles that may be of interest. **Table 6.3** lists several reasons why people may decide to read a particular paper. While all of these reasons have some validity, only readers with previous understanding and interest in the subject are likely to devote the energy necessary to complete the reading task. In fact, a paper that appears to disprove a strongly held belief will generate the most attention in the reader.

Table 6.3

Why Read a Particular Article?

It is an area of science or practice with which you are already quite familiar and have an active interest.
  • The title suggests the paper supports your bias.
  • The title suggests it may disprove your belief.
It appears to be an area in which you know little, and want to know more.
It could it provide a solution for a clinical issue you are currently facing.
You know nothing about the subject but have a desire to increase your knowledge.
It was assigned to you to be read.

A reader may also be interested in a paper that appears to support the reader's bias. Such papers provide only mild interest, as no personal challenge is apparent. Also, a researcher who is "assigned" to read a paper will read it, but without a personal commitment to the content. The exercise will increase critical reading skills but will not likely change understanding of the subject. It can, of course, provide the background for paper selection in the future and should be encouraged when time and effort are available (as in structured classroom learning or at a journal club).

Organization of Research Papers

Research papers are rigidly constructed. Science editors require that submitted papers conform to universal guidelines and style. This is fortunate for the reader, as this predictable organization allows a consistent approach to reading and evaluating a research paper. All research papers will include a title and abstract, as well as the following separate sections: introduction (or background), methods, results, discussion, and conclusions. Additional information will include a list of references or endnotes, institutional affiliation of the authors, if the material has been presented elsewhere, and grant support (if any). This organization scheme is summarized in **Table 6.4**. The names of the separate parts may differ across journals, but there is

Table 6.4

Organization of Research Papers

Title
  Authors
  Affiliation and author contact information
  Grant support (conflict of interest)
  Previous presentation of data (if appropriate)
Abstract
  Introduction (background or hypothesis)
  Setting or subjects
  Methods
  Results
  Major conclusions
Introduction
  Background information
  Statement of study purpose or hypothesis
Methods
  Details of study
  Statistical tests chosen and decided level for significance
Results
  Summary of all results
  Figures
  Tables
Discussion
  Background
  Limitations

(Continues)

Table 6.4 (Continued)

Differences from previous similar studies
Supporting evidence from other studies
Meaning of results
Speculation of importance (or lack thereof)
Future work recommendations
References
Additional contributors not qualifying as primary authors
Audience discussion (if a report of a conference presentation)

an expectation of similar content. Details of this standard organization and other useful information about scientific publications can be found at the Web site of the International Committee of Medical Journal Editors (www.icmje.org). Specific journals may have slightly different requirements for content organization, and these details can be found in the journal section called "Instructions for Authors," often published in the January issue or on the journal's home page. In addition, other important requirements such as listing of authors' institutional affiliations, reporting of conflict of interests, formatting requirements, and qualifications to be included as an author are detailed.

What Is in a Title?

Often, the most helpful part of a paper is the title. This is what attracts a reader in the first place, and it is also where search engines look for keywords and for topics. A poor title may hide an important experiment from the reader or may not even accurately identify the subject matter. The best titles will tell you a great deal about the study and allow quick dismissal or inclusion for further attention. Some titles offer little useful information but only whet your appetite. The efficient reader prefers the most descriptive titles. For instance, a paper entitled "Mechanical ventilation guided by esophageal pressure in acute lung injury" tells the reader in general what this paper is about.[3] However, it does not tell the reader the study was in human subjects. Also missing is the fact that the study is a randomized, prospective, controlled study that demonstrated better oxygenation and pulmonary compliance when PEEP was applied guided by esophageal pressure rather than proximal airway pressure. Also not included in this title is fact that no important clinical outcome benefit (survival or length of stay) was seen. While it is unlikely that all of these facts would appear in a title, some additional information could have saved the reader time in ferreting out these details. This same title could be used for a paper studying laboratory animals, not humans, and it could have been a review article or an editorial. Whether to read this article or not requires more attention and further investigation to decide. If the title had been "Outcome of mechanical ventilation guided by esophageal pressure in patients with ARDS: a randomized, controlled study," even the casual reader would immediately have a better understanding of the content of this paper.

The Abstract

After the title, the abstract is the most important part of the paper to examine. Many journals require a structured abstract with separate subheadings, allowing you to quickly identify the important parts of the study. Most structured abstracts contain the following sections: background (or hypothesis), methods, results, and conclusions. While some people will read the abstract from the beginning, an efficient reader will begin with the abstract conclusions first. This section should provide the most important facts found in the study, which can then help you decide whether to read the entire abstract and, ultimately, the paper. Abstracts of most science papers are available online for free and can be identified and viewed with most search engines. Many bibliographic databases limit the number of words reported in an abstract, so some of the details of the paper will be omitted from the electronic abstract. Extraordinarily long abstracts may be truncated at a specific word limit (usually 250–300 words) and will be missing important parts of the abstract. This is unfortunate and limits your ability to screen papers by electronic abstract alone.

The abstract conclusion highlights the important results from the experiment. In the example presented above, the statement "a ventilator strategy using esophageal pressures to estimate the transpulmonary pressure significantly improves oxygenation and compliance" should attract the acute care respiratory therapist's attention and identify the need for more information. The abstract is not read in order, and the next section of interest will be the abstract methods. This section of the abstract clearly indicates that this is a study of humans with ARDS and it was prospective and randomized—qualities that significantly enhance the strength of the experimental data obtained. A reader with a prior background understanding of how difficult it is to measure esophageal pressure accurately is most likely to want to read more about the study than is presented in the abstract. After quickly reviewing the abstract results section, the question "Why was the study terminated prematurely?" can be answered only by a more detailed analysis of the entire paper.

To recap: a structured abstract often helps you decide if you should read the entire paper. Reading the abstract conclusion first may allow you to reject the paper, or it may lead to an increased interest in the details of the experiment. The abstract methods section may answer the question why *not* to read the paper, or it may strengthen your interest in learning more details of the study. The abstract introduction or background may provide a useful overview of the problem, but it will not help the critical reader who will want to proceed to the actual article for further details. When reading the body of the paper, it is often helpful to have a copy of the abstract physically (or electronically) at hand to compare to the more expanded sections to confirm that the relevant information is consistent in both places. You will also find it useful to note any questions that were raised to be sure you find answers when reading the full paper.

How to Read the Actual Paper

Once you decide to read a paper, you will want to begin with the methods section. The abstract should have provided you with an understanding of the results, but it is important to examine the methods section carefully to determine if the study could answer the research question posed. You should determine the hypotheses being tested with the experiment. An explicit statement of the implied hypotheses will allow you to judge the potential for success of the experiment and assess if correct statistical methods were used. The methods section should provide the details needed to understand the experiment and describe the procedures with enough detail that someone else could exactly repeat the study. If this is not true and significant details are missing, you should note these and continue to search other parts of the paper to determine if these details of the experimental design can be ascertained. Some details may be found hidden in the results section, and occasionally in the discussion. If important details are not found and they may have affected the outcome of the experiment, you should consider writing a "letter to the editor" identifying these deficiencies and describing how they may have affected the reported results. This critical response often elicits an author's response acknowledging the issues or providing further information clarifying the experiment. The ability to question an author publicly and receive a published response is the heart of the scientific reporting that uses challenge and refinement to create new ideas and move knowledge forward.

Next read the results section, with careful attention to the figures and tables. Each element of data described in the methods section should be reported in the results, either in the text or in figures or tables. No interpretations of the data should be reported in the results section, but statistical analysis and probabilities of difference should be reported here. To understand the choice of a statistical test requires understanding of the hypothesis being tested. Although not a required part of the paper, a simple declarative statement of the hypothesis is very helpful in understanding the experiment and evaluating its results, as mentioned above. In the example paper referred to above, the reader could deduce that one hypothesis being tested was: "In ventilating patients with ARDS or ALI, PEEP guided by esophageal pressure rather than by the ARDSnet guidelines will result in a higher oxygenation index (at 24, 48, or 72 hours)." An appropriate statistical test for this hypothesis might be a Student t test, which is used to compare group average differences of continuous, numeric variables.

As mentioned above, a critical reader should decide if the statistical test and level of significance are appropriate for the experiment as described. In complex studies with unusual statistical analyses, the editor of the journal usually employs a statistician to verify that the correct test is chosen and the analysis accurate. Sometimes one of the authors is a statistician, suggesting that a complex analysis was chosen and performed in a suitable way. This may not help your understanding of the test but may reassure you that appropriate statistical oversight was applied. As a rule of thumb, if a study needs a highly complex analysis to achieve mathematical significance, then the clinical utility of the study results is probably not very important.

If the methods and results sections don't indicate what the hypotheses being tested were, the introduction (or background) section may provide clues. You should read this section at this time or earlier if ferreting out the hypotheses. By this time, the value of further investigation (or not) of the paper should be apparent to you. Either there are glaring problems with the study that must be answered, or it is to be accepted as valid, at least on some points. To continue the reading process, read the discussion next. Here the rules are less rigid; comparative analysis of others' work and speculation is usually permitted. The author should self-report shortcomings and limitations in the study and attempt to explain why his or her results might be different from those reported by others. No new data should be revealed in this section, and no information from the other sections should be repeated. Often this section ends with a brief restatement of the major conclusions. Some journals require a separate conclusion section. The conclusions here should be only those actually tested in the study and confirmed to be valid by statistical analysis, and they are often identical to those in the abstract.

When you have completed reading part or most of the article, you should "file" it in memory and make it available for use later. "Memory" can be your cortex or an actual physical location. An organized filing system is very useful at this point to allow information retrieval in the future.

Summary

The process of acquiring new information and creating knowledge is complex and depends heavily on reading scientific reports. It is necessary to develop a reading method aimed at efficiently deciding to stop reading a paper as rapidly as possible. The rigid and predictable structure of scientific writing helps with this task.

Questions

True or False

1. If your study idea has already been published, you should abandon it.
2. A literature review is necessary only if you do not know anything about your study problem.
3. One good reason to perform the literature review is to see how other researchers designed similar studies.
4. Three good sources of information for a literature review are books, journal articles, and the Internet.
5. Books are the best source of information because they are themselves based on literature reviews.

Multiple Choice

1. In which section of a published research article would you find a brief overview of the study?
   a. Abstract
   b. Introduction
   c. Methods
   d. Results
   e. Discussion/Conclusion

2. In which section would you find a description of the statistical analysis?
a. Abstract
b. Introduction
c. Methods
d. Results
e. Discussion/Conclusion
3. In which section would you expect to find the authors' interpretation of the experimental data?
a. Abstract
b. Introduction
c. Methods
d. Results
e. Discussion/Conclusion
4. Where would you find a statement about the research problem or a hypothesis?
a. Abstract
b. Introduction
c. Methods
d. Results
e. Discussion/Conclusion
5. In which section would you find any p values associated with statistical tests?
a. Abstract
b. Introduction
c. Methods
d. Results
e. Discussion/Conclusion

References

1. SearchMedica: Professional Medical Search. (2009). About Us. Accessed July 13, 2009. Available at: http://searchmedica.com/content/about_us/about_us.ftl.
2. National Guideline Clearinghouse. (2009). About NGC. Accessed July 13, 2009. Available at: http://www.guideline.gov/about/about.aspx.
3. Talmor D, Sarge T, Malhotra A, O'Donnell CR, Ritz R, Lisbon A, Novack V, Loring SH. Mechanical ventilation guided by esophageal pressure in acute lung injury. *N Engl J Med.* 2008;359:2095–2104.

CHAPTER 7

Designing the Experiment

Sampling of subjects or devices for observations and choice of an appropriate research design are two links in the logical chain of the research process. That process began with the definition and delimitation of a problem, a review of the literature (prior knowledge on the subject), identification of the research variables, and the translation of the research problem into a hypothesis. At this point, the investigator must specify the population of interest, decide whether and how to choose a sample, and choose a research design appropriate to the research question.

Samples and Populations

The following terms are used frequently in this chapter:

- *Population:* The entire collection of cases as defined by a set of criteria.
- *Accessible population*: The collection of cases as defined by the criteria and that are available to the investigator.
- *Target population*: The entire collection of cases to which research results (observations or conclusions) are intended to be generalized.
- *Sample*: A subset of the population.

The rationale for making observations on a sample instead of the entire population is conservation of time and money. If a sample is in fact representative of the population from which it is drawn, then measurements from the sample can be validly generalized to the whole population. In contrast, poor sampling methods can cause sample bias, and the sample will not represent the population. A classically cited case is the presidential voting poll of the *Literary Digest* for the 1936 election. A sample of 12 million persons was selected from telephone directories and automobile registration lists. Of the 21% who returned the voting preference card (Republican or Democratic preference), 57% indicated they would vote for the Republican candidate, Alf Landon. As events turned out, the Democrat Franklin D. Roosevelt was elected by a landslide. Sample size did not make up for the selection bias inherent in the sampling technique. The bias was caused by selecting the sample from telephone directories and automobile lists, which were not representative of the voting population in 1936. The survey mechanism used led to a further self-selection bias, known as *volunteerism*: the 21% returning the survey cards may not have been typical of the entire group receiving cards, because volunteers are not necessarily representative of a whole group.

The example of the *Literary Digest* sampling method underscores the difference between the accessible and target populations. If we consider the accessible population to be those on automobile lists and telephone directories, then the target population was intended to be the general voting public. In fact, the accessible population differed from the target population to which the *Literary Digest* wished to generalize its findings. The actual target population was those who possessed cars and telephones, which in 1936 was not the entire voting population.

The distinction of accessible and target populations clearly applies to medical research. Suppose pulmonary function measures are performed in a research study on a sample of inpatient asthmatics, of a certain age and with certain airway reactivity, selected at a large metropolitan public hospital. The accessible population is the group of defined asthmatics at the public hospital. These patients may not be typical of all such asthmatics, since nutritional status and compliance with prescribed treatment often varies with income and education level. Also, a hospitalized group is usually more severe, and a university hospital, if this is such, may see more complex and serious cases. Do the results on the indicated accessible population generalize to outpatients, to private practices, or to different socioeconomic levels? Finding an accessible population, representative of the population of interest, is frequently difficult.

The following points and recommendations apply to selecting samples for a research study:

- Populations are defined by the researcher and should be clearly specified. For instance, all asthmatics with a positive reaction to some standard antigen challenge, and under the age of 12 years, constitute an identifiable group.
- Populations need not be large in number. For example, all Eskimos who inhale smoked tobacco make up a small population.
- The accessible population from which a sample is drawn should be clearly described by a researcher in publishing a study, since the accessible population determines the true target population.
- Sample size does affect the precision of estimates, given a certain magnitude of treatment effect, and formulas exist for estimating sample size needed to achieve certain risks of error and precision. With correct sampling techniques, however, probabilities for correct research conclusions can be obtained with very small sample sizes.

Methods of Obtaining a Sample

There are two general classes of sampling: non-probability and probability sampling.

Non-probability sampling occurs when nonrandom methods are used to select a sample from the accessible population. For example, the first 20 patients having arterial blood gas measurements are selected for a study of heparin's effect on measured $Paco_2$. This is a sample of convenience or accidental sample.

Probability sampling is based on random selection, so that a random sample is obtained. Random sampling allows the researcher to specify the probability that each unit in the defined population will be chosen. Because of that fact, the probability of values obtained from the sample can be known. For example, if a sample mean is 10, we can know the probability that the population value is between 8 and 12, if a form of random sampling is used. Thus, probability sampling is essential to the use of inferential statistics in testing hypotheses. There are four types of random sampling methods usually distinguished.

Simple random sampling occurs when every unit in the population has an equal and independent chance of being selected. This is achieved if every unit in the population is numbered, and then a sample is selected by using a table of random numbers. The list of numbered units is the *sampling frame*. **Table 7.1** illustrates the selection of a simple random sample using random digits. Let the accessible population be the frame in Table 7.1, giving the list of patients' initials numbered 1 to 20. To obtain a simple random sample of five from the population, enter the table of random numbers blindly and sequentially choose the first five numbers between 1 and 20. For instance, beginning with 08, in row 3, column 2, the first five non-repeating random digits between 1 and 20 are 08, 14, 13, 15, and 18. The selected sample is indicated by bold type in the table.

Stratified sampling is useful when the population is or needs to be subdivided into strata. A sample is selected by randomly choosing a specified number from each stratum, using a method such as that described for simple random sampling. A stratified sample can preserve the proportions found in strata of the population, a procedure known as *proportional* stratified sampling.

Systematic sampling is a procedure that, despite its name, ensures a random sample. Briefly, let the population size be N, and the desired sample size n. The sampling interval,

Table 7.1

Selection of a Simple Random Sample (Bold Numbers) Using a Small Set of Random Digits
(taken from a larger table in a statistics textbook or from a computer routine)

Random Digits					
20	15	03	10	26	05
13	06	32	12	11	02
12	**08**	**14**	**13**	21	14
15	**18**	09	20	09	04
22	03	07	05	11	20
18	12	15	28	24	17

Sampling Frame				
1. J.W	5. J.S.	9. A.R.	**13. V.D.**	17. B.H.
2. A.C.	6. T.S.	10. M.W.	**14. R.D.**	**18. J.T.**
3. D.X.	7. L.W.	11. H.D.	**15. J.R.**	19. J.E.
4. B.T	**8. E.D.**	12. W.C.	16. D.M.	20. J.Y.

K, is simply *N/n*. The first unit is randomly chosen between 1 and *K,* and then every *K*th subject or unit is chosen until a sample of size *n* is obtained. For example, if the population size is 50 and a sample of size 5 is desired, then $K = N/n = 50/5 = 10$. A random number between 1 and 10 is chosen, such as 6. Then units 6, 16, 26, 36, and 46 are selected from the sampling frame.

Cluster sampling is necessary when sampling units occur in intact groups or clusters. For example, if the sampling frame is made up of allergists or practices with asthmatic patients, a cluster sample of these asthmatics is obtained by randomly selecting the desired number of clusters (the allergist, with practice) and then incorporating *all* asthmatic patients in each practice chosen to enter the study.

The list of potential research subjects for a sample usually specifies the accessible population. Be aware that a narrowly defined accessible population limits the ability to generalize results to an equally narrowly defined target population.

When evaluating treatment techniques, mixing populations with no plan can blur results or give false results. For instance, intermittent positive pressure breathing (IPPB) treatments may have different results in a population of abdominal surgery postoperative patients with no history of lung pathology versus a population of diagnosed emphysema subjects. If we wish to study both groups in one investigation, then stratified random sampling would be useful.

Finally, sampling from a population is the basis for inferential statistics. We *infer* from the statistic value in the sample to the population value (parameter). We expect that a sample statistic will differ from the actual population parameter due to sampling error. Knowing the probability of a sample, since it is randomly drawn, allows us to know the probability of any difference between the sample and population values. The following mnemonic helps to relate the terms *statistic* and *parameter:* sample is to population as statistic is to parameter. A statistic is a measure from a sample, and a parameter is a measure from an entire population.

Basic Concepts of Research Design

The research design is the plan or organization for manipulating, observing, and controlling variables in a research question. In this chapter, such plans will be diagrammatically presented using a simple notation for convenience and conciseness. We define the terms involved as follows:

- *Variable*: An entity that can take on different values. Examples are height, weight, and blood pressure.
- *Independent variable*: A variable that is manipulated; the treatment.
- *Dependent variable*: A variable that is measured; the outcome variable of the treatment.
- *Nuisance variables:* Extraneous (usually uncontrollable) variables, also called confounding variables, which can affect the dependent variable.
- *Placebo:* A treatment designed to appear exactly like a comparison treatment, but which has no active component; a presumably inert substance or process to allow a comparison control. In the simplest situation, the research problem is to decide if a change in *X,* the independent variable, causes a corresponding change in *Y*, the dependent variable. Is there a relationship

between *X* and *Y*? In most clinical research, this question is not easy to answer because many other factors, termed nuisance variables, may affect the dependent variable. Age, for instance, influences pulmonary function measures.

In a two-group design, inherent group differences can affect outcomes. For example, more-intelligent health science students may do well with computer-based instruction, while less-intelligent students may not. Are results due to the instruction or to inherent aptitude? Perhaps the treatment group is consciously or unconsciously handled or evaluated differently, causing more motivation for them to do well. Of course, the change may be caused by the treatment itself, and the lack of change may mean a treatment is ineffective. The advantage of a probability sample is that we can quantify the probability of sampling error—that is, the probability of random fluctuation in the measured, dependent variable. For instance, with random sampling we can determine the probability that an observed difference between a treatment and control group is due to chance. If the probability that the effect is due to chance is low, then we may conclude that the difference is due to the treatment and not caused by sampling or random error.

The major challenge dealt with by research design is that of *control*. John Stuart Mill, in *A System of Logic*, stated the Law of the Single Variable:[1] If two situations are equal except for one factor, any difference between the situations is attributable to that factor. In the life sciences, holding all factors constant except for the factor (treatment) under investigation is practically impossible. Instead, randomization and probability theory replace the control of absolute equality, at least in the strongest research designs. There are generally two categories of research designs, experimental and non-experimental.

Experimental Designs

Scientific experiments have three characteristics:

1. Manipulation of an independent (treatment) variable
2. Control of all other variables except for the dependent (outcome) variable
3. Observation of the change, if any, in the dependent variable

A research design that plans for manipulation, observation, and control is thus an experimental research design—that is, a plan for a scientific experiment. This will not be the case in non-experimental research design, which we consider subsequently.

The major purpose of a research design, especially in clinical research, is *control* of potential nuisance variables. There are four methods of control commonly used in experimental research design:

1. Random selection of sample and random assignment to groups
2. Matching of subjects between groups or grouping of subjects based on a nuisance variable to achieve homogeneity (e.g., grouping based on age or weight)
3. Inclusion of a nuisance variable as a treatment variable
4. Statistical removal of a nuisance variable through analysis of covariance

The first three methods are of *experimental* control, whereas the last is a *statistical* control. The advantage of the first method, randomization, is that random or chance assignment can be expected to even out any nuisance variables for all groups, whether a nuisance variable is known in advance or not. The second method of control is frequently seen when subjects are used as their own controls in a before-and-after study, or in studies of paired twins. A blocking design, termed a randomized block, will be illustrated when presenting common designs.

Experimental research designs are distinguished from the weakest to the strongest, on the basis of the amount of control employed, using the following terms:

- *Pre-experimental:* These designs are characterized by little or no control of extraneous nuisance variables. Such a design is often useful for a pilot study.
- *Quasi-experimental:* These designs lack full control of all variables, but there is an effort to compensate with other controls. Usually, randomization is lacking, perhaps because of ethical constraints in choosing or assigning subjects to treatment.
- *True experimental:* These designs provide full control of variables by one or more of the methods previously described.

The differences among these three classes of design will be clarified with specific examples.

Pre-Experimental Designs

In a single-group, pre-experimental design, the outcome variable is measured, the treatment is given, and then the outcome variable is measured again to see if any change occurred. This is sometimes called the *pre-test/post-test* design. If there are two groups, no pre-test measurement is conducted. The control group receives placebo treatment, and the outcome is measured (**Figure 7.1**).

Pre-experimental designs are considered weak because of poor control of nuisance variables. In the one-group design, we cannot conclude that a change in the treatment caused a change in outcome. Would the same result be seen with placebo? Perhaps the change is simply because the study subjects know they are being studied (known as the "Hawthorne effect"). The weakness is that no comparison to a group *without* the treatment is available. In the two-group case, if a difference exists in outcome with and without the experimental treatment, how do we know that the difference was not there *before* the treatment was given (inherent group differences)? In both designs seen in Figure 7.1, no random assignment is present to guarantee equivalence of the two groups in the second case and representativeness of the population in the first. However, such designs can be very useful for initial or "pilot" studies.

Quasi-Experimental Designs (Case Control)

Case control designs are often used in retrospective studies. *Retrospective* studies are those in which all the events of interest occur prior to the onset of the study, and findings are based on past records. Comparisons are made between individuals with a particular condition (the cases) and individuals without the condition (the controls). Cases and controls can be made more

Figure 7.1

Pre-experimental designs.

One Group, Pre-Test/Post- Test

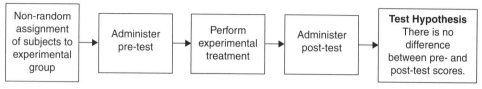

Two Groups, Post- Test Only

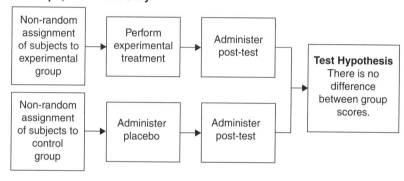

comparable by matching them on characteristics known to be strongly related to the condition of interest such as age, gender, race, and socioeconomic status.

In the design in **Figure 7.2**, groups have not been randomly assigned, but there is compensation for the lack of control usually achieved with randomization. There is a comparison group, and subjects are measured before treatment or placebo. Any inherent group difference with regard to the dependent variable can be detected with the pre-test, and equivalence of the experimental and control groups can be verified before any manipulation. Although such a design is stronger than the pre-experimental designs considered, the lack of randomization causes this design to be classed as quasi-experimental. There is no true control of potential differences. For example, suppose drug X and blood pressure were independent and dependent variables, respectively. The pre-test may show there is no difference between the two groups before the treatment, which is important. But the experimental group may be older and respond differently to the drug than younger subjects. Therefore, a difference may be seen *after* treatment that is partially due to age, or perhaps no difference may be seen if older subjects do not respond to the drug. Although the drug may be effective for younger people, it could be described as ineffective, and the pre-test would not necessarily reveal this possibility. As we will see in the next section, random assignment of subjects to the two groups would have caused such differences as age to cancel out. However, the design in Figure 7.2 will be useful when intact groups prevent random assignment. Subsequent designs will illustrate how a nuisance factor such as age can be blocked out or incorporated as a separate treatment variable.

Figure 7.2

Quasi-experimental design (case control).

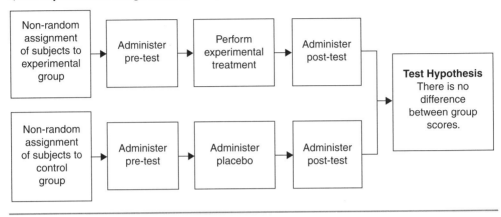

True Experimental Designs (Randomized Control)

The greatest degree of control occurs with true experimental designs. In the randomized, post-test-only design, any inherent differences such as age, sex, or weight that could affect the dependent variable are presumed to be averaged out between the experimental and control groups. If the two groups are made equivalent by randomization, then a pre-test is not needed to determine equivalence (**Figure 7.3**).

The same design can be modified to match, or pair, the subjects in the two groups (**Figure 7.4**). The extreme example is a study using twins, where a twin in the experimental group is

Figure 7.3

True experimental design (randomized control).

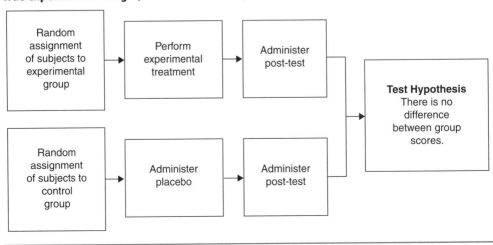

matched to a twin in the control group. Other forms of matching include pairing of subjects on suspected or known nuisance variables. For instance, a subject in the 30- to 40-year age range in the experimental group has a corresponding, matched subject in the control group.

The matched subjects design also includes the case where subjects are used as their own controls. The entire group of subjects first receives placebo, and the dependent variable is measured. Then, the entire group receives treatment, and again the dependent variable is measured. Subjects are essentially matched to themselves (**Figure 7.5**).

Figure 7.4

Modified true experimental design (matched control subjects).

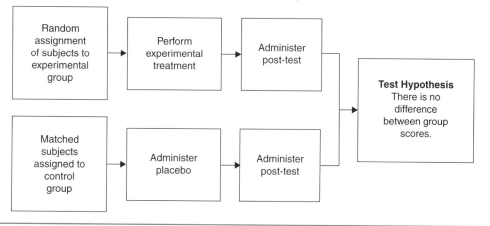

Figure 7.5

Modified true experimental design (subjects are their own controls; used only if the order of treatment is not important).

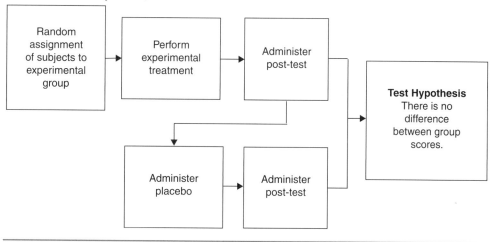

To guard against any residual or learning effect from the order of the treatment and placebo sequence, a *crossover* design may be used (**Figure 7.6**). Half of the group receives treatment, then placebo, while the other half receives the reverse order. The entire group still receives the treatment and the placebo, and is measured on the dependent variable.

The type of research design can affect which statistical test is used for making a conclusion regarding the research hypothesis. For instance, with two matched groups (as in Figures 7.4 and 7.5), a paired t test is required. If the groups are different (i.e., not paired as in Figures 7.2 and 7.3), then an unpaired t test is used.

Analysis of Variance

Analysis of variance (ANOVA) is a general statistical technique that applies to a number of experimental designs. A *completely randomized one-way ANOVA* is diagrammed in **Table 7.2**.

Figure 7.6

Modified true experimental design (subjects crossover; used when the order of treatment may affect outcome).

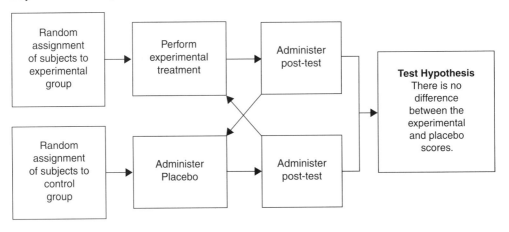

Table 7.2

One-Way (or One-Factor) Analysis of Variance (ANOVA)

Experimental Factor (Independent Variable)			
Level 1	**Level 2**	**Level 3**	**Level n**
subject 1	subject 1	subject 1	subject 1
subject 2	subject 2	subject 2	subject 2
. . .	. . .	. . .	. . .
subject n	subject n	subject n	subject n

The advantage of this design over those considered previously is that more than two groups can be used. For example, instead of comparing an experimental treatment with placebo, we can investigate three or more dosage levels of the experimental treatment, the independent variable, by using three or more groups of subjects in the experiment. **Table 7.3** illustrates this with the example of the effects of different levels of positive end expiratory pressure (PEEP) during mechanical ventilation on patients' arterial oxygen tension. Subjects are different in different groups, and they are randomly assigned to groups. Differences among the groups can be detected with a single statistical test, the *F* test (discussed later). In the design in Table 7.2, there is only *one* independent variable with *n* levels, and there is only one dependent variable being measured.

A modification of one-way ANOVA allows for homogeneous blocks of subjects to be incorporated in the design, which is termed a *randomized block design*. The design is diagrammed in **Table 7.4**. In addition to the *n* levels of the treatment variable, there are blocks, which are groups of subjects who are homogeneous on some trait or traits.

For example, if the independent variable is a bronchodilator, the dependent variable is forced expiratory volume at one second (FEV_1), and we suspect that age can affect the dependent variable even using all males. The design minimizes the effect of age, the nuisance variable, by blocking on age. Subjects might be grouped into blocks with homogeneous ages (**Table 7.5**). For instance, block 1 is 20 to 29 years old, block 2 is 30 to 39 years old, and so forth.

Subjects within a block are then randomly assigned to the *n* treatment groups. The number of subjects within blocks should be equal. Homogeneity may also be achieved in animal studies

Table 7.3

Example of One-Way ANOVA Comparing Arterial Oxygen Tensions

		PEEP Level	
5 cm H₂O	**10 cm H₂O**	**5 cm H₂O**	**20 cm H₂O**
78 torr	100 torr	120 torr	65 torr
99 torr	105 torr	101 torr	57 torr
67 torr	87 torr	116 torr	88 torr

Table 7.4

Randomized Block ANOVA

	Experimental Factor (Independent Variable)			
	Level 1	**Level 2**	**Level 3**	**Level *n***
Block 1	subjects	subjects	subjects	subjects
Block 2	subjects	subjects	subjects	subjects
Block 3	. . .	. . .	. . .	. . .
Block *n*	subjects	subjects	subjects	subjects
	mean 1	mean 2	mean 3	mean *n*

Table 7.5

Example of a Randomized Block ANOVA Design

Bronchodilator Drug

	Dosage 1	Dosage 2	Dosage 3
age 20–29	mean FEV_1	mean FEV_1	mean FEV_1
age 30–39	mean FEV_1	mean FEV_1	mean FEV_1
age 40–49	mean FEV_1	mean FEV_1	mean FEV_1

by use of littermates within a given block. A special case of blocking is to have a single subject in each block, with *repeated measures* of the subject for each treatment level. The order of treatment levels is randomized for each subject, and the subject should be in the same condition when each treatment level is experienced—that is, any residual effects from the previous treatment level must have ended before a new treatment level begins. When it is desirable to have the same group of subjects undergo two or more treatment levels, the randomized block used as a repeated measures design can be very useful.

The randomized block design is most appropriate when there is greater variability among blocks than *within* blocks and when this variability makes a difference in the dependent variable. The creation of blocks allows the researcher to isolate the effect of the independent variable and statistically remove the variability in the dependent variable due to the nuisance (blocking) factor.

A *completely randomized factorial* design can be understood as an extension of the previous two designs. This design is diagrammed in **Table 7.6**. The term *factorial* experiment indicates that more than one independent variable is being investigated. Table 7.6 illustrates the design for a 2 × 3 factorial. Each number refers to the number of levels of an independent variable. For example, in Table 7.6, which shows a 2 × 3 design, there are two levels of factor 1 and three levels of factor 3. In a 2 × 4 × 2 scheme, there are three independent variables, with two, four, and two levels, respectively.

Notice that the treatment variables are "crossed"—that is, all combinations of treatments can be considered. Subjects are randomly assigned to treatment combinations, or cells, with different subjects in different cells. The advantage of a factorial design lies in the economy of investigating more than one treatment variable in a single study. The design allows the

Table 7.6

A Two-Factor ANOVA Design

Factor 1

		Level 1	Level 2
Factor 2	**Level 1**	subjects	subjects
	Level 2	subjects	subjects
	Level 3	subjects	subjects

investigator to analyze statistically the effect of each treatment variable, and in particular to detect any *interaction* between the treatment variables.

An example is helpful to illustrate both a factorial design as well as the concept and importance of interaction. **Table 7.7** gives a 2×2 factorial design in which the two independent variables are drug dosage and weight. There are two levels of each independent variable. The dependent (measured) variable is change in systolic pressure. First, consider the mean values for 10-mg and 20-mg dosages, calculated as $(25 + 10) \div 2 = 17.5$ and $(23 + 14) \div 2 = 18.5$. There is little difference (17.5 mm Hg compared with 18.5 mm Hg). There is a larger difference between fat and thin subjects: $(25 + 23) \div 2 = 24$ mm Hg compared with $(10 + 14) \div 2 = 12$ mm Hg. If we had looked at the independent variables (drug dosage and weight) in two *separate* studies, we might have concluded that there is no difference in 10- and 20-mg dosages, and there is a difference between fat and thin subjects. By combining the independent variables in *one* study, we find they *affect each other*—that is, there is interaction between drug dosage and body weight.

Interaction can be defined as the situation in which one treatment gives different results under different levels of the other treatment. The graph in **Figure 7.7** illustrates this. Results with the two dosage levels are graphed at each level of body weight. The measured variable, change in systolic pressure, is on the vertical axis. Points on the graph are the factorial cell entries. We see that the 20-mg dose gives a larger change in systolic pressure than the 10-mg dose for thin subjects. But the reverse is true for fat subjects. This is interaction: levels of drug dosage give different results at different levels of body weight. The numbers in the factorial cells show the same result, but the graph is more striking. This result, which is clearly important, would not have been detected in two separate studies.

In a factorial design, we distinguish the effect of each treatment variable (main effects) from the interaction effect. Whether main effects or interaction effects are significant is decided statistically. If interaction *is* present, main effects must be interpreted with qualification. In general, when the graph in Figure 7.7 shows parallel lines, there is no interaction between treatment variables. When the lines are not parallel, whether they cross or not, interaction is present, and statistical testing determines if this interaction is significant.

Validity of Research Designs

The primary rationale for a research design, particularly an experimental design, is *control,* to answer correctly the question: Is X related to Y? Experimental validity is concerned with the

Table 7.7

An Example of Two-Way ANOVA with Interaction

		Drug	
		10 mg	**20 mg**
Weight	**Fat**	25 mm Hg	23 mm Hg
	Thin	10 mm Hg	14 mm Hg

Note: Cells contain mean values for change in systolic blood pressure.

Figure 7.7

Illustration of an interaction effect.

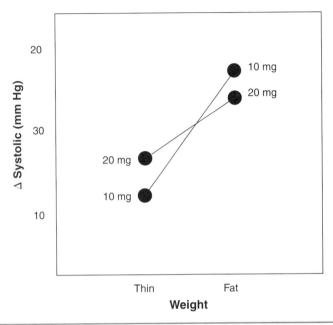

correctness of conclusions in a research design and is differentiated into internal and external validity.

- *Internal validity:* The extent to which we are correct in our conclusion concerning the relation of independent and dependent variables.
- *External validity:* The extent to which we are correct in generalizing the conclusions from sample results to the population.

Internal validity includes the specific question of *statistical conclusion validity*, since inappropriate statistical analysis or failure to meet the assumptions of statistical tests is so widespread in the medical literature, as well as in other fields.

Threats to internal validity exist and challenge any study. Completely eliminating all potential threats is often impossible (because of practical constraints or the nature of the question). The researcher, as well as the consumer of research, should be aware of the following extraneous factors that can cause incorrect conclusions or inaccurate generalizations.

- *Threats to internal validity*
  - *History and maturation:* The passage of time introduces the possibility of events affecting subjects, or of changes in the subjects themselves, that may affect the dependent variable.

For example, news of a stock market crash might worry some subjects and raise their average blood pressure, or change in seasons may affect the severity of asthma episodes as much as an experimental drug.

- *Instrument change:* Measurements obtained can be affected by changes in instruments. For example, bias caused by friction building up in a water-seal spirometer can change later measurements.
- *Mortality:* Any loss of subjects, whether voluntary or through death, can seriously affect research results. For example, if less-severe asthmatics lose motivation to continue in a treatment, then the results may be inaccurately poor or even indicate no effect of treatment.
- *Threats to external validity*
  - *Population validity:* The accessible population is not equivalent to the intended target population. The possibility of this occurs when volunteers are used, because volunteers may not typify the entire population. Volunteerism leads to a self-selection bias and is an inherent difficulty in survey research.
  - *Hawthorne effect:* The awareness of being in a study can alter a subject's responses or behavior, even in medical patients. Psychosomatic effects are quite real, as evidenced by stress ulcers. The effect is named for a study that took place in the Hawthorne plant of the Western Electric Company. No matter what treatment was employed, productivity rose! There was a positive response to perceived attention. Subjects not in such a study may not respond similarly, and this limits the ability to generalize beyond the study.
  - *Experimenter effect:* Investigators can also bias results by consciously or unconsciously conveying expectations or motivating subjects to respond to treatment more than to placebo. A double-blind approach helps to control this, since the investigator does not know whether a subject receives treatment or placebo. With an investigator causing bias in the results, the conclusion cannot be generalized.

These are by no means exhaustive lists of threats to internal and external validity. The threats given, however, can easily occur in medical or clinical research. The term *validity* used to denote experimental validity is not the same as measurement validity. The latter refers to an instrument measuring what it is intended to measure.

Non-Experimental Study Designs

Non-experimental research designs do not directly manipulate or control an independent variable. The main activity is observation. This design is often necessary when the researcher must use intact groups. Such groups are created or defined on the basis of inherent traits or traits that are acquired in the course of natural events. Such traits are termed attribute variables. Examples include smokers and nonsmokers, second graders in a school, patients having neuromuscular diseases, all 20-year-olds, subjects requiring mechanical ventilatory support, males, and so on. The *experimental* variable that is manipulated is replaced by an *attribute* variable or trait in non-experimental research designs. Comparison or control groups can be identified in some cases, defined by the presence or absence of the trait being investigated.

Non-experimental research designs lack the manipulation and control of experimental designs. Groups remain intact when it is not feasible or ethical to manipulate the trait defining the group. Naturally occurring traits, such as age, sex, or presence of disease, obviously cannot be assigned to subjects. With other traits, such as smoking, random allocation to smoking or not smoking is not considered ethical. Ethical considerations will often require the use of non-experimental design studies in medical research. Are we ethical in withholding a possibly beneficial or superior treatment for the sake of a placebo control? Can we decide who receives ventilatory support and who does not, among patients who meet criteria for mechanical ventilation? A very well known medical experiment did use an experimental design and randomly assigned placebo versus vaccine: the 1954 experiment to determine effectiveness of the Salk polio vaccine.[2] There was discussion at the time concerning the ethics of giving placebo to children who might contract polio. However, part of the research *did* use a randomized placebo control method, and as a result the researchers were able to conclude that the Salk vaccine was effective. By contrast, using non-experimental methods, it has been impossible to determine conclusively that smoking causes lung cancer.

There is no well established and widely agreed upon classification scheme for the different types of non-experimental research. In addition, terms associated with non-experimental research—for example, *ex post facto*, *retrospective*, *prospective*, and *cohort*—are also used in different ways among individual writers and in various fields of research such as the behavioral sciences (education, psychology, sociology) or clinical medicine (epidemiological research). With this realization in mind, I offer a description of the major types of non-experimental research, using labels that are acceptable among medical research methodologists. The types of non-experimental research to be presented are the *prospective study*, the *retrospective study*, the *case study*, the *survey*, and the *correlational study*. Non-experimental designs can be very useful and are often the best possibility for medically related research, especially in allied health fields. The following types of non-experimental research suggest that clinical practice can be a fertile source of research information to begin putting health care on a scientific basis.

With non-experimental research, control can be a major hindrance to drawing conclusions. One solution is to match intact groups on certain variables, or use analysis of covariance to statistically equate groups on given variables. Another approach is to incorporate nuisance variables into an analysis of variance design to examine or control their influence.

Retrospective Studies

Retrospective studies attempt to reason from a present effect, or consequence in a population, back to antecedent causes. For example, a retrospective study on lung cancer would identify cases of lung cancer, identify a comparable group based on age, sex, or other characteristics, and then determine what variables were prevalent in the lung cancer group that are not in the control group. Another example is a retrospective study to identify antecedents of breast cancer by profiling and taking extensive histories on subjects with breast cancer. The idea is to find a common characteristic in those subjects with the disease. That characteristic is then interpreted as a risk factor. Causality is almost impossible to establish in such studies; instead, we identify functional relationships among variables.

Prospective Studies

Prospective studies attempt to reason from a present antecedent or event in a population to future consequences or effects. A good example is a study on complications of assisted ventilation. Suppose records were kept of complications (mainstem intubation, pneumothorax, and so on) in a group of patients requiring assisted ventilation. The data from such a study could be used in quantifying relative frequencies of common complications.

The term *cohort* has also been used to describe a group of subjects who are followed prospectively, or forward, in time. The defining feature of cohort research is that the group is followed forward from antecedent to outcome. Terms such as *development* or *follow-up* have also been used to describe studies in which an intact group or cohort is followed longitudinally over time.

The terms *prospective* and *retrospective* are properly used in reference to the chronological direction in which a group is followed. *Prospective* describes a study where the group of subjects is tracked in the forward direction. *Retrospective* applies when a group is followed in a backward (retro) direction. These terms have been misapplied to describe the direction in which the data are collected. For example, a researcher wishes to study the complications of mechanical ventilation in a homogeneous group of chronic obstructive pulmonary disease (COPD) patients. Suppose that all such patients who require mechanical ventilation next year are identified for inclusion. If the researcher plans now to follow such a group, then observations can be made from the time of commitment until discontinuance of the ventilator occurs. In contrast, if the researcher decides now to investigate the same group of patients from five years ago, then subjects as well as complications will have to be gleaned from past medical records. Regardless of whether we start collecting data now or review old records, we are following the group in a forward direction, from ventilator commitment to discontinuance. Such a study is prospective, whether the data are obtained at the time of ventilatory support or afterward. In other words, it is not the chronology of data collection but the direction of population pursuit (forward versus backward) that distinguishes prospective from retrospective studies.

Case Studies

The case study usually provides a description of a single subject, with a treatment or trait (e.g., disease state) that is unusual, rare, atypical, or experimental. Case studies often provide good teaching examples.

Surveys

A survey typically gathers information on a large group of subjects or units by either written or oral questionnaires, or even on-site inspection. A sample survey based on random methods can give very good information on populations, as evidenced by political polls and quality control techniques that use random checking. A manpower survey in a particular state can indicate what proportions of health care practitioners are registered, certified, or on-the-job trained. Problems with survey questionnaires include response rate and self-selection bias (volunteerism). Unambiguous wording, clear-cut and non-overlapping answer choices, a brief, clear introduction that motivates the reader to respond, and an uncomplicated format help to obtain accurate and adequate responses. Pilot testing of a questionnaire to eliminate ambiguities is essential. This is done by administering a small number of questionnaires to volunteers who can provide some feedback on the clarity and appropriateness of the questions.

Correlational Studies

For a technologically oriented field, correlational studies are very useful and provide information on the presence and strength of a relation between two variables. For example, we might ask if there is a correlation between mid-maximal expiratory flows and Pao_2. We would select a group of subjects who are homogeneous in representing a population, and then in each subject measure the mid-maximal flow and the Pao_2. Then the pairs of measurements from each subject are statistically analyzed to determine the strength or absence of correlation between the two variables (flow and Pao_2).

The term *correlation* means that two variables co-vary. Covariance means that when one variable changes, the other variable is also likely to change (in the same or opposite direction). *Correlation does not imply causality.* Both variables may be caused by a third variable, and they will co-vary simultaneously.

Actually, any two variables can be analyzed for the presence of correlation. For example, a suspected relationship between degree of sunspot activity and brightness of the northern lights might be analyzed using a correlation study. Generally, theory should suggest the possibility of a relationship between two variables. This occurs usually when there is a cause-effect relation, or if two variables already coexist in the same subject. Examples of the latter include situations in which the same entity is measured by two different instruments and one uses a correlation study to examine the accuracy of one instrument against the other, or where physiological variables such as heart rate and blood pressure exist in the same subject.

Questions

Definitions

Define the following terms:

- Assessable population
- Target population
- Sample
- Variable
- Independent variable
- Dependent variable
- Nuisance or confounding variable
- Placebo
- Hawthorne effect

True or False

1. Random sampling is essential for descriptive statistics but not for inferential statistics used in hypothesis testing.
2. In simple random sampling, every unit in the population has an equal chance of being selected.
3. The Law of the Single Factor states that if two situations are equal except for one factor, any difference between the situations is attributable to that factor.
4. Pre-experimental research designs are preferred because there is full control of nuisance variables.
5. The pre-test/post-test design is classified as pre-experimental.
6. The case control design is considered quasi-experimental.
7. The randomized control design is the only true experimental design.
8. One advantage of ANOVA is that more than two groups can be compared at a time.

Multiple Choice

1. Which of the following non-experimental designs attempts to reason from current effects back to antecedent causes?
   a. Retrospective study
   b. Prospective study
   c. Case study
   d. Survey
   e. Correlational study
2. Which type of study seeks information on the strength of a relation between two variables?
   a. Retrospective study
   b. Prospective study
   c. Case study
   d. Survey
   e. Correlational study
3. Which type of study attempts to reason from a present event to future effects?
   a. Retrospective study
   b. Prospective study
   c. Case study
   d. Survey
   e. Correlational study
4. Which type of study usually provides a description of a single subject that is unusual and provides a good teaching example?
   a. Retrospective study
   b. Prospective study
   c. Case study
   d. Survey
   e. Correlational study

5. Which type of study gathers information from groups of subjects using questionnaires?
   a. Retrospective study
   b. Prospective study
   c. Case study
   d. Survey
   e. Correlational study

References

1. Mill JS. (1843). *A System of Logic: Ratiocinative and Inductive*. Honolulu: University Press of the Pacific.
2. Meldrum M. A calculated risk: the Salk polio vaccine field trials of 1954. *BMJ*. 1998;317(7167): 1233–1236.

Section III

Conducting the Study

CHAPTER 8

Steps to Implementation

Devising a comprehensive plan should be the first step of any research project. Having a plan will avoid many problems during the actual study. Although the details of formulating a research plan have been discussed earlier, I cannot emphasize enough that careful, detailed planning should be completed long before the study begins.

Writing the Study Protocol

Three major benefits accrue from a *written* research plan. First, the process of writing it out will help you clarify the goals of the study and methods of investigation. The realization that problems in approach or analysis exist may not occur until ideas are committed to paper. Second, you often must present a plan to obtain permission or approval to proceed with the study. You may need to seek permission from a funding source, institutional review board, department manager, or student adviser before beginning a study. Third, the research plan, or *protocol*, as it is often called, provides an operational guide for the entire research team. Successful coordination of study personnel is all but impossible without a detailed protocol. For these reasons, a properly formulated proposal is an essential first step in the research process.

Creating a General Plan

Organizing the plan takes a good deal of thought. Considering the following questions will help you place the plan in proper perspective:

- What is the primary goal of the study?
- What makes this particular study important?
- What has previous research shown in this area?
- How is the study to be carried out?

Concise answers to these questions will help you clarify the objective and methods. The research protocol is a map of the path the project is to follow. It must be written in language comprehensible to all team members and should clearly delineate the role of each participant. It should make clear that the study will produce valid results and that an interpretation will flow easily from results obtained.

A well-written protocol addresses several issues. First, it should place special emphasis on the criteria for selection of the experimental population sample. It also should clearly specify which factors will be used to classify subjects into groups and must define the criteria for treatment. Here is a general outline you can follow:

1. *List the study's specific aims.* Include a statement of what goals are to be accomplished and the hypothesis to be tested. Condense the broad research topic into a concise problem statement.
2. *State clearly the primary significance of the study.* By this time you should have completed your literature review. Evaluate your project in light of the published data. Show how your study will fill in knowledge gaps. Relate the specific study objectives to long-term goals. For example, your study objective might be to assess the accuracy of oxygen analyzers when using concentrations below 21%. The long-term goal of such a study would be to ensure the safety of providing subatmospheric oxygen levels to children with hypoplastic left heart syndrome.
3. *Cite any preliminary studies you may have undertaken.* Show that preliminary experiments have demonstrated the feasibility of methods you intend to use for the current study. This is also the place to state the qualifications (as needed) of all your co-investigators. For example, if you are studying the contamination rate of nebulizers in the home, you'll want to state that you have a microbiologist on your team.
4. *Specifically state the experimental design.* Consider innovative procedures, advantages and disadvantages of methods used, limitations of the methods or study design, anticipated difficulties, alternative approaches in case of experimental obstacles, sequence of experimental events (make a flow chart if necessary), and procedures used to analyze the data. Don't be discouraged if several revisions are required to get the plan right. And always consult your mentor.

The IRB Study Protocol Outline

If you are planning a study involving human subjects, you will have to create the study protocol using a detailed format specified by your hospital's institutional review board (IRB). An example of the format is as follows:

1. *Name of investigator/co-investigator(s).* The principal investigator (or a co-investigator) must be a member of the hospital staff in all studies that involve therapeutic interventions or that alter medical care.
2. *Title of project.* All projects must have a title without abbreviations. This title must appear on all pages of the consent form.
3. *Introduction.* Describe how this study relates to previous studies in the field (including pertinent references) and the significance of the study. Mention relevant laboratory and/or animal studies.

4. *Purpose, specific aims, and hypotheses.* State clearly what you hope to learn from the research.
5. *Study design.* This is where you inform the IRB of the specific nature of the procedures to be carried out on human subjects in sufficient detail to permit evaluation of the risks. You should provide information that will allow the IRB to confirm the claim that methods employed will enable the investigator to evaluate the hypothesis posed and to collect valid data. The study design and specific procedures must contain the information needed in the consent form and allow the evaluation of the consent form.

The following section goes into more detail about what to include in the description of study design. You'll want to include a brief discussion of specific procedures, population, financial considerations, risks and benefits, and the consent form.

Specific Procedures

Explain in detail all procedures to be performed on human subjects for purposes of research. Fully explain any uncommon medical procedures. Distinguishing between the usual patient care and any experimental procedures is important. The protocol should indicate what changes in medical care will occur as a result of the study, how care will be managed, and by whom. Provide a tentative time schedule for various procedures showing what a subject might expect regarding how long each aspect of the study will take, the frequency and timing of ancillary procedures (i.e., "standard of care" treatments), and the expected duration of discomfort. Present complicated studies using a simple flow chart to enhance the narrative description. Indicate the location of the study, including laboratories for special testing. In studies involving the use of a placebo or "washout" period, the protocol and the consent form must discuss what will happen if the subject's condition deteriorates.

Population

Indicate the source and means of identifying patients/subjects and control subjects, as well as the number of subjects to be studied. If the study involves patients whose care is the responsibility of departments or special care areas other than that of the responsible investigator, you need to specify that the department or special care area has approved the protocol. Protocols must be precise as well as concise in defining a study population and the mechanism whereby the population will be contacted. If you are soliciting subjects through paid advertising, the IRB must approve the ad copy. Give specific justification for the use of subject groups with compromised ability to give consent.

Prisoners

For prisoners, conditions of confinement, penury, and parole may constitute significant duress.

Minors

Informed consent is required from a responsible parent or guardian for minors aged 17 or under. In studies involving older children, particularly those 13 and above, the investigator is urged, in addition, to obtain assent of the minor on the consent form. You may wish to use a separate "consent form" for minors able to follow it. Consents need to be written very carefully if a minor is to also sign. Any child capable of signing his or her name should do so. For studies involving young children, it may be desirable for one of the parents to be present during an investigational procedure.

Legally Incompetent People

Studies involving legally incompetent individuals will require the signature of a legal guardian and not the next of kin. When competency is in question, the responsible physician will assist in assessing the patient's competency. *Signature of spouse or next of kin does not constitute agreement to participate in research studies unless the person is a legal guardian.*

Unconscious Patients

Unconscious patients may not be used in research studies unless there is no alternative method of approved or generally accepted therapy that provides an equal or greater benefit. The investigator and an independent physician must make the determination in writing for the medical record and sign the consent form, if:

1. The study offers potential benefit to the patient.
2. The patient's condition is life threatening.
3. There is inability to communicate with the patient.
4. There is insufficient time to obtain consent from a legal representative or there is no legal representative.
5. The next of kin are informed, and agree to the study and sign the consent. However, this does not constitute informed consent. When able the subject has the right to withdraw consent.

House Staff, Students, and Employees

When directly solicited to participate in a study, staff, students, and employees must be informed that their participation in a study or refusal to do so will in no way influence their grades or subsequent recommendations. Medical students on a clerkship should not be asked to take part in experimental procedures conducted by a service while the student is on that service. Hospital employees must never be made to feel that their job, promotion, salary, or status in any way depends on participation in research studies.

Financial Considerations

Compensation to Subjects

Experimental subjects may be reasonably reimbursed for their time, their expenses, and the degree of discomfort they may experience during an investigation. Amounts must be specifically stated in both the protocol and consent form and justified in the protocol. Payments should never be so large as to induce a subject to submit to experimentation that they might otherwise reject. Payments totaling $600 (subject to IRB regulations) or more per year will result in a 1099 tax form being sent to the subject. Compensation should never be considered as a benefit of the study.

Extra Costs Incurred for Purposes of the Study

The IRB is concerned about the cost accounting of research studies, so investigators are required to address the problem of extra costs incurred because of the research project. If the patient/subject will incur costs due to the research, you must state such costs on the consent form. It is illegal to charge non-therapeutic studies to the patient or third-party payers.

Examples of procedures in this category are: radiographic studies done solely for research purposes; additional anesthesia time in a surgical procedure that includes research procedures; techniques/drugs for which there is no benefit; investigational devices (the FDA classifies investigational devices as to whether or not they can be charged for; many are chargeable); and drugs (drugs being used under an IND number may not be charged to patients or third-party payers). The protocol and consent form must include a statement regarding the responsibility for costs.

Risks and Benefits

Discuss the risks and potential benefits, if any, of the proposed study to the patient/subject, his or her family, and/or society, as well as an analysis of the risk/benefit ratio. Risk analysis includes an estimation of both the probability of an adverse event and the severity of consequences if it should occur.

A discussion of precautions to minimize risks is appropriate so that the IRB can ascertain the true risks of procedures to be performed. Precautions range from those applicable to a group, such as the exclusion of pregnant or possibly pregnant women from a study, to those applicable to an individual subject, such as the presence of an emergency cart in studies in which a patient may be subject to arrhythmias.

Offer justification for the proposed study. How significant is the new knowledge being sought in relation to the potential risks in carrying out the research?

A study involving children requires the identification of any special risks that may apply.

Consent Form

The consent form should express to the patient/subject the realistic expectations of participation in the research study, avoiding inducement by raising false hopes. Write the consent form in simple, non-technical lay terms and avoid medical jargon. A person with an eighth-grade education should be able to understand the consent form. The consent form is written in the first person (e.g., "I understand that I am being asked to voluntarily participate in a study"). Consent forms for studies involving minors should read "I/my child" when appropriate and be modified depending on the age of the child and the child's ability to understand. Do not include listings of inclusion or exclusion criteria on the consent form. The following section discusses what should be included in a consent form.

Purpose of the Study and Individual Participation

Provide a clear and concise statement of the purpose of the research study and why the individual is being asked to voluntarily participate in the study. Identify the participation of normal individuals as control subjects. For patients who have an identifiable responsible physician, you must include a statement in the consent form that the physician has given approval to contact this patient for possible participation in a study.

Study and Procedures

Describe the study and procedures to be performed. Identify or separate routine management or therapeutic procedures from procedures being carried out solely for investigational purposes. If a placebo is to be used, identify this and define a placebo early in the description of a study or in stating the purpose of a study. Include a statement indicating reasonable expectations of time commitment. If blood is being collected as part of the study, indicate the amount of blood in lay terms (teaspoons/tablespoons) as well as risks involved, and explain what will be done with the blood. Consent forms are most often returned for revisions due to the lack of a clear statement separating routine care from research.

Risks and Benefits

Include an assessment of the possible risks and discomforts of each procedure, as well as degree of risk. Describe any possible drug side effects and state whether they are rare or common. Where appropriate, discuss possible side effects. Explain expected benefits clearly. Indicate distinctions between personal and societal benefits. The consent form must address the worsening of a condition or lack of response in treatment protocols or in protocols involving a medical intervention. This means you must include criteria for stopping a study, particularly if a study involves a placebo or a "washout" period. In many protocols that state "there may be a benefit" it would be more appropriate to state "there may or may not be a benefit." Where appropriate, include a statement regarding compensation and medical care in the event of research injury.

Alternatives and Withdrawal

State alternatives, including non-participation, if a new diagnostic or therapeutic procedure is being used. Discussion of the alternatives must be fair and should balance the alternatives against the proposed experimental therapy or procedures. The patient must be informed that he or she may withdraw from the study at any time.

Treatment After the Study

Discuss treatment or management after completion of the study in studies that involve therapeutic interventions.

Financial Considerations (Cost Responsibility Statement)

When appropriate, the consent statement must indicate compensation to subjects. You must spell out extra costs that may be incurred as part of participation in the study. Otherwise, indicate that no extra costs are involved. Include a statement in the consent form to acknowledge that third-party payers may or may not cover the expense of some procedures and hospitalization involving research studies. It is mandatory that cost responsibility for usual routine care be separated from cost of research procedures. When appropriate, add a line to the "cost statement" in the consent form, such as "I should check with my insurance carrier to determine what my coverage will be."

Confidentiality Statement
Include this statement in the final paragraph of the consent form.

Identification of Persons Obtaining Consent
Identify the persons obtaining consent, providing both work and home phone numbers. In all studies involving therapeutic interventions or significant risk, the principal investigator, physician co-investigator, or a specific research nurse shall obtain consent. Technicians and "floor nurses" may not obtain consent. Note that the principal investigator is required to co-sign the consent document within two weeks from the date consent is obtained from the subject.

As you can see, a study involving human subjects can be very complex. That is why most novice researchers start with device evaluation studies that can be performed outside of patient care areas.

Funding

Funding should never be an obstacle for the novice researcher beginning with a small project. Most studies produced in health care departments require no special funds, with the possible exception of some overtime for the staff involved. If the study is an evaluation of a new device on the market, the manufacturer is usually glad to give you free samples to test, assuming your protocol is convincing. After all, when you publish your results the manufacturer will get free advertisement.

Major clinical studies are generally funded by government grants, but health insurance agencies, nongovernmental public institutions, the pharmaceutical industry, and the medical equipment industry also support clinical studies. The educational credentials required to obtain research grants may be quite demanding. Successful researchers, through their protocols and grant applications, are able to demonstrate their abilities to:

- Think clearly and logically
- Express logical thought concisely
- Discriminate between the significant ant the inconsequential
- Display technical prowess
- Handle abstract thought
- Analyze data objectively and accurately
- Interpret results confidently and conservatively

Data Collection

One of the most important considerations for clinical studies is the method used for data collection. You must describe how and by whom the data will be recorded. Data collection is the most time-consuming and expensive step in the research process. If the data are misplaced or cannot be understood when it is time to analyze the study results, the project is ruined.

The Laboratory Notebook

Good scientists keep a notebook that represents the permanent written record of all activities related to the research project. The act of writing in the notebook causes the scientist to stop and think about what is being done, encouraging "good science." And you never know, you may discover something useful that you want to patent. The patent system in the United States rewards the "first person" who invents a new product. The laboratory notebook helps you prove you were first.

The information in the notebook is used for several purposes. Most important, it records the experimental data and observations that will be used later to make conclusions. Everything you do and the sequence in which you did it should be recorded, because you often can not determine what will be important later. Include drawings of experimental setups and flow diagrams of the sequence of events. Include tables of measurements and descriptions of procedures. Problems and limitations encountered are just as important to record as the successful experimental outcomes. See **Table 8.1** for more ideas. There is also a wealth of ideas for keeping notebooks available on the Internet.

The guiding principle for note keeping is to write with enough detail and clarity that some scientist in the future could pick up the notebook, repeat the work based on the descriptions, and make the same observations. If fact, that scientist in the future might just be you after you have forgotten what you did!

A professional laboratory notebook is bound with specially printed pages (**Figure 8.1**). You can purchase notebooks at university bookstores, through the mail, or through the Internet (see, for example, www.laboratorynotebooks.com). Look for features like sequentially pre-printed numbered pages, spaces for you to sign and date, and instructions on how to use the journal to record your observations. Also look for pages with blue-lined grids for easy drawing. Some notebooks have special copy features; copy drawings on a light copier setting, and the grid pattern fades away for preparing manuscript drawings. Never use a loose-leaf notebook or a three-ring binder to use as a notebook. Never use a legal pad or any glued-together notebook. Buy a notebook with pages as secure as possible—a bound or sewn notebook. Otherwise, pages will get accidentally torn out or out of order. Mead brand composition books are acceptable if you can't find a true laboratory notebook. Buy only notebooks with white pages—the lines can be colored blue or black. Make all entries in ink and cross errors out rather than erasing. Search the Internet for "advice on keeping a laboratory notebook" or "writing the laboratory notebook" for much useful guidance.

Specialized Data Collection Forms

Sometimes data collection is easier on specially made forms instead of in the laboratory notebook. This is certainly true if other people in other locations will be collecting the data. The best way to make forms is to use a spreadsheet program like Microsoft Excel to design a form you can print on paper. You can make the form look any way you want *and* build in equations to summarize the data (e.g., calculate sums, means, and standard deviations). You can even do graphing and statistical analysis within Excel, although dedicated statistical software is easier

Table 8.1

Keeping a Laboratory Notebook

- Keep detailed records of the concepts, test results, and other information related to the experiment. You can start from the very first moment you think of an idea.
- Enter ideas, calculations. and experimental results into the notebook as soon as possible, preferably the same date they occur.
- Make all entries in the notebook in permanent black ink and be sure to make them as legible and complete as possible. Do not use abbreviations, code names, or product codes without defining them clearly.
- Draw a line through all errors. *Do not erase.*
- Do not skip pages or leave empty spaces at the bottom of a page. If you wish to start an entry on a new page, draw a line through any unused portion of the previous page. Never tear out or remove a page from the notebook.
- You can buy a specially printed laboratory notebook or make one yourself. Use a bound notebook, because the pages cannot be added or subtracted without that being evident.
- Number all your pages consecutively. Draw a line across any blank pages or portion of a page left. Start a new notebook when yours is full. Assign each notebook a consecutive number.
- Keep your notebooks in a secure location and make records of when you take or return your notebooks from that spot.
- Use a header for each entry with the following information–date, project number, subject, participant(s).
- The more details, the better. Make sure that you have all the information you will need when writing up the results later.
- Make records of everything. Include all your tests, not just the successful ones. Add all your sketches, measurements, and computations.
- All loose material, such as drawings, data collection forms, printouts, photographs, etc., should be signed, dated, and cross-referenced to a particular notebook entry.
- If you can, tape or staple the loose material into the body of the appropriate notebook entry.
- Anything else, such as samples, models, and prototypes, should be carefully labeled with a date and cross-referenced to notebook entries. Keep all of it.

to use. But for that, you can either export the data from Excel or simply cut and paste the data from Excel into the statistics program. You can use different worksheets (i.e., tabs) within a workbook for your laboratory notes, illustrations, and so on.

Computers

You can hardly be a scientist in today's world without some computer skills. At minimum, you need to know how to type, how to use word-processing and spreadsheet software, and preferably how to use statistical and database software. You need to know the basics of how to store data in files and how to make backup files. Get some experience with the Internet and have an e-mail address. The Internet provides a way to access a whole world of information, not only for literature searches, but to get help with every aspect of research. In addition, many journals

Figure 8.1

Example of a page from a laboratory notebook.

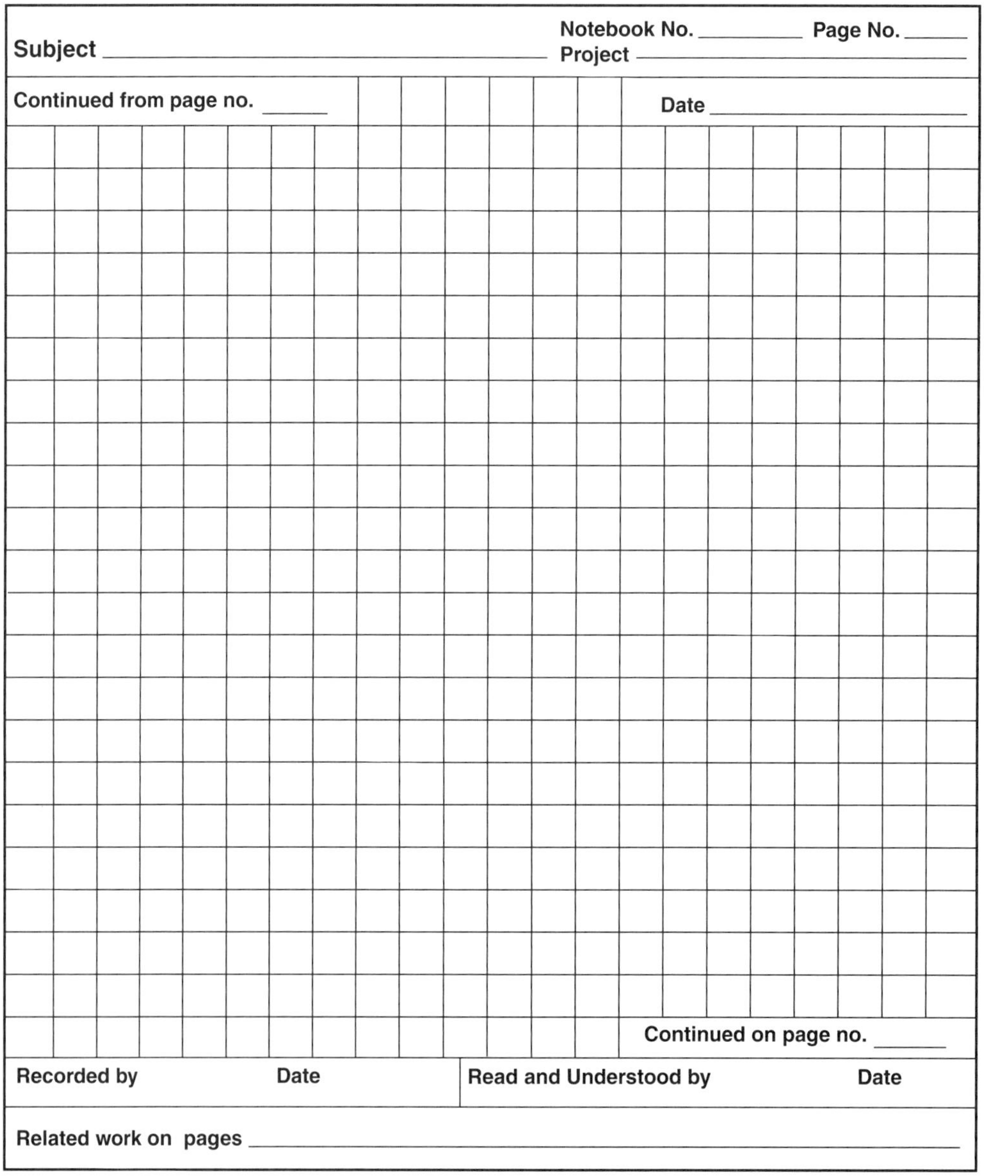

| Subject _____ | Notebook No. _____ Page No. _____ |
| Project _____ |

| Continued from page no. _____ | | | | | | | | Date _____ |

(grid of cells)

Continued on page no. _____

| Recorded by | Date | Read and Understood by | Date |

Related work on pages _____

are now accepting electronic submissions of abstracts and papers. And don't forget that help from your colleagues or mentors is just an e-mail away.

One area of computing that merits special attention is the use of personal digital assistants (PDAs). These little handheld computers can be used to collect data in the laboratory or on patient care divisions much more conveniently than paper forms. They are designed to share or "upload" their data with your desktop computer where you would normally perform the data analysis. PDAs can be programmed with forms, spreadsheets, and even databases with minimal effort. They can even be connected to specialized sensing devices to automatically record signals from experiments. These little gadgets can really make your life easier.

Questions

True or False

1. One of the major reasons for writing a study protocol is that it is required to obtain permission from the IRB.
2. Most IRBs will allow the use of any type of outline for a protocol so long as it includes both methods and a risk/benefit analysis.
3. Funding should never be an obstacle for the novice researcher beginning with a small project.
4. A laboratory notebook is no longer necessary now that computers can perform statistical analyses.
5. An IRB protocol will require a statement about any financial compensation to study subjects.
6. A description of risks and benefits can be omitted if the study subjects are prisoners.
7. The consent form should be written in a technical style so the subject's referring physician can interpret the feasibility of the study.
8. You should record everything you do and the sequence of events in a laboratory notebook because you cannot always tell what will be important later.

CHAPTER 9

Making Measurements

M easurements are made either by *direct comparison* with a standard or by *indirect comparison* using a calibrated system. Measurements of length and weight are examples of the direct comparison of an object with an accepted standard (e.g., a ruler or standard mass). The monitors in an intensive care unit typically employ indirect comparison. They convert some physical quantity, like pressure, to an intermediate variable, like voltage, through a relation previously established by comparison to a standard. Ideally, the standard should be traceable (through three or four generations of calibration copies) to the prototype kept by the National Institute of Standards and Technology (formerly the National Bureau of Standards).

Basic Measurement Theory

Every measurement is assumed to have errors. Even standards are simply the best estimate of a true value made from many carefully controlled measurements. Errors fall into two categories: systematic and random.

Systematic errors occur in a predictable manner and cause measurements to consistently under- or overestimate the true value. They can be constant over the range of input values, proportional to the input value, or both. Systematic errors are not affected by repeated measurements but can be reduced by proper calibration.

Random errors occur in an unpredictable manner due to uncontrollable factors. They cause measurements to both over- and underestimate the true value. As the number of repeated measurements of the same quantity increases, random errors tend to sum to zero. Random errors often exhibit a normal or Gaussian distribution. This assumption, along with the Central Limit Theorem of statistics, provides the basis for establishing the probability of a given measurement value and hence our confidence in the reliability of our observations.

The effects of measurement errors may be expressed as

$$\text{measured value} = \text{true value} + (\text{systematic error} + \text{random error})$$

The observed measurement is seen as the sum of the true value and the measurement errors. The goal is to identify and minimize the measurement errors. Calibration does not improve random error.

Accuracy

Accuracy is usually defined as the maximum difference between a measured value and the true value (what we have called error above) and is often expressed as a percentage of the true value:

$$\text{accuracy}\,(\%) = \frac{\text{measured value} - \text{true value}}{\text{true value}} \times 100$$

Some authors talk about accuracy as reflecting only systematic error. They define accuracy as the difference between the true value and the mean value of a large number of repeated measurements (which is the definition of *bias* in statistics). Equipment manufacturers generally include systematic and random errors in their "accuracy" specifications as the worst-case estimate for a given reading.

Accuracy is commonly expressed as a percentage of the full-scale reading (**Figure 9.1A**), indicating a constant error. For example, suppose a device with a scale of 0 to 100 has a stated accuracy of plus or minus 2% (written as ±2%). Two percent of 100 is 2. This means that if the device is used to measure a known true value of 80, the expected error would be ±2, so the instrument's reading would be somewhere between 78 and 82. Alternatively, the accuracy specification might be stated as a percentage of the reading (**Figure 9.1B**), indicating a proportional error. In this case, 2% of the known value is $0.02 \times 80 = 1.6$, so the reading would lie somewhere between 78.4 and 81.6. Sometimes the accuracy specification includes both full-scale and proportional components (**Figure 9.1C**). If the accuracy specification does not state which type it is, we usually assume it to be a percentage of full scale.

Unfortunately, the common usage of the term *accuracy* is counterintuitive. An instrument that is considered highly accurate will have a low value for its accuracy rating and vice versa. The terms *inaccuracy* and *total error* are more descriptive. Manufacturers do not use these terms, however, because they are afraid doing so will make their products seem defective.

Error specifications indicate how far the instrument's reading is expected to be from the true value. Inferring the true value from the instrument's reading is not the same problem. For a more detailed discussion, see the section entitled "Interpreting Manufacturers' Error Specifications" in Chapter 10.

Precision

Repeated measurements of the same quantity result in small differences among the observed values because of random error. *Precision* is defined as the degree of consistency among repeated results. It is quantified with statistical indexes such as variance, standard deviation, and confidence interval (described in the section on basic statistical concepts). As with the term *accuracy,* the common usage of the term *precision* is counterintuitive. A measurement considered to be highly precise has a small deviation from the true value and vice versa.

Precision should not be confused with *resolution*, defined as the smallest incremental quantity that can be measured. Resolution is an inherent but often overlooked limitation of digital displays. A digital display changes only when the measured value varies by some minimum amount. Any variation less than this threshold is ignored. For example, digital pressure monitors on ventilators display increments of 1.0 cm H_2O. When used to make repeated

Figure 9.1

Various conventions used to express instrument inaccuracy specifications.

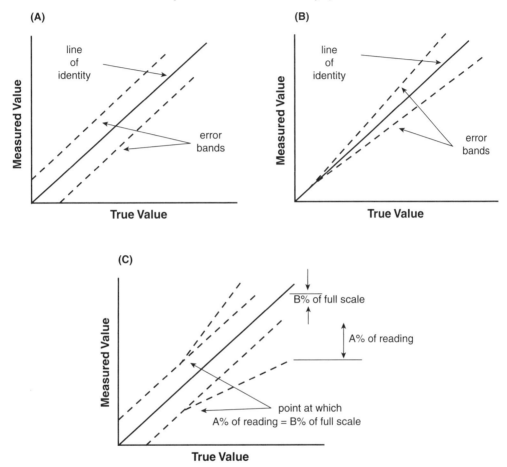

The line of identity represents a perfect match between measured and true values, or zero error. The error bands show the range of measured values expected above or below each true value. In other words, the vertical distance from the error band to the line of identity is the expected measurement error. (A) Error expressed as plus or minus *X* percent of full scale. (B) Error expressed as plus or minus *X* percent of the reading. (C) Error expressed as percent of full scale or percent of reading, whichever is greater.

measurements of, for example, the baseline airway pressure level, they may give very precise (i.e., unvarying) readings. But they do not have the resolution to detect the small changes in pressure (less than 1.0 cm H_2O) caused by small inspiratory efforts or vibrating condensation in the patient circuit (see the discussion of range error in the section on sources of bias, next). If these phenomena were of interest, such a measuring device would be inaccurate.

Inaccuracy, Bias, and Imprecision

To avoid any confusion regarding nomenclature, the term *inaccuracy* is used hereafter to mean the total error of a measurement, *bias* to mean systematic error, and *imprecision* to mean random error. Therefore, a highly inaccurate measurement is one that is highly biased and/or highly imprecise. Thus,

inaccuracy = total error = measured value – true value = bias + imprecision

If the inaccuracy for a given measurement is a positive number, we say that the measured value overestimates the true value and vice versa. We interpret an inaccuracy specification as meaning that any measurement of a known value will be within the given range with a given probability. The effects of bias and imprecision on measurements are illustrated in **Figure 9.2.**

As we said earlier, random errors are usually assumed to exhibit a normal or Gaussian distribution. This property allows us to make probability statements about measurement accuracy. **Figure 9.3** illustrates this concept.

Figure 9.2

An illustration of the effects of bias and imprecision (systematic and random errors) using the analogy of target practice on a rifle range.

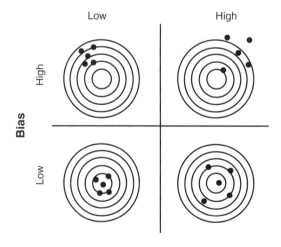

When bias is low, measurements group around the true value (represented here as bullet holes clustered around the bull's eye on bottom two targets). When imprecision is low, the cluster is tight, showing that the random errors of repeated measurements (or rifle shots) is small (top and bottom targets on left). The ideal situation is for both bias and imprecision to be low (bottom left target).

Figure 9.3

Measured values expressed in the form of a Gaussian frequency distribution.

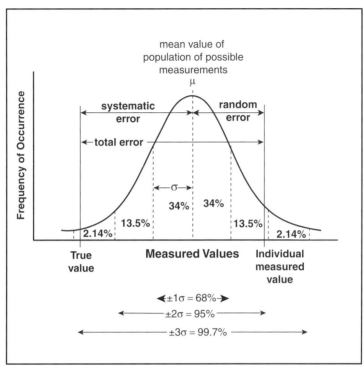

The difference between the true value and an individual measured value is the sum of both systematic and random errors. The random errors are what make the measured values appear Gaussian. That is, most random errors are small and clustered near the mean value, m. The assumption of a Gaussian distribution allows us to predict, for example, that 95% of measurements will lie within plus or minus 2 standard deviations, s, of the mean. See the chapter on Basic Statistical Concepts for a more detailed explanation of frequency distributions.

Linearity

A device is linear if a plot of the measured values versus the true values can be fitted with a straight line. For a linear device, the ratio of the output to the input (referred to as the *static sensitivity*) remains constant over the operating range of the measurement device. Linearity is desirable because once the system is calibrated with at least one known input, unknown input values will be accurately measured over the linear range.

The linearity (or rather nonlinearity) specification for a system can be assessed by first fitting the best straight line to the device's output (measured) values over the range of acceptable input values. The "best" straight line is determined by using the statistical procedure known as least-squares regression analysis. The resulting line will have the form of $Y = a + bX$. The value Y in the equation is the estimated mean value of repeated measurements of the true value of X. The parameter a in the equation is the estimate for the y intercept (the point where the regression line crosses the Y axis in the plot). The parameter b is the slope of the line (slope = the change in Y for a unit change in X). Together, they give estimates of constant and proportional systematic errors, respectively.

The linearity specification for an instrument is usually defined as the maximum observed deviation (vertical distance from the measured value to the line) from the regression line expressed as a percentage of full scale or of the reading, similar to accuracy (**Figure 9.4**). Remember that the linearity specification is relative to the best straight line through the data, while accuracy is relative to the line of identity. For a device with negligible systematic error, the specification for linearity is equivalent to a specification for accuracy, because the straight line that best fits the data is the line of identity. Thus, some commercial instruments give only a linearity specification and not an accuracy specification. In contrast, an accuracy specification but not a linearity specification may be given if linear behavior of the device is implied by a fixed sensitivity specification.

Calibration

Calibration is the process of adjusting the output of a device to match a known input so that the systematic error is minimized. *Calibration verification* is the process of measuring a known value with a calibrated device and making a judgment of whether or not the observed error is acceptable for future measurements.

Figure 9.4

Illustration of linearity specification.

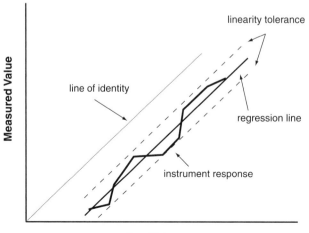

For a linear measurement system, calibration can be a simple two-step procedure. First the readout is adjusted to read zero while no input signal is applied to the instrument. (A modification of this procedure is to select a known input having a low value on the scale, such as the use of 21% oxygen during the calibration of an oxygen analyzer.) Next, the sensitivity (also called gain or slope) is set by applying a known value at the upper end of the scale (such as 100% oxygen for an oxygen analyzer) and adjusting the readout to this value (**Figure 9.5**). If the instrument has good linearity, the readouts for all inputs between these two points will be accurate. If the instrument is not very linear, and it will be used for only a part of its measurement range, it should be calibrated for just that limited range. In other words, you would select two calibration points that represent the maximum and minimum values that the instrument will be expected to measure. For example, suppose you had a flow meter that was linear up to 20 L/min but became nonlinear at higher flows. If you were only interested in using it to measure flows between 8 and 12 L/min, you would calibrate it using known flows of 5 and 15 L/min.

Sources of Bias (Systematic Error)

If the zero point of an instrument is not set correctly but the gain is correct, the instrument will be biased; this is known as *constant error* or *offset error*. The readings will be low or high over the entire scale (**Figure 9.6A**). *Drift error* is a form of time-dependent offset error in which the changes occur over time.

Proportional error refers to when the zero point is set correctly but the gain is wrong. In this case bias will be dependent on (i.e., proportional to) the input level. The higher the true input value, the more error there is in the measured value (**Figure 9.6B**).

Figure 9.5

The two-point calibration procedure.

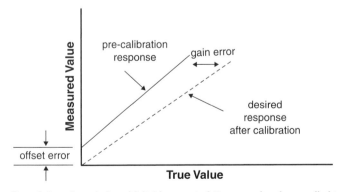

First the offset is adjusted, then the gain (sensitivity) is corrected. For example, when applied to a flow sensor, the offset error would be corrected by occluding the meter so there was no flow and adjusting the readout to zero. Then, the sensor is exposed to a known flow, for example 10 L/min, and the readout is adjusted (using a separate gain control) to read 10 L/min.

Range error occurs when the true value of the input signal is outside the operating range of the instrument (**Figure 9.6C**). Signals that are either below or above the calibrated scale values will be clipped (the true value changes but the readout does not). In the worst case, the instrument may be damaged when exposed to over-range conditions.

If an instrument gives a different reading for a given input value depending upon whether the input is increasing or decreasing, the device is said to show *hysteresis* (**Figure 9.6D**).

Figure 9.6

Common sources of measurement error.

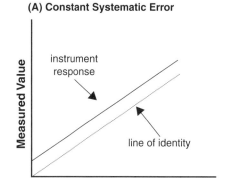

(A) Constant Systematic Error

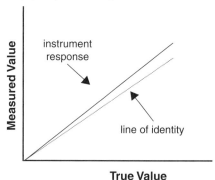

(B) Proportional Systematic Error

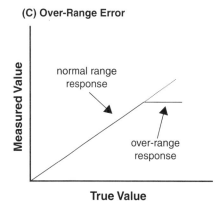

(C) Over-Range Error

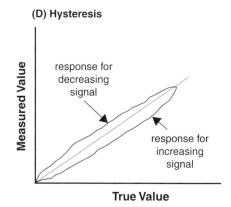

(D) Hysteresis

(A) Constant systematic error in which the instrument reading is always higher than the true value.
(B) Proportional systematic error in which the instrument reading is higher than the true value and the error gets larger as the reading gets higher. (C) Range error can occur when measurements are made outside the instrument's calibration level, resulting in "clipping" the signal. The example shown is an over-range error. Beyond the instrument's highest level the readout may stay constant even though the true value increases.
(D) Hysteresis, where the instrument reads too low as the signal increases and too high as the signal decreases.

Response time is a measure of how long it takes a device to respond to a step change (i.e., an instantaneous change from one constant value to another) in the input. There are two accepted methods for stating response time. The first is to simply give the *time constant*, which is the time required for a device to read 63% of the step change. For example, if an oxygen analyzer giving a stable reading in room air is suddenly exposed to 100% oxygen, the time constant is the time required for the meter to read 50% ($0.63 \times [100 - 21] \approx 50$). Alternatively, response can be expressed as the time necessary to reach 90% of the step change (sometimes modified as the time to go from 10% to 90%). For example, a 90% response time of about 100 milliseconds is required for breath-by-breath analysis of respiratory gas concentrations. Slow response times can cause errors during calibration if you do not allow enough time for the instrument to stabilize at the known values. For practical purposes, it takes about five time constants to reach a steady-state value. The relation among measured value, time, and the time constant is given by:

$$measured\ value = 100(1 - e^{-t/\tau})$$

where the measured value is expressed as a percentage of the steady-state value, e is the base of natural logarithms (approximately equal to 2.72), t is time, and τ is the time constant expressed in units of time (the same units as t).

Frequency response is a measure of an instrument's ability to accurately measure an oscillating signal. Measurements will generally either underestimate (attenuate) or overestimate (amplify) the true signal amplitude as the frequency increases (**Figure 9.7**). A system will generally follow an oscillating signal faithfully at low frequencies but amplify the signal as the frequency increases due to *resonance*. Resonance is a property of any oscillating mechanical system that has both inertia and elastance. It occurs when the potential and kinetic energies of these components are stored and released in synchrony (as in a pendulum). The frequency at which this occurs is called the resonant frequency or natural frequency. At higher frequencies, the system will attenuate the signal.

It can be shown mathematically (through Fourier analysis) that any complex signal waveform can be constructed by combining sine waves at different frequencies, amplitudes, and phases (**Figure 9.8**).

A system is said to be *damped* when some of the signal component frequencies are attenuated. A *critically damped* system is one that follows a step-change input with maximum velocity but does not overshoot (Figure 9.7). An *optimally damped* system will measure all signal frequencies within the working range with equal amplitude. Such a system is said to have a "flat" response, meaning that the amplitude distortion is less than $\pm 2\%$ up to 66% of the undamped resonant frequency. A device that is tuned for a given frequency range may exhibit errors in the magnitude and timing of the measured signal if used at higher frequencies. Frequency response problems are especially evident for pressure and flow measurements and with instruments like analog meter readouts and strip chart recorders.

A basic axiom of measurement theory is that the measurement process inevitably alters the characteristics of the measured quantity. Therefore, some measurement error will always be present; this is referred to as *loading error*. For example, placing a pneumotachometer in a flow stream changes the flow rate because of the added resistance. Also, when electronic devices are coupled, unrecognized electronic loading can occur and can be quite serious.

Figure 9.7

The top two graphs show the response to a square wave input of three different blood pressure transducers with different damping. The bottom two graphs show how damping affects the measurement of blood pressure.

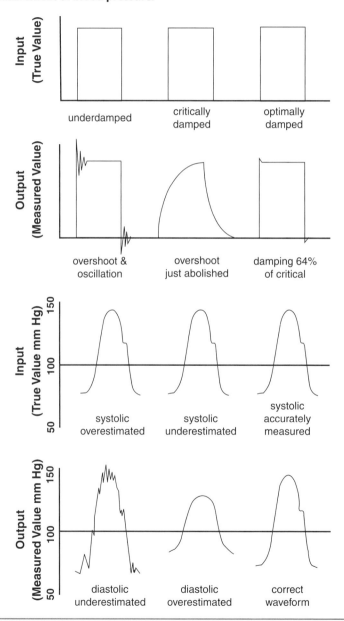

Figure 9.8

A complex signal waveform can be constructed by combining simple sine waves.

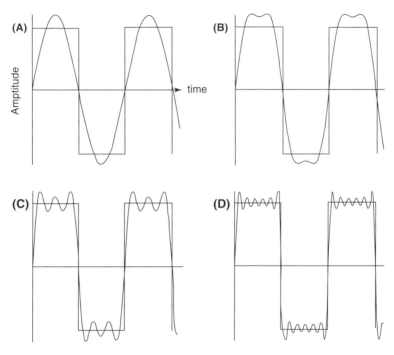

In this example, a rectangular waveform is "built up" by adding harmonics of different amplitudes. Harmonics are sinusoids whose frequencies are multiples of the main or fundamental frequency. The amplitudes of the harmonics decrease as their frequency increases. (A) The rectangular waveform is first approximated by a sine wave at the same frequency (i.e., the first harmonic). (B) Summation of the first and third harmonics. (C) Summation of first, third, and fifth harmonics. (D) Summation of the first, third, fifth, ninth, and eleventh harmonics. As more harmonics are added, the waveform becomes more rectangular. On the other hand, if a rectangular waveform is damped, it becomes more rounded as harmonics are filtered out.

If a measurement system is used under significantly different *environmental conditions* (like pressure or temperature) than those under which it is calibrated and no correction is made, systematic errors result. A typical example is the effect of barometric pressure, humidity, or anesthetic gases on polarographic oxygen analyzers.

Operator errors are the result of between-observer variations in measurement technique and within-observer habits (such as always holding your head to one side while reading a needle and scale, causing parallax). Human observers also exhibit what is known as "digit preference." Anytime an observer must read a scale, a guess must be made as to the last digit of the measurement. Most people tend to prefer some digits over others. For example, a blood pressure of 117/89 mm Hg is rarely recorded. Observers tend to prefer terminal digits of 0 and 5. Thus, readings such as 120/85 mm Hg are far more commonly recorded. The way observers round numbers and select significant digits can also introduce error.

Sources of Imprecision (Random Error)

Noise

All measurements are subject to some degree of minor, rapidly changing disturbance caused by a variety of environmental factors. This is called noise. It may be difficult to trace and is not reduced by calibration. Noise distortions, however, are usually considered to occur randomly. That means their effects should cancel out if enough repeated measurements are made. Noise can be particularly disturbing with weak signals that are highly amplified. The noise is amplified along with the signal, such that a limit is eventually placed on the sensitivity of the measurement. For example, an electrocardiographic (ECG) signal may be contaminated with intercostal electromyographic (EMG) signals of equal amplitude along with noise from electrochemical activity between the skin and the electrode. On the way to the amplifier, the signal is subject to electrostatic and electromagnetic noise (at 60 Hz) from nearby power lines. Radio frequency noise may be added from surgical diathermy or radio transmitters. Physical movement of the electrode cable changes its capacitance and may add low-frequency noise. The most common form of electrical noise is called *thermal* or *Johnson noise*, caused by the random motions of electrons in conductors.

The efficiency with which a signal can be distinguished from background noise is defined as the signal-to-noise ratio, using a logarithmic bel scale. One bel is a ratio of 10:1. Two bels is 100:1. A more convenient unit is the decibel, which is one-tenth of a bel:

$$\text{decibel (dB)} = 10 \log_{10}(P_2/P_1)$$

where P_1 is input power and P_2 is output power. Thus, a ratio of 100:1 is 20 dB.

Nonlinearity

Nonlinearity is considered to cause imprecision because it will introduce an unpredictable error that varies over the operating range, depending on the level of the input signal (in contrast to proportional error that is predictable). Errors due to nonlinearity can be minimized by calibrating at two points within the range in which most measurements will be made.

Operator Errors

Human errors during measurement can also introduce imprecision. For example, variations in readings given by different observers may be caused by reading a dial at different angles, failing to judge the exact reading consistently, or slight variations in preparing transducers or samples.

Measuring Specific Variables

In this section, we will review the standard techniques for measuring some of the variables common to research in pulmonary medicine and related disciplines.

Pressure

Perhaps the most fundamental measurement in respiratory mechanics is the measurement of pressure. *Absolute pressure* refers to the absolute force per unit area exerted by a fluid. *Gauge pressure* is the pressure of interest referred to local atmospheric pressure. The difference, therefore, between absolute pressure and gauge pressure is the local atmospheric pressure on that particular day. Steady-state pressures are easily measured by a variety of devices; the measurement of a pressure that varies with time is far more complicated.

U-Tube Manometer

This device consists of a U-shaped tube (usually glass or clear plastic) filled with a liquid (e.g., water for most purposes, but perhaps mercury for measuring higher pressures or oil for smaller pressures). A scale is attached to measure the height of one liquid surface with respect to the other (**Figure 9.9**). If one leg of the manometer is attached to a source of pressure and the other leg is open to atmospheric pressure, the liquid will rise in the leg with the lower pressure and fall in the leg with the higher pressure. The distance between the levels is a measure of gauge pressure (e.g., in cm H_2O or mm Hg). This device is good only for measuring static pressures and is often used to calibrate other types of pressure sensors.

Bourdon-Type Pressure Gauges

Bourdon-tube gauges are available for reliable static pressure measurements. Basically, they employ a curved tube with a shape that changes under an applied pressure difference. This shape change is mechanically coupled to the rotation of a shaft; a needle attached to this shaft gives the pressure reading on a dial (**Figure 9.10**). The mechanical components are cumbersome and the dynamic response relatively slow compared with the usual methods for dynamic pressure measurements. This type of gauge is commonly used on compressed gas cylinders. Some mechanical ventilators use a variation of this type of gauge for measuring airway pressures. Bourdon-tube gauges tend to go out of calibration easily.

Diaphragm Pressure Gauges

Two different arrangements exist for measuring pressures by means of detecting the deflection of a metal diaphragm under an imposed pressure loading. In one type, a thin circular metal plate with clamped edges deflects under an applied pressure loading. The engineering theories of plate deflection can be used to relate the displacement at the center of the plate to the pressure difference applied. The deflection can be measured by strain gauges bonded to the surface of the diaphragm (**Figure 9.11**).

Figure 9.9

The U-tube manometer. The height, *h*, indicates that the measured pressure, P_0, is 60 cm H_2O above atmospheric pressure, P_{atm}.

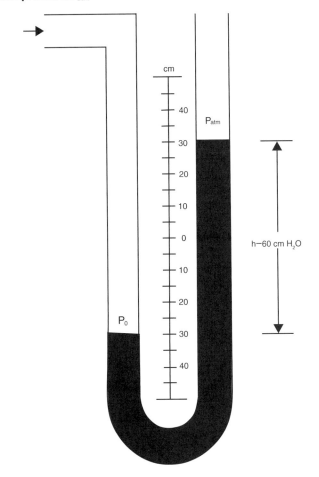

The strain gauge is an element with an electrical resistance that changes as it is deformed. Continuously measuring the voltage drop across a circuit containing this resistance (the "bridge") is equivalent to continuously measuring the displacement of the diaphragm. The second method for measuring the displacement involves the fact that movement of a magnetic core between two coils changes the magnetic coupling between the coils, and therefore changes the voltage output of the secondary coil. In this case, there has to be a signal input to the primary coil—the carrier—and a means to decode the signal that appears in the secondary coil. With either of these methods, the displacements of the diaphragm are generally small and the

Figure 9.10

The Bourdon-tube pressure gauge.

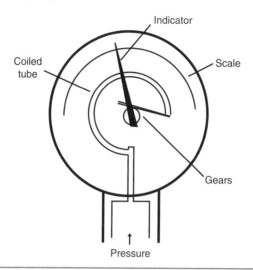

Figure 9.11

Diaphragm pressure gauges.

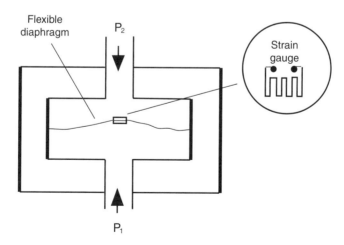

The diaphragm is clamped at the edges and deflects under applied pressure load ($P_1 - P_2$). The magnitude of the load is detected by the elongation or compression of the strain gauge.

diaphragms used are extremely thin and light. Therefore the dynamic response of the solid components of the device is very good. The frequency response, however, may be limited by the fluid in the connecting tube and in the chambers of the gauge.

Piezoelectric Crystals

Very small pressure gauges can now be constructed of piezoelectric crystals. A piezoelectric substance, when stressed or deformed, produces a potential difference (voltage drop) across the crystal. Sensing this voltage therefore measures the deformation of the crystal. Because there are essentially no moving parts, this device is very good for both static and dynamic pressure measurements. Piezoelectric pressure sensors are used in most modern medical equipment, including ventilators.

Flow

Several types of flow-measuring devices are available; again, the determination of which to use depends upon whether one wants to measure steady flows or time-varying (unsteady) flows. In respiratory mechanics we are generally interested in flow into and out of the airways and in how this changes lung volume. We therefore speak of volume as if it flows; flows are expressed in liters per minute, for example. This shorthand notation overlooks an important physical fact: gases flow; volumes do not. When we speak of a *volume flow* of so many liters per minute, what we are really saying is that the mass of gas that has exited from the lung over that time would occupy a volume of so many liters *at some specific temperature and pressure*. Thus, flow measurements require accurate temperature and pressure measurements to be accurate.

In terms of the frequency response required from flow-measuring instrumentation, studies of the usual maneuvers performed in pulmonary function laboratories show that flow from humans can have significant frequency components up to 60 Hz. This approaches the limits of the available instrumentation.

Rotameters

The rotameter is commonly used to measure steady flow. In the pulmonary laboratory, it finds its greatest use in calibrating other devices. Essentially, it is a tapered vertical tube containing a float (**Figure 9.12**). The float rises as flow rate is increased, thereby increasing the cross-sectional area through which flow can occur. Volume flow is then directly proportional to this open area. Because the float is stationary, its weight is then balanced by the pressure of the gas on its surfaces and the drag caused by the flow going past it. The scale is usually calibrated in terms of liters per minute of volume flow, but the specific temperature and pressure conditions that prevail on that day must be recorded.

Pneumotachometers

Pneumotachometers are devices designed to produce a pressure drop when exposed to a given flow. The pressure drop is measured and flow is then inferred from the pressure measurement. Pneumotachometers are the workhorses of respiratory research flow measurements. They are

Figure 9.12

A rotameter.

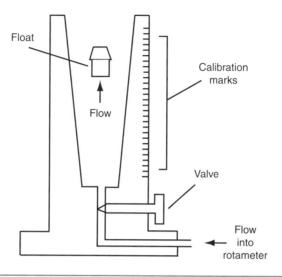

of two basic types (**Figure 9.13**), the capillary bed (Fleisch) type and the screen (Silverman) type. The basic principle behind the bed of packed capillary tubes (or other close-packed channels) is that the tubes are of such small diameter that near their center the flow is essentially one-dimensional and relatively steady. The Poiseuille equation for steady flow through a

Figure 9.13

Pneumotachometers.

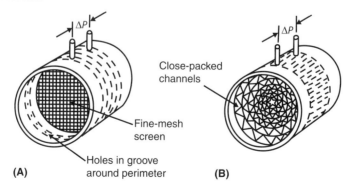

(A) Silverman or screen type. (B) Fleish or capillary tube type.

pipe shows that the pressure drop (P) is linearly related to the volume flow rate. This concept works well for steady or slowly changing flows. However, if a sinusoidal flow is generated (for example, with a piston pump), one finds that the frequency range over which a Fleisch pneumotachometer faithfully records the flow is limited.

Screen-type pneumotachometers rely on a fine mesh screen to produce a pressure drop related to flow through the screen. Their frequency response is better than that of the capillary-type pneumotachometers, but they generate much more turbulence in the flow and hence more noise in the pressure signal. Pneumotachometers may be heated to prevent condensation of exhaled water vapor and subsequent obstruction of the channels for flow.

A modification of the Silverman pneumotach involves the use of a solid membrane of plastic instead of a screen. There is a cut in the membrane creating a flap. The flap deforms and creates a hole in the membrane as flow passes through the pneumotach. This design is often used to make inexpensive, disposable sensors that are not affected by condensation (such as in ventilator circuits), which would ruin the calibration of a screen pneumotach.

Hot Wire Methods

This type of flow detector depends on the principles of hot wire anemometry. A heated wire is placed across the channel of a cylinder, much like that of a pneumotachometer. Electrical heating is supplied, and either the wire temperature or temperature of the flowing gas is monitored. Flow across the wire produces a cooling effect. The degree of cooling can be measured and calibrated to provide an indicator of flow. Because the heat is taken up by molecules of the gas, this is a direct measurement of *mass flow* rather than volume flow.

Vane Transducers

For relatively steady flows, the displacement of a mechanical device such as a rotor or a disk may be used to measure flow (**Figure 9.14**). In the device shown, the gas strikes the vanes and a fixed quantity of gas is contained in each section, much like people passing through a revolving door. As the vane turns, the gas is delivered to the outlet; the rotations are counted and the appropriate flow rate is displayed on some scale. In this case, the rate measured is the volume occupied by the gas; the rate of mass flow depends upon the density (and therefore the composition, temperature, and pressure) of the gas. These devices are not used for the measurement of flows that vary rapidly in time (such as during a forced vital capacity maneuver). However, they are commonly used for such things as measuring spontaneous tidal volumes on patients at the bedside.

Turbine Flowmeters

For these meters the float is replaced by a vaned disk or turbine wheel. The viscosity or drag generated by the flow spins the wheel. A magnetic probe in the body senses the number of vanes rotating by in a given time, much like the cruise control detects engine rpm and therefore vehicle speed in an automobile. These meters are somewhat better in their transient response than those discussed earlier and occasionally are used to measure time-varying flows. Again, the relationship between rotational speed and mass flow depends on gas viscosity and density, and hence on local temperature and pressure.

Figure 9.14

A typical vane flow transducer. The example shown is a Wright Respirometer.

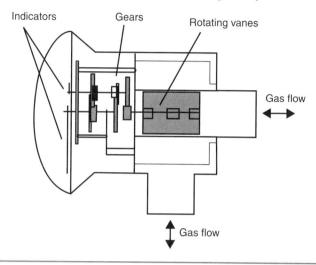

Ultrasonic Transducers

Ultrasonic flowmeters consist of two piezoelectric transducers separated by a known distance and electrical circuitry to generate and then detect high-frequency sound waves. In some designs, the transducers are mounted axially. In others, the wave crosses the flow at a shallow angle to the axis. Each transducer is alternately used as a transmitter and then a receiver, and the time of transit for the sound wave measured. Waves traveling in the direction of fluid flow arrive more quickly than sound waves traveling against the flow. From the differences in transit time the flow velocity can be computed. In general, these devices are capable of use in unsteady flow conditions. Their signal at zero flow (the baseline), however, tends to drift over time, making them relatively unreliable.

Volume

Spirometer

One of the first, and the simplest, methods to track changes in lung volume is to collect gases in a spirometer, an inverted, counterbalanced can with a water seal (**Figure 9.15**). Because the spirometer is at a different temperature than the lungs, the spirometer volume changes must be corrected for temperature to represent changes in lung volume. The spirometer gives only a relative measure of volume in that it detects *volume changes*. In addition, because of the mechanics of the spirometer and the mechanical linkages to the drum and pen on which volume change is recorded, its dynamic response is not optimal. In fact, the frequency response deteriorates at around 4 Hz.

Figure 9.15

Water seal spirometer.

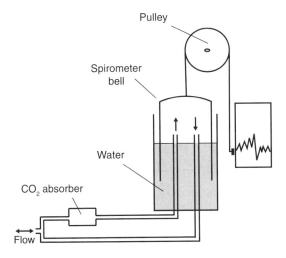

Tracer Gas

Methods for determining *absolute volume* frequently make use of tracer gases. An inert gas (such as helium) not usually present in the respiratory system and not highly soluble in blood can be introduced to a closed system such as a spirometer. The amount introduced is known. If the subject respires the gas mixture until a uniform concentration exists in the closed system, conservation of mass together with a measurement of the concentration gives the volume of the subject's lungs *that exchanges gas with the system:* any blebs or obstructed areas that contain air but do not receive the gas are not included in this measurement.

A variant of this process employs pure oxygen in the closed system and uses the nitrogen present in the subject's lungs as the tracer gas. This is known as the nitrogen washout method, and again measures only the volume of gas in the subject that exchanges gases with the environment.

Plethysmograph

Most of the literature of traditional respiratory mechanics fails to distinguish between the volume flow of gas out of the lung and the rate of change of lung volume. Consider a simple syringe whose outlet is closed by a stopcock. Pressure on the plunger will change the volume of gas in the syringe because of gas compression; however, no gas flows out of the syringe. If the stopcock is opened a crack, and if one pushes slowly and gently on the plunger, gas will flow without much change in the pressure in the syringe—that is, without much gas compression. The volume of gas exiting the syringe will be very close to the volume change in the syringe itself. If instead one attempts to force the plunger, gas compression occurs, and the volume in the syringe decreases to a greater amount than can be explained by the amount of air that has exited. In fact, this gas compression makes possible a measurement of lung volume by a process called body plethysmography. You may gain some insight into how plethysmographs function by a simplified discussion employing the relationships among pressure, temperature, and density of ideal gases.

In the most common type of plethysmograph, the pressure plethysmograph (**Figure 9.16**), there is a rigid box around the subject, a mouthpiece to breathe through, and pressure taps at the mouth end of the mouthpiece and in the box itself. The box is attached to a small piston pump with a known stroke volume. In addition, there is a shutter at the subject's mouth that can be electronically closed. In the diagram, we assume that the lung behaves as a single compartment—that is, that the pressure is the same everywhere within the lung. When the gases in the subject and in the box are at the same constant temperature, the gases will obey Boyle's law:

$$PV = \text{constant}$$

Furthermore, the total volume inside the box is constant, so that small changes in lung volume (dV_L) and box volume (dV_B) must be equal and opposite:

$$dV_L = -dV_B$$

Figure 9.16

Pressure type plethysmograph.

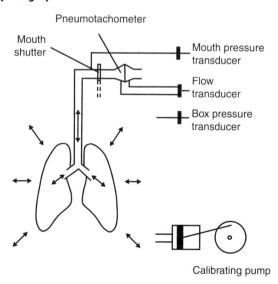

When the shutter is closed and the gas in the subject's lungs is compressed and expanded by panting against the closed shutter, changes in pressure and volume occur in both the lung (P_L, V_L) and in the box (P_B, V_B). These changes must be related by:

$$\frac{dP_B}{dP_L} = \frac{P_B}{V_B} \times \frac{V_L}{P_L}$$

If one has previously quantified the relationship between changes in box pressure and volume by changing the box volume with the piston pump, the calibration factor (P_B/V_B) is known. Thus one can measure the absolute volume of the lung by measuring pressure and its changes in the lung (that is, mouth pressure) and box during the occlusion maneuver.

Volume (V) measurements are commonly derived from flow ($\dot{V}$) measurement. This is possible because, mathematically, volume can be expressed as the integral of flow between two point in time (t):

$$V = \int \dot{V}\, dt$$

In the simplest case, if flow is constant, then volume = flow × time. Conversely, flow is the derivative of volume:

$$\dot{V} = \frac{dV}{dt}$$

Again, the simplest case is when flow is constant such that volume is simply the change in volume divided by the change in time.

In some cases, volume measurements can also be derived only from pressure measurements. Ventilators are often evaluated by connecting them to a simulated lung consisting simply of a rigid-walled container. As gas enters the container from the ventilator, the pressure inside the container rises. The internal energy also increases so that the temperature of the gas increases. If the container is a perfect insulator, the gas will not lose heat during the process, and an *adiabatic* compression is said to occur. The pressure change is a function of the quantity of gas added (measured in moles) and the change in temperature. Therefore, a simulated volume measurement can be made by measuring the pressure inside the container. The equation relating volume and pressure for an adiabatic compression is:

$$V = P\left(\frac{V_c}{1.9P_B}\right)$$

where V is the simulated volume measurement, which is proportional to the pressure measurement (L); P is the pressure change, above ambient barometric pressure, inside the container (cm H_2O); V_c is the fixed volume of container (L); and P_B is the barometric pressure (mm Hg).

Sometimes the container is filled with fine copper wool (very thin copper wire, densely packed). This material provides a huge surface area for heat exchange and acts like a thermal buffer. The effect is that the temperature inside the container remains relatively constant as pressure increases. This process is known as an *isothermal* compression. The equation relating volume and pressure for an isothermal compression is:

$$V = P\left(\frac{V_c}{1.36P_B}\right)$$

In practice, a pressure transducer is connected to the container, and the output calibrated to read volume using a calibrated syringe to inject known volumes into the container. The fixed volume of the container can be selected to simulate adult, pediatric, and neonatal patients (**Table 9.1**). Note that both of the equations above can be solved for *V/P*, which is the simulated compliance of the lung model.

Humidity

In some experiments we need to measure the amount of water vapor present in a gas sample. Of all the physical quantities measured in a pulmonary function laboratory, humidity is probably the most difficult to measure accurately. Errors on the order of 2% are at the leading edge of the available technology.

Table 9.1

Example Parameters for Rigid Wall Lung Simulator

	Premature Infant	Infant	Toddler	Small Child	Child	Adolescent	Adult
Age	24–36 weeks	36 weeks– 1 year	1–3 years	4–5 years	6–12 years	13–18 years	>18 years
Respiratory rate (breaths/ min)	30–60	25–40	20–35	20–30	18–25	12–18	12–16
Tidal volume	4–6	5–8	5–8	6–9	7–10	7–10	7–10
Resistance (cm H_2O/L/s)	150.0	40.0	30.0	25.0	20.0	15.0	10.0
Compliance (mL/cmH_2O)	0.5	8.0	15.0	20.0	30.0	40.0	50.0
Simulator volume (L)*	0.527	8.434	15.814	21.085	31.628	42.171	52.714

*Volume of a rigid-walled container required to achieve specified compliance when filled with wire wool (2% by volume) at normal atmospheric pressure (760 mm Hg). Changes in atmospheric pressure will change the simulated compliance of the container so that some method of adjusting volume may be necessary to keep within the specified tolerance for compliance of ±5%.

The gold standard is the absorption method, by which the gas sample of interest is introduced into a chamber containing a desiccant and the amount of water extracted is determined by the change in weight. This method is not, however, rapid or practical, particularly for measurements over time. To perform repeated experiments at reasonable time intervals, some indirect measure of humidity must be used. For serial measurements at fairly large time intervals, the dew-point hygrometer has long sufficed. In this method, the gas is cooled while its pressure is maintained constant. Some method must be provided for determining the temperature at which condensation first appears. This may involve a polished metal mirror that is visually observed, or in a sophisticated hygrometer it may be a quartz crystal oscillated at its resonant frequency. In the latter case, as water condenses on the crystal, its weight increases and the resonant frequency changes. This change can be detected. The temperature at which the condensate forms is related to, but generally not equal to, the dew-point temperature of the air. The dew point in turn is a measure of humidity in that it is the temperature at which the amount of water vapor present fully saturates the volume of air in contact with it. The discrepancy between the condensation and dew-point temperatures occurs because the appearance of the droplets is affected by the nature of the surface, any contaminants that may form nuclei for condensation, and other factors.

Perhaps the most practical methods for determining humidity are those based on capacitance changes. A capacitor is a circuit device consisting of two metal plates separated by a dielectric layer that acts as an insulator. When the two plates are electrically charged, a voltage difference is produced that depends upon how well the dielectric material avoids becoming polarized. In capacitance humidity sensors, the dielectric material is one that can absorb water. Because water polarizes so readily, this changes the dielectric constant of the sandwiched material and therefore changes the output of the sensor. Currently, the best sensors have employed a polymer as the dielectric material. Unfortunately, at high relative humidity such as that encountered in the respiratory system, the sensors tend to be unstable. In addition, the sensors are very sensitive to temperature changes and the results must be correlated with local temperature. Thus, truly dynamic humidity measurements are still difficult to make.

Humidity sensors are calibrated by exposing them to the air above a saturated salt solution. This is because the relative humidity above the solutions can be predicted (**Table 9.2**).

Table 9.2

Relative Humidity (%) in Air Above Saturated Salt Solutions as a Function of Solution Temperature

	20°C	25°C	30°C	35°C
Lithium chloride (LiCl)	12.4	12.0	11.8	11.7
Sodium chloride (NaCl)	75.5	75.8	75.6	75.5
Potassium sulfate (K$_2$SO$_4$)	97.2	96.9	96.6	96.4

One procedure for calibration is as follows:

1. Select a salt that will provide the desired humidity calibration level). LiCl salt will provide a low calibration point, NaCl (table salt) will provide a midrange calibration point, and K_2SO_4 will provide the high calibration point. Pour approximately 20 mL dry salt into a 100-mL beaker. Add enough pure distilled water (do not use deionized water) to just cover the salt (no standing water above the salt).
2. Stir the moistened salt.
3. Cover the beaker with plastic and allow to sit for at least 24 hours.
4. Check that there is some undissolved salt with a clear saturated salt solution above it. If not, add more water and stir. If all the salt is dissolved (because too much water was added initially), add more salt and wait another 24 hours.
5. Place the humidity sensor in the beaker approximately 20 mm above the solution. Do not let the sensor touch the solution.
6. Cover the beaker, making sure to seal tightly around the cable. Let stand for about two hours so that the humidity level reaches a steady state.
7. Note the room temperature and calibrate the output of the humidity sensor according to Table 9.2.
8. Repeat steps 5 through 7 to get a calibration at three points using the three salts.

Signal Processing

The transducers mentioned all provide some sort of signal together with some noise. Some of them, such as the inductance-coupled pressure transducer or the strain gauge transducer, require some electrical input to be operated upon to produce an electrical output. All of these signals must be processed in some fashion to be useful. For many of the mechanical meters, processing may be done internally in terms of the connections inside the meter to pointers and scales. This internal mechanical processing may limit the frequency response or damp out unwanted or excessive oscillations. Thus, not all signal processing is electrical.

Several particularly prevalent methods of signal processing need to be mentioned. The first is amplification. Small signals often need to be boosted to be used by other electrical equipment. In contrast, some very large signals occasionally need to be reduced. Both of these processes, oddly enough, are referred to as *amplification*. The *gain* is the ratio of the output signal to the input signal amplitude. If the gain is greater than 1, we have what we traditionally think of as amplification. If the gain is less than 1, the device is still said to be an amplifier, but it really is an attenuator. Given what was said about Fourier analysis, we obviously want the gain to be constant over the frequency range of interest. Just as important, amplification should not introduce a phase shift into the signal.

Signals also can be filtered. A *filter* is a device that removes certain frequency components from the signal. If it removes high-frequency components, it is called a low-pass filter. If it removes low-frequency components, it is a high-pass filter. If it removes low and high components, it is referred to as a band-pass filter. Filtering can be accomplished either electronically or mathematically from data that have been taken without a filter. Generally, pulmonary function laboratories use low-pass filters to get rid of noise and other signals at high frequency. This makes sense because if most of our devices distort signals at higher frequency, it is just as well to remove these frequencies from the signals we are trying to analyze. In contrast, signals of interest totally unknown to us may be present in the frequencies we are eliminating. The frequency at which the filter starts to attenuate the signal by a given amount is called the *corner frequency* and is generally specified on the filter. Another characteristic of importance is the *roll-off,* or the rate of attenuation. It is generally specified in terms of decibels (dB) per decade. The higher the roll-off, the more effective the filter is in removing frequencies near the corner frequency. This ensures that these frequencies will be nearly totally eliminated rather than merely phase shifted and somewhat reduced in amplitude. The names of the types of filters (Butterworth, Bessel, Chebyshev) refer to the mathematical relationship between amount of attenuation and frequency.

Recording and Display Devices

An oscilloscope is a cathode ray tube on which a voltage can be displayed versus time or versus a second voltage. For monitoring purposes, signals may be observed on the oscilloscope and may even be photographed on its face to provide a permanent record. Alternatively, the signal may be sent directly to a strip chart recorder or to a plotter. However, the dynamics of the pen systems will generally preclude accurate recording of signals that vary rapidly in time.

Signals may also be recorded by computer. In this case, the sampling rate at which the computer acquires the data is important. A continuous signal presented to a computer is recorded at fixed increments in time at the sampling interval. This is called *analog-to-digital conversion* because a signal continuous in time (analog signal) is represented in the computer by the discrete sample values obtained at certain time points (digital representation). This conversion is not as straightforward as it seems. In particular, if the sampling rate is too slow, a phenomenon known as *aliasing* occurs. The higher-frequency components of the signal are shifted to appear as lower-frequency components, and the representation of the signal is consequently distorted. In order to avoid aliasing, the sampling interval must be less than half the period for the highest frequency component of the signal. Thus, if the signal is expected to have a component of 50 Hz, one must sample at least 100 samples per second. The software may or may not support a sampling rate fast enough for the experimenter's purposes. In addition, the converters in various computers differ in the range of input voltage expected and in how these signals are represented in the computer's memory. These details are important for any given application.

Perhaps the best way to set up a laboratory for making measurements is to purchase a computer-based system that combines sensors with signal processing hardware and special software making it easy to capture, view, and analyze measurement data. One of the most popular systems is called LabVIEW by National Instruments, Inc. You can learn more about this product at www.ni.com/labview.

Questions

Definitions

Define the following terms:

- Systematic errors
- Random errors
- Accuracy
- Precision
- Resolution
- Calibration
- Calibration verification

True or False

1. A U-tube manometer is used for measuring humidity.
2. A pneumotachometer is used to measure gas flow.
3. A rotameter is used to calibrate pressure sensors.
4. A hot-wire anemometer senses changes in fluid volume.
5. A spirometer is used to measure changes in gas volume.
6. A dew-point hygrometer is used to determine the humidity of a gas sample.
7. Calibration reduces systematic errors but not random errors.

Multiple Choice

1. The ideal situation for a measurement is to have:
    a. High bias and low imprecision
    b. Low imprecision and low bias
    c. High imprecision and high bias
    d. Low bias and high imprecision
2. All of the following are true about a highly linear measurement device except:
    a. The ratio of the output to the input remains constant over the operating range.
    b. The linearity specification can be assessed using least-squares regression.
    c. The linearity specification is defined as the maximum deviation from the regression line.
    d. Linearity is desirable because the system does not have to be calibrated.
3. The two-point calibration procedure involves:
    a. Adjusting the sensitivity and the linearity
    b. Adjusting the offset and the gain
    c. Measuring a known quantity and reducing the random error
    d. Decreasing both bias and imprecision

4. Which of the following sources of bias occur if the zero point is not set correctly?
   a. Constant error
   b. Proportional error
   c. Range error
   d. Hysteresis
   e. Frequency response
   f. Noise

5. Which source of error can be caused by electromagnetic radiation?
   a. Constant error
   b. Proportional error
   c. Range error
   d. Hysteresis
   e. Frequency response
   f. Noise

6. Which source of error is due to an improperly set sensitivity?
   a. Constant error
   b. Proportional error
   c. Range error
   d. Hysteresis
   e. Frequency response
   f. Noise

7. What type of error would you expect if the needle on the measurement device went off the scale?
   a. Constant error
   b. Proportional error
   c. Range error
   d. Hysteresis
   e. Frequency response
   f. Noise

8. If the instrument gives a different reading for a given input value depending upon whether the input is increasing or decreasing, the device is said to show:
   a. Constant error
   b. Proportional error
   c. Range error
   d. Hysteresis
   e. Frequency response
   f. Noise

9. If the signal is moving faster than the measuring device is capable of following, what type of error would you expect?
   a. Constant error
   b. Proportional error
   c. Range error
   d. Hysteresis
   e. Frequency response

CHAPTER 10

Basic Statistical Concepts

S tatistical analysis of the numbers generated by observation and measurement in a research study is usually one of the most intimidating topics for an investigator. Unfortunately, inappropriate statistical analyses sometimes appear in published studies. The goal of this chapter is to provide a clear overview of the meaning and use of common statistical techniques. Emphasis is on the concepts and correct use of statistics more than the math. For this reason, simplified data sets are used, and calculations are included only to the extent necessary to discuss the concepts. The purpose of this chapter is to help you to be an educated consumer of research publications first, and to help you become a researcher second. However, this chapter and the next will give you enough information to understand published research articles and even to perform some basic statistical analyses on a computer. Beyond that, you really need to study formal statistical textbooks if you want to understand the theory.

Preliminary Concepts

Statistics is a branch of mathematics dealing with the collection, analysis, interpretation, and presentation of masses of numerical data. *Biostatistics* is the application of statistics to the fields of medicine and biology. Historically, the term *statistic* referred to numbers derived from affairs of state, such as number of births or deaths, or average age expectancies. Such numbers form the basis for what are called *descriptive statistics* of today, which include frequency distributions, measures of central tendency (mean, median, and mode), measures of variability (variance, standard deviation, and coefficient of variation), standard scores, and various correlation coefficients.

In the mid-1600s the *theory of probability* was developed and applied to games of chance by mathematicians Blaise Pascal and Jacques Bernoulli. In 1812, Pierre-Simon Laplace applied the theory of probability to the distribution of errors of observation, and a few years later Adolphe Quételet used probability models to describe social and biological phenomena—for example, height or chest circumference distributions.

The application of probability theory to descriptive statistics led to *inferential statistics*. This area of statistics allows us to test hypotheses; that is, we can obtain the probability of getting the observed results by random chance and decide whether the treatment made a difference. Inferential statistics include parametric statistics (those based on specific distributions such as the normal and t-distributions) and non-parametric tests (those that do not assume the data are distributed in any particular fashion).

Definition of Terms

The following terms are used frequently in this chapter:

- *Population:* Collection of data or objects (usually infinite or otherwise not measurable) that describes some phenomenon of interest.
- *Sample:* Subset of a population that is accessible for measurement.
- *Variable:* Characteristic or entity that can take on different values. Examples are temperature, class size, and political party.
- *Qualitative variable:* Categorical variable not placed on a meaningful number scale. An example is the variable gender, which generally has two values, male and female. Any assignment of numbers to these two values is arbitrary and arithmetically meaningless.
- *Quantitative variable:* One that is measurable using a meaningful scale of numbers. Both temperature and class size are quantitative variables.
- *Discrete variable:* Quantitative variable with gaps or interruptions in the values it may assume. An example is any *integer* variable, such as class size, number of hospital beds, or number of children per family. We have 1 child, not 1.5 or 1.82.
- *Continuous variable:* Quantitative variable that can take on any value, including fractional ones, in a given range of values. An example is temperature or pH. Between a pH of 7.41 and 7.42, we can have 7.411, or 7.4115. Every value is theoretically possible and limited by instrumentation or application.

The distinctions between discrete and continuous variables, as well as between quantitative and qualitative, are fundamental to a presentation of statistics. Such distinctions determine the appropriateness of particular statistics in both descriptive and inferential statistics. Their meaning will be further clarified by their use in applications.

Levels of Measurement

Statistics involves the manipulation and graphic presentation of numbers. The process of assigning numbers to things (variables) is termed *measurement,* and the numbers that result are termed *data.* However, the arithmetic properties of numbers may not apply to the variables measured. The problem can be illustrated with some examples. Numbers (0, 1, 2, …) have the following properties:

- *Distinguishability:* 0, 1, 2, and so on, are different numbers.
- *Ranking (greater than or less than):* 1 is less than 2. If 1 is less than 2, and 2 is less than 3, 1 is less than 3.
- *Equal intervals:* Between 1 and 2, we assume the same distance as between 3 and 4. Therefore, $2 - 1 = 4 - 3$.

When numbers are applied to variables, these properties may or may not hold. For example, consider the qualitative variable gender, which can be assigned a 1 for male and a 2 for female. The only numerical property that applies is distinguishability. Although 1 is less than 2, we would not dare suggest any inequality in the two values (male, female) of the variable. Nor is there any meaning to the equal interval between 1 and 2 when applied to gender.

Levels of measurement are used to show the differences and extent to which numerical properties apply in objects that are measured. Different statistical analyses of numbers require, or assume, the presence of certain numerical properties. Otherwise, the analysis is inappropriate, invalid, and sometimes meaningless. The following levels of measurement are illustrated with examples.

Nominal

Data measured at the nominal level consist of named categories without any particular order to them. Numbers are used here to name or distinguish the categories and are purely arbitrary.

Variable: political party
Values: Republican = 1, Democrat = 2

Ordinal

Data measured on the ordinal level consist of discrete categories that have an order to them. No implication of equal intervals between numbers is made. Some variables do not admit of more precise measurement than simple ordering.

Variable: pain
Values: none = 0, mild = 1, moderate = 2, severe = 3, excruciating = 4

Continuous (Interval)

Data measured at the continuous level can assume any value, rather than just whole numbers. In addition, we assume that equal, uniform intervals between numbers represent equal intervals in the variable being measured. An example is the Celsius scale of temperature, where the distance between 2 and 4 degrees is the same as the distance between 8 and 10 degrees.

Variable: temperature
Values: the centigrade scale, originating at $-273°$

Continuous (Ratio)

The mathematically strongest level is the ratio, where numbers represent equal intervals and start with zero. The existence of a zero value allows ratio statements, such as "4 is twice 2." Examples are provided by any absolute scale or variable that has no negative numbers (less than zero) in its scale of measurement; these include height, weight, pH, blood pressure, and temperature measured on the Kelvin scale.

Variable: temperature
Values: the Kelvin scale, originating at $0°$

The order of the levels given is from the weakest to the strongest, where strength refers to the level of mathematical manipulation. A nominal level permits counting frequencies. An ordinal level allows use of the algebra of inequalities. Interval and ratio levels allow multiplication and division. Higher levels preserve and include the properties of lower levels. A variable that allows ratio measurement can always be reduced to a more primitive level of measurement, as seen with temperature, using an interval (Celsius) and ratio (Kelvin) level. We could also use an ordinal level with temperature by devising the following scale:

0   Cold
1   Lukewarm
2   Warm
3   Hot
4   Extremely hot

We could even categorize temperature, and use numbers arbitrarily with no ranking indicated, for a nominal level:

Hot   1
Warm   2
Cold   3

Although higher levels of measurement can be reduced to lower levels, the reverse is not necessarily true unless the numerical properties of higher levels apply to the values of the variable. The variable *pain* cannot be measured above an ordinal level at this time. The lower, or more primitive, the level of measurement, the more restricted and less mathematically sophisticated is the statistical analysis.

Statistics and Parameters

The term *statistic* refers to a measure made on a sample and is denoted by Roman letters, such as X or s. The term *parameter* refers to a measure made on a population and is denoted by Greek letters, such as α or β. This distinction will be very important when discussing inferential statistics.

Significant Figures

By convention, the number of digits used to express a measured number is a rough indication of the error. For example, if a measurement is reported as being 35.2 cm, you would assume that the true length was between 34.15 and 35.24 cm (the error is about 0.05 cm). The last digit (2) in the reported measurement is uncertain, although we can reliably state that it is either a 1 or 2. The digit to the right of 2, however, can be any number (0, 1, 2, 3, 4, 5, 6, 7, 8, 9). If the measurement is reported as 35.20 cm, it would indicate that the error is even less (0.005 cm). The number of reliably known digits in a measurement is referred to as the number of *significant figures*. Thus, the number 35.2 cm has three significant figures, and the number 35.20 has four. The numbers 35.2 cm and 0.352 m are the same quantities, both having three significant figures and expressing the same degree of accuracy. The use of significant figures to indicate the accuracy of a result is not as precise as giving the actual error, but it is sufficient for some purposes.

Zeros as Significant Figures

Final zeros to the right of the decimal point that are used to indicate accuracy are significant:

170.0	four significant figures
28.600	five significant figures
0.30	two significant figures

For numbers less than one, zeros between the decimal point and the first digit *are not* significant:

0.09	one significant figure
0.00010	two significant figures

Zeros between digits *are* significant:

10.5	three significant figures
0.8070	four significant figures
6000.01	six significant figures

If a number is written with no decimal point, the final zeros may or may not be significant. For instance, the distance between the earth and the sun might be written as 92,900,000 miles, although the accuracy may be only ±5,000 miles. Only the first zero after the 9 is significant. On the other hand, a value of 50 mL measured with a graduated cylinder would be expected to have two significant figures owing to the greater accuracy of the measurement device. To avoid ambiguity, numbers are often written as powers of 10 (using scientific notation), making all digits significant. Using this convention, 92,900,000 miles would be written 9.290×10^7, indicating that there are four significant figures.

Calculations Using Significant Figures

The least precise measurement used in a calculation determines the number of significant figures in the answer. Thus, $73.5 + 0.418 = 73.9$ rather than 73.918, since the least precise number (73.5) is accurate to only one decimal place. Similarly, $0.394 - 0.3862 = 0.0078$, which is approximately 0.008 with only one significant digit, since the least precise number (0.394) is precise to only the nearest one-thousandth (even though it has three significant figures).

For multiplication or division, the product or quotient has the same number of significant figures as the term with the fewest significant figures. As an example, in $28.08 \times 4.6/79.4 = 1.6268$, the term with the fewest significant figures is 4.6. Because this number has two significant figures, the result should be rounded off to 1.6.

Rounding

The results of mathematical computations are often rounded off to specific numbers of significant figures. Rounding is done so that you do not infer accuracy in the result that was not present in the measurements. The following rules are universally accepted and will ensure bias-free reporting of results (the number of significant figures desired should be determined first).

- If the final digits of a number are 0, 1, 2, 3, or 4, the numbers are rounded down (dropped, and the preceding figure is retained unaltered). For example, 3.51 is rounded to 3.5.
- If the final digits are 5, 6, 7, 8, or 9, the numbers are rounded up (dropped, and the preceding figure is increased by one). For example, 3.58 is rounded to 3.6.

Descriptive Statistics

Although open to both misapplication and misinterpretation, statistics can provide us with the meaning in a data set. A data set is simply the list or group of numbers that results from measurement. Descriptive statistics offers a variety of methods for organizing data and reducing a large set of numbers to a few, informative numbers that will *describe* the data.

Data Representation

When a data set is obtained, it should be organized for inspection through use of a frequency distribution, which can represent the data both numerically and graphically. Regardless of how sophisticated the data analysis will be, taking a look at the data is one of the most useful and simplest procedures to suggest further analysis and prevent inappropriate analysis.

In representing data, we distinguish a frequency distribution from a grouped frequency distribution. In a *frequency distribution*, the data are ordered from the minimum to the maximum value, and the frequency of occurrence is given for each value of the variable. With a *grouped frequency distribution*, values of the variable are grouped into classes. For example, if values range from 1 to 100, a frequency distribution that could be an ordered list of 100 different values is not practical or helpful. Usually 10 to 20 is a desirable number of classes.

Table 10.1 illustrates both an ungrouped and grouped frequency distribution. In constructing a frequency distribution, we first find the minimum and maximum values of the variable, list the values in order, tally the number of occurrences for each value in the ordered list, and calculate the percentage and cumulative percentages. The percentage is obtained from the frequency divided by the total number of values. The cumulative percentage accumulates the percentage of each value. For example, the value of 3 occurs three times, or 15%, ([3/20] × 100). The values of 2 and 3 account for 25% of the total observations in the distribution.

In the ungrouped frequency distribution, the class interval is actually one. Every value between the minimum and maximum is included. If the range of values is extremely large, group values into classes and represent the frequency of each class, as shown in Table 10.1, for the same data set. The ability to "see" information in the numbers is lost with more than 20 intervals, and many prefer 10 to 12 intervals.

The goal of constructing a frequency distribution is to allow inspection of the data by summarizing, organizing, and simplifying the data *without misrepresenting the data.* A frequency distribution allows you to observe patterns or trends and to begin extracting information about the numbers. In Table 10.1 we see that values of the variable tend to occur most frequently in the middle range, and to be relatively infrequent at extreme values (the "tails" of the distribution). The frequency marks indicate this distribution. The percentage column shows the largest percentages for the middle values of 4 and 5. We also see that the cumulative percentage grows most rapidly in the middle range. As we add the value of 4, the cumulative percentage jumps from 25% to 45%, and adding 5 brings it to 70%. Almost three-fourths of the values are included at that point. A researcher would want to know how values distribute,

Table 10.1

Frequency Distributions, Ungrouped and Grouped Data

Data set: (6, 5, 3, 7, 3, 2, 4, 6, 5, 4, 6, 4, 3, 2, 8, 7, 4, 5, 5, 5)

Ungrouped Frequency Distribution

Value	Frequency	Percentage	Cumulative Percentage
2	2	10	10
3	3	15	25
4	4	20	45
5	5	25	70
6	3	15	85
7	2	10	95
8	1	5	100
Total	20	100	

Grouped Frequency Distribution

Value	Frequency	Percentage	Cumulative Percentage
2–3	5	25	25
4–5	9	45	70
6–7	5	25	95
8–9	1	5	100
Total	20	100	

and this may be of significance for interpreting results. If the frequency of values tended to be high at low values and more infrequent at high values, we would say that the distribution was skewed. If the variable was test scores, then such a distribution tells us that the test was difficult, the students were poorly prepared, the students were lacking in ability, or all three!

If we wish to see, literally, how the data distribute, then graphic presentation of the frequency distribution is possible. The most basic forms are the histogram, the frequency and percentage polygon, and the cumulative percentage or ogive curve.

- *Histogram:* A bar graph in which the height of the bar indicates the frequency of occurrence of a value or class of values.
- *Frequency polygon:* A graph in which a point indicates the frequency of a value, and the points are connected to form a broken line (hence a polygon).
- *Percentage:* The numerical frequency on the Y-axis is replaced with the percentage of occurrence in this form of the polygon.
- *Percentile:* A percentile is the value of a variable in a data set below which a certain percent of observations fall. So the 10th percentile is the value below which 10 percent of the observations may be found. The 25th percentile is known as the first quartile, the 50th percentile as the median or second quartile, and the 75th percentile as the third quartile. The data between the 25th and 75th percentiles is called the interquartile range, or the middle 50 percent. There are at least 20 different ways to calculate percentiles described in the literature, but all definitions yield similar results when the number of observations is large. You can calculate percentiles for a data set and create a percentiles plot using an Excel spreadsheet. **Table 10.2** shows the procedure using the data from Table 10.1. The table is formatted this way so that it can be used for making a percentiles plot. To do so, create an XY (scatter) plot with column D on the horizontal axis and column E on the vertical axis (**Figure 10.1**). Note that Figure 10.1 shows some horizontal rows of dots. These dots represent the fact that there are duplicate values in the data set. The length of the rows gives the approximate percentage of duplicates. For example, the dashed lines in Figure 10.1 show that 75% of data are below the value of 6 (i.e., 6 is the 75th percentile) and 50% of the data are below the value of 5 (the median value of the data set). Thus, the value of 5 occurs 25% of the time (ie, 75% − 50% = 25%), which is confirmed by the fact that there are five 5s out of 20 data points in all (i.e., 5 ÷ 20 = 0.25 or 25%)
- *Cumulative percentage curve:* This graph plots the cumulative percentage on the Y-axis against the values of the variable on the X-axis. The curve then describes the rate of accumulation for the values of the variable.

In using graphs, the horizontal axis is often referred to as the X-axis and is the abscissa, whereas the vertical axis may be referred to as the Y-axis, or the ordinate.

Figure 10.2 shows a histogram for the data set used in Table 10.1. Here the variable, $X,$ is assumed to be continuous, so that the bars are joined at their bases, and the *real limits* of the variable values are indicated on the horizontal axis. The first bar is for the value 2, but if X is in fact a continuous variable, then X could have any value, so that 2 has a *width* on the real number line of 1.5 to 2.5. Alternatively, if X were a discrete variable, then the bars could be separated, and the numbers on the horizontal axis would most likely be whole numbers, or integers. Bar

Table 10.2

Excel Spreadsheet Example of Data Layout for Calculating Percentiles and Creating a Percentiles Plot

	A	B	C	D	E
1	**Raw Data**	**Sorted in Ascending Order**	**Ranked**	**Cumulative Fraction**	**Percentile**
2	5	2	1	5	2.00
3	2	2	2	10	2.90
4	5	3	3	15	3.00
5	6	3	4	20	3.00
6	6	3	5	25	3.75
7	7	4	6	30	4.00
8	5	4	7	35	4.00
9	4	4	8	40	4.00
10	8	4	9	45	4.55
11	6	5	10	50	5.00
12	5	5	11	55	5.00
13	3	5	12	60	5.00
14	4	5	13	65	5.00
15	4	5	14	70	5.30
16	3	6	15	75	6.00
17	5	6	16	80	6.00
18	2	6	17	85	6.15
19	3	7	18	90	7.00
20	4	7	19	95	7.05
21	7	8	20	100	8.00

Note: The cumulative fraction (see column D) of each value expressed as a percent (e.g., $100\% \times rank/n$, where n = number of data points. For example, cell D3 is, $=100*C3/C21$, where C3 is the cell's numerical rank and cell C21 is the highest rank which is equal to the number of data points in the array. The percentile (see column E) is calculated using the percentile formula in Excel, which is $=PERCENTILE(array,k)$. This gives the kth percentile of the values in the array (range of cells containing the data). The value of k in this formula must be between 0 and 1. For example, we could calculate the value in the data set that represents the 50th percentile as: $=PERCENTILE(B2:B21,0.50)$, which gives the value 5. In this formula, the array or range of data for which the percentile is calculated resides in cells B2 to B21 (we could also have used unsorted data in the array A2 to A21 for this calculation). The values in column E are calculated using the values in column D. For example, cell E3 has this formula, $=PERCENTILE(B2:B21,D3/100)$, and cell E4 has this formula, $=PERCENTILE(B2:B21,D4/100)$.

Figure 10.1

Percentiles plot of data from Table 10.1.

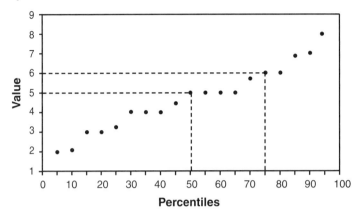

graphs are appropriate when representing the frequencies of the categories with a qualitative variable, or the frequencies of values with a quantitative but discrete variable. For example, the discrete variable, number of children per family, could be shown with a histogram.

One good way to display a frequency distribution is with a pie chart (**Figure 10.3**). This way of representing the contribution of various parts to the whole was invented by Florence Nightingale, a pioneer in the fields of nursing and outcomes research.

Figure 10.2

Histogram and frequency polygon for a continuous variable, *X*.

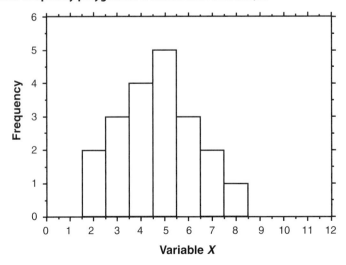

Figure 10.3

Frequency distribution displayed as a pie chart.

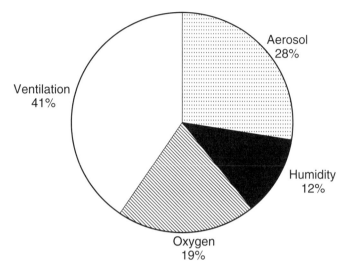

Each area represents a percentage of the total. In this example, various therapies are shown as percentages of the total workload.

Figure 10.4 shows a percentiles plot of some real data for billable days of mechanical ventilation in a hospital. This graph shows the percentile values along the horizontal axis and the actual values of the data on the vertical axis. The value of a percentiles plot is that it summarizes complex raw data in a way that makes intuitive sense. For example, the top graph in Figure 10.4 shows the number of ventilators used daily for a number of months. But we cannot predict how many ventilators we need to own and how many we may need to rent. The percentiles plot in the bottom graph shows that 85% of the time, we use fewer than 50 ventilators. Thus, if we purchase 50 ventilators we can expect to need rentals no more than 15% of the time.

The graphic representation of a distribution of data is associated with a number of terms used to describe the *distributional form*—that is, the shape of the distribution. Thus, we can characterize an entire distribution with a single term. These terms are illustrated in **Figure 10.5**. The smooth curves in Figure 10.5 actually indicate that we have a continuous variable; every value can occur with some frequency along the horizontal axis, which gives the variable values. If we take the histogram in Figure 10.2 and make the class widths smaller and smaller, a smooth curve will ultimately result. Unless a variable is discrete or qualitative, we can represent the distribution of its values with such smooth, or continuous, curves. This is convenient for explanatory presentations of many statistical concepts and will be used later in this chapter.

The form of the curve in Figure 10.5A is often referred to as *normal*. It is symmetrical and bell-shaped. However, it is a normal curve only if it represents a mathematical function known as the normal or Gaussian function, and this cannot be determined from inspection. A rectangular shape as in Figure 10.5B results from a uniformly distributed variable such as the

Figure 10.4

Percentiles plot.

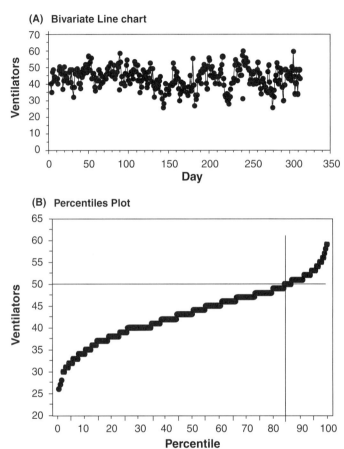

(A) Bivariate Line chart

(B) Percentiles Plot

(A) This bivariate line chart shows ventilator usage (number of ventilators per day on the vertical axis) over a range of several months (days on horizontal axis). (B) This percentiles plot shows the percentile (or percent of the days) that a given number of ventilators or less is used. The lines intersecting the plot show that 85% of the time, less than 50 ventilators are in use.

frequency of values in a deck of cards. Skewness is seen in Figures 10.5C and 10.5D, which show that values of the variable occur more frequently at either end of a distribution. A bimodal distribution, as in Figure 10.5E, occurs when there is no single most-frequent value. For instance, if there are high and low clusters of IQ values in a large group, we could see a bimodal or, more generally, a multimodal distribution. Figure 10.5F illustrates kurtosis, the peakedness or flatness of the distribution.

Figure 10.5

Illustration of various distribution shapes.

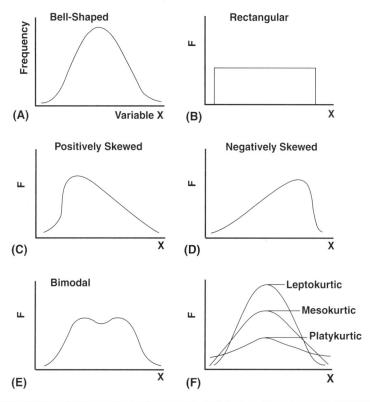

Measures of the Typical Value of a Set of Numbers

Three statistics are used to represent the typical value (also called the central tendency) in a distribution of values. Each statistic is a single number or an index that characterizes the center, or average value, of the whole set of data. These statistics are the mean, the median, and the mode.

The Summation Operator

Summation is a mathematical operation common in statistical calculations. The summation operator is denoted by the Greek capital letter sigma (Σ) and simply indicates addition over values of a variable. The general representation of the operator is $\sum_{i=1}^{n} X_i$, which is read "the summation of X_i for i equal 1 to n." Summation simply means to add the values of X_1 through X_n:

$$\sum_{i=1}^{n} X_i = X_1 + X_2 + \ldots + X_n$$

The subscripted variable, X_i, which is read "X sub i," is used to denote specific values of the variable. For instance, X_1 is one value of X_i, X_2 another, and so on. An example should make the use of the summation operator clear. Let the variable X have three values, each of which is given by a subscripted variable: $X_1 = 3$, $X_2 = 4$, $X_3 = 2$. Then,

$$\sum_{i=1}^{3} X_i = X_1 + X_2 + X_3 = 3 + 4 + 2 = 9$$

The Mean

The mean is the sum of all the observations divided by the number of observations. The symbol for the sample mean is $\overline{X}$. The symbol for the population mean is μ. The formula for the mean represents the definition in briefer form:

$$\overline{X} = \frac{\sum_{i=1}^{n} X_i}{n}$$

where X is the variable and there are n values. For example, let us use the above values of X (3, 4, and 6) so that $n = 3$. Then the mean is:

$$\overline{X} = \frac{(3 + 4 + 2)}{3} = 3.0$$

The Median

The median is the 50th percentile of a distribution, or the point that divides the distribution into equal halves. The median is the value below which 50% of the observations occur. For grouped observations, a formula is used to find the exact value of the median. For an *odd* number of observations, the median is the value that is equal to $(n + 1) \div 2$, where n is the number of observations. For example, if we have 1, 3, 5, 6, and 7 as our data, n is 5. The median is $(5 + 1) \div 2 = 5$, the third value. Notice that this formula gives the number of the observation, not its value.

With an *even* number of observations, the median is equal to the sum of two middle values divided by 2. For example, if we have 1, 3, 5, 6, 7, and 9 as data, the median is $(5 + 6) \div 2 = 5.5$. This formula gives the value of the observation that divides the data set.

The Mode

The mode is the most frequently occurring observation in the distribution. The mode is found by inspection, or counting. In Table 10.1 the mode is the value 5, which occurs 5 times. In a histogram, the mode is the highest bar.

Interpretation and Application

The mean is the most sophisticated measure of central tendency, is influenced by every value in the distribution, and assumes at least an interval level of measurement to perform addition and division. The mean is inappropriate for a qualitative variable with a nominal or ordinal level of measurement. What sense is there in calculating the mean of political affiliations, which have the values 1, 2, and 3 for Republican, Democrat, and other? Of course, we could calculate a number, but it is inappropriate for the variable. The mean is termed an *interval* statistic.

The median is considered an *ordinal* statistic and is less sophisticated than the mean. The median requires only ranking of numbers, not equal intervals. If a single value skews the value of the mean, the median may give a more typical representation of the data than the mean. For instance, if salaries range from $10,000 to $14,000, and one person earns $25,000, then the mean will be increased, or skewed, while the median will probably better represent the average salary.

The mode is a *nominal* statistic, since it requires only a nominal level of measurement. The qualitative variable, political affiliation, is a good example for using the mode to typify the observations. Which category occurs most frequently with the qualitative variable? With only a nominal level, we cannot (at least appropriately) calculate a median or a mean.

Measures of Dispersion

Most research studies provide at least two descriptive statistics: one measure of central tendency and one measure of dispersion. Measures of dispersion indicate the variability, or how spread out, the data are and include the range, variance, standard deviation, and coefficient of variation. The need for a measure of central tendency *and* dispersion to characterize a distribution more fully is seen in **Figure 10.6**. We have two different distributions of pH values, both with the same mean. Although both center on the same value, they do not "distribute" the same. The range and variability are different. If we had only the mean (7.40) to characterize the data, we would conclude that the distributions are the same. But while they are the same with regard to their central tendency, they are quite different in their dispersion. Note that pH is a continuous variable and measurable at a ratio level (there are a true zero and equal intervals).

Range

The range is the distance between the smallest and the largest values of the variable. Range = $X_{max} - X_{min}$, where X_{max} and X_{min} are the maximum and minimum values in the distribution. The

Figure 10.6

Two distributions of pH values with the same mean but different amounts of dispersion.

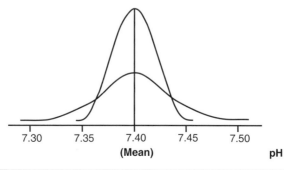

| 7.30 | 7.35 | 7.40 | 7.45 | 7.50 |

(Mean)   pH

range is the simplest measure of dispersion and is very informative to a researcher. Although the range is the actual distance between the smallest and largest values, the actual minimum and maximum values themselves are usually more informative.

Variance and Standard Deviation

The variance is a measure of how different the values in a set of numbers are from each other. It is calculated as the average squared deviation of the values from the mean. The standard deviation is the square root of the variance. The standard deviation has the same units as the original measurements, while the variance does not. There is a difference in the equation for the variance, depending on whether we have a sample with n observations or a population with the total collection of N observations. For a *sample*,

$$S^2 = \frac{\sum_{i=1}^{n} (X_i - \overline{X})^2}{n-1}$$

For the *population*,

$$\sigma^2 = \frac{\sum_{i=1}^{n} (X_i - \mu)^2}{n}$$

We use Roman letters, S^2 and $\overline{X}$, for the variance and mean with a *sample*, but Greek letters, σ^2 and μ, to indicate the *population* variance and mean. The use of $(n-1)$ when calculating sample variance is needed to obtain an unbiased estimate of the true population variance from the sample values. With a large n, such as 100, the numerical difference between n and $n-1$ tends to diminish, and use of $n-1$ does not greatly affect the calculation of the variance. Further explanation of biased estimators and the reason for using $n-1$ can be found in statistical textbooks.

As a squared value, the variance is always a positive number. By taking the square root, we have the standard deviation, which is then the *average deviation* from the mean. The larger the variance and standard deviation are, the more dispersed are our values. For example, in Figure 10.6 the narrower distribution of pH values might have a standard deviation of 0.02, while the wider distribution may be 0.05.

When testing hypotheses and estimating sample sizes, it is often necessary to calculate a *pooled standard deviation* (S_p):

$$S_P = \sqrt{\frac{(n_1 - 1)S_1^2 + (n_2 - 1)S_2^2}{n_1 + n_2 - 2}}$$

where S_p is the pooled standard deviation, S_1^2 is the variance of the first sample, S_2^2 is the variance of the second sample, and n_1 and n_2 are the two sample sizes.

Coefficient of Variation

The coefficient of variation expresses the standard deviation as a percentage of the mean. The equation for the coefficient of variation is:

$$CV(\%) = 100\% \left(\frac{S}{\overline{X}} \right)$$

where CV is the coefficient of variation expressed as a percentage, S is the sample standard deviation, and $\overline{X}$ is the sample mean.

The coefficient of variation is not useful as a single value, but it is applicable when we wish to *compare* the dispersion of observations—for example, with two different instruments or methods intended to measure the same variable. This statistic can also be helpful in comparing the dispersion of values at high and low values of a variable. For example, the dispersion of measured values is large at low creatinine levels but shrinks at higher creatinine levels. The data suggest that an instrument to measure creatinine has more random error (dispersion is greater) at the low range of creatinine values.

Standard Scores

A standard score, or z score, is a deviation from the mean expressed in units of standard deviations:

$$z = \frac{X - \overline{X}}{S}$$

where z is the z score, X is an individual value from the data set, $\overline{X}$ is the mean value of the data set, and S is the standard deviation of the data set. A z score of $+2.0$ means that the value of X is two standard deviations above the mean. A z score of $+1.6$ is likewise 1.6 standard deviations above the mean. Standard scores offer a way to express raw values in terms of their distance from the mean value, using standard deviation units.

The data set (2, 3, 5, 6) has a mean value of 4.0 and a standard deviation of 1.83. Calculating the z or standard score for the raw value of 2 is as follows:

$$z = \frac{2 - 4.0}{1.83} = -1.09$$

This value of z indicates that the value of 2 is 1.09 standard deviations *below* (indicated by the negative sign) the mean. Standard scores will be useful when obtaining percentages and probabilities with certain well-known distributions such as the normal.

Propagation of Errors in Calculations

Frequently, a physical quantity of interest is not measured directly but rather is a function of one or more measurements made from an experiment. For example, resistance and compliance of the respiratory system are not measured directly but are calculated from measurements of pressure, volume, and flow. In such cases, the bias and imprecision of the calculated parameter depends on the bias and imprecision of the measurements. Given two or more variables (e.g., X and Y) and their means and standard deviations (e.g., $\overline{X}$, $\overline{Y}$ and S_x, S_y), we are interested in estimating the mean and standard deviation of a calculated parameter Z (e.g., $\overline{Z}$ and S_z). For this, the following equations have been suggested.

Sum or difference: Let $Z = X \pm Y$, then:

$$\overline{Z} = \overline{X} + \overline{Y}$$

$$S_Z = \sqrt{S_X^2 + S_Y^2}$$

Linear combination: Let $Z = a + bX + cY + \ldots$, then:

$$\overline{Z} = a + b\overline{X} + c\overline{Y} + \ldots$$

$$S_Z = \sqrt{(bS_X)^2 + (cS_Y)^2} + \ldots$$

Product or quotient: Let $Z = X \times Y$ or $Z = X/Y$, then:

$$\overline{Z} = \overline{X} \times \overline{Y} \text{ or } \frac{\overline{X}}{\overline{Y}}$$

$$S_Z = \overline{Z} \sqrt{\left(\frac{S_x}{\overline{X}}\right)^2 + \left(\frac{S_Y}{\overline{Y}}\right)^2}$$

General product: Let $Z = \alpha X^a Y^b \ldots$, then:

$$\overline{Z} = \overline{X}^a \overline{Y}^b \ldots$$

$$S_Z = \overline{Z} \sqrt{\left(\frac{aS_x}{\overline{X}}\right)^2 + \left(\frac{bS_Y}{\overline{Y}}\right)^2} + \ldots$$

Logarithmic function: Let $Z = a \log x$, then:

$$\overline{Z} = a \log \overline{X}$$

$$S_Z = \frac{aS_X}{\overline{X}}$$

Correlation and Regression

A coefficient of correlation is a descriptive measure of the degree of relationship or association between two variables. This is the first statistic that involves *two* variables. The concept of correlation implies that two variables co-vary. That is, a change in variable X is associated with a change in variable *Y*. The most common correlation coefficient with a continuous variable measurable on an interval level is the Pearson product-moment correlation coefficient (the Pearson *r*). Another basic assumption of the Pearson *r* is linearity: the relation of the two variables is linear. Visual inspection of a plot of coordinate points for the *X* and *Y* variables is necessary to confirm linearity or to determine nonlinearity. Such a plot is called a *scattergram* and is illustrated in **Figure 10.7** for both a linear (A) and a curvilinear (B) relationship between two variables.

In Figure 10.7B, the Pearson *r* value would erroneously underestimate the degree of relation between *X* and *Y* because of its nonlinear nature. Calculation of the *r* value without inspection of the scattergram in Figure 10.7B could have led you to conclude that *X* and *Y* have a weak relationship, or none at all, when in truth they are clearly related.

The Pearson *r* statistic ranges in value from −1.0 through 0 to +1.0 and indicates two aspects of a correlation, the *magnitude* and the *direction*. **Figure 10.8** illustrates some possible values for a Pearson *r* and their meanings. A positive value indicates a positive or direct relation: *Y* increases as *X* increases (Figure 10.8A). A negative value for *r* indicates an inverse relation: *Y* decreases as *X* increases (Figure 10.8B). The closer the absolute value is to 1.0, the stronger and more perfect the relation (Figure 10.8C), while a value approaching zero indicates a lack of relationship, as in Figure 10.8D. In Figure 10.8D, low values of *X* are seen to correspond to high and low values of *Y*. The same is true for high values of *X*. Thus there is no systematic co-varying suggesting *X* and *Y* are related.

As a rule of thumb, the correlation between *X* and *Y* is considered *weak* if the absolute value of *r* is between 0 and 0.5, *moderate* between 0.5 and 0.8, and *strong* between 0.8 and 1.0.

When there is a linear relationship between two variables, we often wish to use the value of one variable (which may be easy to measure) to predict the value of the other variable (which we cannot easily measure). Of course, both variables had to be measured at some time to establish the presence of a correlation and prediction equation. The procedure is called

Figure 10.7

Illustration of scattergrams for both linear (left) and curvilinear (right) relations between the variables *X* and *Y*.

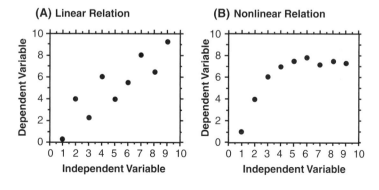

Figure 10.8

Illustration of four Pearson *r* values, indicating varying strengths of relation between variables *X* and *Y*.

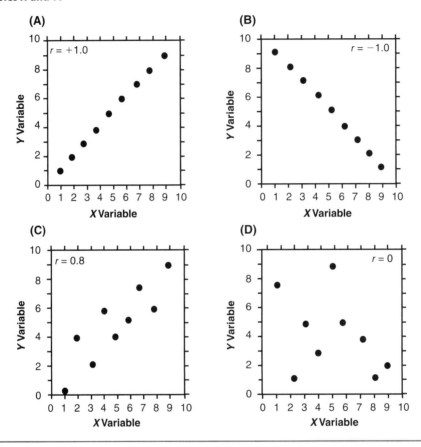

least-squares, simple-regression analysis. When we measure *X* and predict *Y*, *Y* is said to be *regressed* on *X*. The term *simple* indicates that *Y* is predicted from only one variable and not several simultaneously, which would involve multiple linear regression. Essentially, a line of best fit is that with the minimum distance to all of the data points. This is referred to as a *least squares* criteria for fitting the line because it is the line that minimizes the squared distance between points on the line and the actual data points on the graph. **Figure 10.9** illustrates this line for the a set of sample data. Such a line can be described with a linear equation of the form $\hat{Y} = a + bX$, where $\hat{Y}$ is the *predicted* value of *Y* for the given value of *X*. The letter *a* stands for the *Y*-intercept (the value of *Y* when *X* equals zero). The letter *b* stands for the slope of the line (the change in *Y* for a given change in *X* or $\Delta Y/\Delta X$).

Figure 10.9

An example of simple linear regression, giving the line of best fit for data.

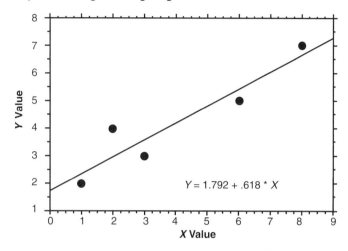

$Y = 1.792 + .618 * X$

Computer programs often give a value for r^2 along with the regression equation as a measure of how well the line fits the data. The r^2 statistic is called the *coefficient of determination*. The value of r^2 ranges from 0 to 1.0 and is interpreted as the proportion of the variation in Y that is explained by the variation in X. To understand what this means, consider that the total difference in Y values relative to their mean value has two components. One component is due to the linear relationship between Y and X. For example, as the independent variable X increases, the dependent variable Y may also increase as predicted by the regression equation. If a perfect correlation existed between the two (i.e., $r = 1.0$ and all of the X, Y points lie on the regression line) then *all* of the variation in Y would be explained by the variation in X (that is, $r^2 = 1.0$). We say that the difference between an individual value of Y and the mean value for Y is "explained" by the variation in X.

However, when less than a perfect correlation exists, some of the measured Y values will lie away from the regression line. This second component in the difference between an individual value of Y and the mean value of Y is the difference between the measured value of Y and its corresponding predicted value, $\hat{Y}$. This difference is "unexplained" by the variation in X values. The value of r^2 can be thought of as the explained difference divided by the total difference. Thus, the worse the correlation, the more the unexplained difference is relative to the total difference, making the explained difference smaller and the value for r^2 smaller.

Measures of correlation exist for lower levels of measurement. The Spearman rank coefficient can be used with ordinal levels of measurement, and the phi coefficient with nominal levels.

Inferential Statistics

Although a sample from a population is economical, we still wish to use the sample measurements (statistics) to *infer* to the population measures (parameters). Inferential statistics offer methods for inference by combining probability with descriptive statistics. Essentially, inferential statistics allow us to make probability statements about unknown population parameters based on the sample statistics. A basic understanding of probability forms the basis for an explanation of inferential statistics.

The Concept of Probability

The probability of an event can be defined as the relative frequency, or proportion, of occurrence of that event out of some total number of events. Since probability is a proportion, it always has values between 0 and 1, inclusively. For example, the probability of obtaining an ace from a deck of well-shuffled cards is 4/52, or 0.077. There are 4 aces (the event) out of a total of 52 cards, or events.

When a frequency distribution gives the relative frequencies of each value of a variable, it is actually a *probability distribution*. The concept of a probability distribution is essential to inferential statistics and can be easily understood by use of a discrete variable.

The distribution of values for a discrete variable is called a *discrete distribution*. Let the discrete variable be the number of heads in five flips of a fair coin. Values of this variable can range from 0 heads to 5 heads. We then perform the sequence of five flips 32 different times, and obtain the frequency distribution in **Table 10.3**. Since probability is simply relative frequency of occurrence, we can obtain the probability of each value of the variable (number of heads in five flips) as shown in Column 3. For instance, the probability of the variable X having the value 0 is 1 out of 32, or 0.03125.

Several helpful mathematical conventions are shown in Table 10.2. First, the uppercase X denotes a *variable*, while the lowercase x denotes the *value* of the variable. Second, the symbol p denotes probability. The expression $P(X = x)$ is read "the probability that the variable X has the value x." Likewise, $P(X \leq x)$ is read "the probability that the variable X is less than or equal to the value x."

Table 10.3

Probability Distribution and Cumulative Probability Distribution for the Number of Heads in Five Flips of a Coin

		$P(X = x)$		$P(X \leq x)$	
X # Heads	Frequency	Ratio	Fraction	Ratio	Fraction
0	1	1/32	0.031	1/32	0.031
1	5	5/32	0.156	6/32	0.188
2	10	10/32	0.313	16/32	0.500
3	10	10/32	0.313	26/32	0.813
4	5	5/32	0.156	31/32	0.969
5	1	1/32	0.031	32/32	1.000
	32	32/32			

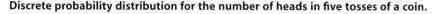

Figure 10.10

Discrete probability distribution for the number of heads in five tosses of a coin.

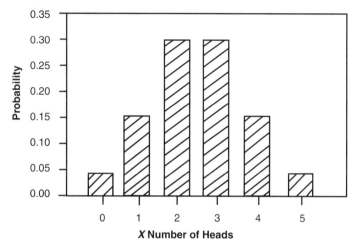

Column 3 gives probabilities of exact values of *X*. Column 4 provides *cumulative* probabilities. For instance, the probability that *X* is less than or equal to 2, $P(X \leq 2)$, is the sum of the probabilities that *X* is equal to 0, *X* is equal to 1, and *X* is equal to 2. The sum of these probabilities is: $1/32 + 5/32 + 10/32 = 16/32$, or 0.50. In other words, half of the values are between 0 and 2.

If we graph the relative frequencies in Table 10.2, we can obtain a visual representation of the probability distribution (**Figure 10.10**). A bar graph is used because we have a discrete variable. The height of a bar indicates how probable or improbable a value is. The values 0 and 5 are rare, or improbable, because they occur infrequently. The most probable events are 2 and 3.

Just as we obtained the cumulative probabilities in the table, we can *sum* the probabilities represented by the height of each bar in Figure 10.10. This is in effect adding up the bars in Figure 10.10. We can obtain cumulative probabilities by summation when we have a discrete variable, but we must use the integration of calculus to "add up" the probabilities when we have a continuous variable. This difference, as well as the similarity, is seen in **Figure 10.11**. In the continuous case, the probability that *X* is less than or equal to 2 is given by the *area under the curve* between 0 and 2. This area is obtained by integration, not summation. The total area under the curve is 1.0, which indicates that there is a 100% likelihood that *X* will have a value between 0 and 5, which it must! Throughout the discussion on inferential statistics, we will use continuous distributions, as in Figure 10.11B, to present or illustrate probabilities. For a continuous probability distribution, the probability of any particular value is zero, and the probability of an interval does not depend on whether or not either of its endpoints is included. For example, in Figure 10.11B, $P(X = 2) = 0$ and $P(X \leq 2) = P(X > 2)$.

The key to obtaining probabilities is to have the probability distribution. Many biological variables such as height, weight, or pH follow a distribution known as the normal distribution.

Figure 10.11

Comparison of cumulative probabilities.

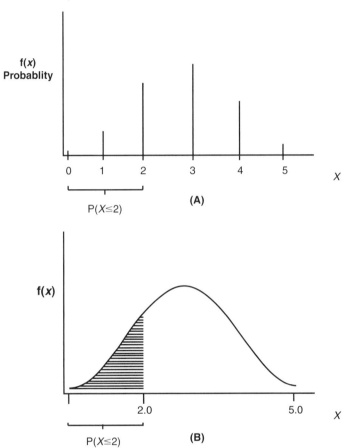

For a discrete distribution (A) and for a continuous distribution (B). The Symbol f(x) means that the values on the vertical axis (probability in these graphs) are a function of the horizontal values of x.

This is a particular distribution described with a certain mathematical function (the Gaussian function), and from which we can obtain probabilities whenever we are willing to assume that a variable follows this distribution. The normal is a continuous, not a discrete, distribution. Other probability distributions will also be used when discussing inferential statistics. First we illustrate the use of the normal distribution for determining probabilities.

The Normal Distribution and Standard Scores

Earlier we defined standard or z scores, and now we will use such scores with the normal distribution. **Figure 10.12** illustrates the areas under the normal curve. In a normally distributed

Figure 10.12

Approximate areas under the normal curve within one, two, and three standard deviations around the mean.

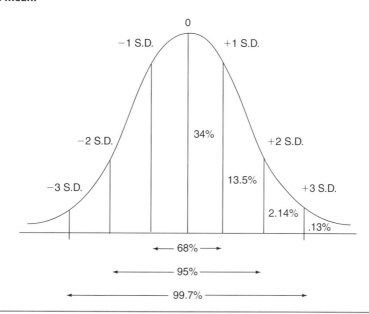

variable, the mean is at the center of the distribution, and therefore, the mean is also the median and the mode. The curve in Figure 10.12 is called a standard normal curve because the areas are indicated for standard deviation units from the mean. Thus, the mean itself, regardless of its value from actual data, is zero standard deviations away from itself. The z score for the mean must always be zero. In other words, points on the curve are actually z scores. Rather than recalculate areas under the curve for particular values of the mean and standard deviation, we use a general form of the curve with standard deviation units.

In a normal curve, approximately 68% of all the values are included in the area around the mean spanning ± 1 standard deviations. The area encompassed by ± 2 standard deviations from the mean corresponds to approximately 95% of the values in the distribution. The interval of ± 3 standard deviations encompasses 99.7% of all the values. Exact areas, which are the probabilities for particular z score values, can be obtained from a table in a statistics book or from a computer program.

An application of z scores and the normal distribution will identify the usefulness of knowing areas under the normal curve. We will use the continuous variable, pH, and assume that its values follow a normal distribution. Further, pH in humans has a population mean of 7.40 and a standard deviation of 0.02. **Figure 10.13** shows the distribution of pH values. Both original units and z scores are given. Since pH is normally distributed, we can say that approximately 95% of the population's values will be between 7.36 and 7.44, because that is a width of ± 2 standard deviations. We could also say that only approximately 2.5% of the population

Figure 10.13

Normal distribution of pH values, with a mean of 7.40 and a standard deviation of 0.02.

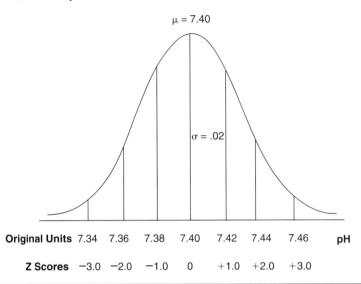

will have a pH greater than 7.44, or the probability that a pH value is above 7.44, $P(\text{pH} > 7.44)$, is less than 0.025. The percentile statement tells what percentage of observations are less than the value of 7.44, and the probability statement gives the proportion of observations above or below a point, depending on the direction of the statement. Notice that we can determine from the distribution which values or range of values are likely, and which are unlikely. If 95% of the values are between 7.36 and 7.44, then values *outside* this range, such as 7.33 or 7.46, are *not* likely. This reasoning is the basis for establishing normal ranges of many clinical variables. An appropriate table or computer gives exact areas under the normal curve for z scores within three standard deviations of the mean.

For example, what is the probability of obtaining a pH value greater than 7.43? First, we need the z score for the value 7.43; that is, $z = (7.43 - 7.40)/0.02 = +1.5$. The value 7.43 then is 1.5 standard deviations above the mean. Now we ask what is the probability of a z score greater than 1.5, $P(\text{pH} > 7.43) = P(z > 1.5)$. The normal curve is symmetrical around the mean, which is a z score of zero. A z score of zero, for example, has a value of 0.50, indicating that half of the total curve area is accumulated at this midpoint.

For a probability of a z score greater than 1.5, we could use a statistical table. Alternatively, we could use Microsoft Excel to do a simple spreadsheet calculation using the cell equation =NORMSDIST(z), where z is the desired number of standard deviations. If we substitute 1.5 for z, the cell evaluates to 0.9332, which indicates that 93.32% of the total area under the normal curve is found between negative infinity and 1.5 standard deviations above the mean. The area remaining under the curve *above* a z score of $+1.5$ will be equal to

1.0 − 0.9332 = 0.0668. These areas corresponding to a z score of +1.5 are illustrated in **Figure 10.14**. The probability of a pH value above 7.43 is 0.0668. Alternatively, we could say that approximately 93% of the population has a pH *less* than 7.43, and 7% above 7.43; or a pH of 7.43 is in the 93rd percentile.

To summarize, if a variable is normally distributed, then we can standardize any value of the variable by calculating a z score. Then we find the probability of a value greater, or less than, the given value from a table or computer program. *Remember that these probabilities will be accurate only if the variable does in fact have a normal distribution.*

Sampling Distributions

Since we defined probability as the relative frequency of an event, we were able to use the frequency distribution of a variable as a probability distribution. We have used a particular probability distribution known as the normal, or Gaussian, distribution. The single most important concept in inferential statistics is that of a sampling distribution of a statistic.

A sampling distribution is the probability distribution of a *statistic*. We assumed that the variable pH has a normal distribution, and then we were able to calculate probabilities from this distribution. A statistic such as the mean, $\overline{X}$, which is calculated from a sample, will also have different possible values in different samples when the samples are randomly drawn from

Figure 10.14

Areas under the normal curve for pH value of 7.43 with a corresponding *z* score of 1.5.

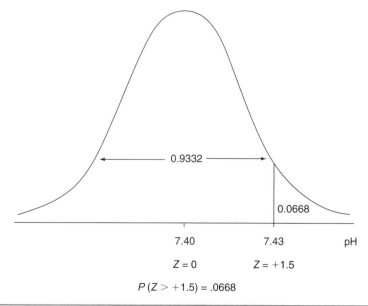

a population. These different possible values of $\bar{X}$ will also have some distribution, called a sampling distribution. The mean, $\bar{X}$, can have a normal or a t distribution, depending on certain conditions, which we will present.

An example of a sampling distribution may clarify this. Suppose that we have the continuous variable National Board Scores, and the distribution of values for the *population* is normal, with a mean, μ, of 100, and a standard deviation, σ, of 15. We have already seen that we can obtain probabilities for particular values of the variable. Now let us take a random sample of size 9, and calculate the sample mean, $\bar{X}$. Then we take another random sample of nine scores and calculate a second $\bar{X}$, and repeat this procedure several thousand times. We would have a *distribution* of different $\bar{X}$ values.

The values are different because of *sampling error*, which is a random error. Even though the population has a mean of 100, our sample means are going to differ more or less from 100 due to random chance. The nine particular scores in a given sample are not likely to have a mean of *exactly* 100. However, the distribution of the sample means does center on 100, which is the original population mean. The mean of the sample means (symbolized as $\mu_{\bar{x}}$) is also 100. Where the population distribution has a standard deviation to describe its variability, the sampling distribution of the mean has a *standard error of the mean* (SEM), which is symbolized by $\sigma_{\bar{x}}$:

$$SEM = \sigma_{\bar{x}} = \frac{\sigma}{\sqrt{n}}$$

where σ is the standard deviation of the population and n is the sample size. If (as is usually the case) σ is unknown, S is substituted in the above equation. The SEM is simply the standard deviation of the values of $\bar{X}$.

We would expect the dispersion of sample means to be less than the dispersion of population values, and indeed, the equation shows that the SEM is smaller than the population standard deviation, σ. In fact, as the sample size increases, the smaller the SEM becomes. Finally, we can convert any specific value of the mean into a standard or z score with

$$z_{\bar{x}} = \frac{\bar{X} - \mu}{\sigma_{\bar{x}}}$$

We divide the difference between the sample mean and the population mean by the standard error of the mean. This quotient gives us the number of standard errors the sample mean is above or below the population mean. Just as with z scores for values of a variable, so we can use this z score for the mean with the normal curve to determine probabilities. For instance, if the population mean is 100 with a standard deviation of 15, what is the probability of obtaining a sample mean of 110 or greater for a sample size of 9? The steps to obtain a probability from the sampling distribution are the same as before:

1. Convert the sample mean value to a z score.
2. Find the probability for the z score from a table or computer program.

The z score for a mean of 110 is

$$z_{\bar{x}} = \frac{\bar{X} - \mu}{\sigma_{\bar{x}}} = \frac{110 - 100}{15 / \sqrt{9}} = +2.0$$

Again using Microsoft Excel we fill a cell with the equation =NORMSDIST(2.0). When we hit the ENTER key, the cell shows the value 0.9772. This means that the area under the normal curve up to a value of 2 standard errors above the mean represents 97.72%. The area remaining in the upper tail of the distribution is $1.0 - 0.9772 = 0.0228$. Thus, the probability of a sample mean of 110.0 or greater is the same as the probability of a z score of 2.0 or greater, which is 0.0228, or 2.28%. We would conclude that a value of 110.0 is not very likely to occur.

Inferential statistics use sampling distributions, which are probability distributions of a statistic, to make conclusions about *population parameters* based on *sample statistics*. Obviously, if we measure an entire population, we have a parameter, and would not need inferential statistics to make a probability statement about that value.

The t Distribution

The use of z scores and the normal distribution are usually based on the assumption that samples sizes are "large" and that we know the sample variance. Large usually means more than 30. However, a large sample size is frequently difficult to obtain in medical research. Therefore, we need another distribution, the t distribution. It looks like the normal distribution but is more spread out. In fact, there is a whole family of t distributions whose shape depends on the "degrees of freedom" (defined for this purpose as one less than the sample size; $n - 1$). The smaller the sample size, the more spread out the distribution looks. However, that will not concern us unless we have to look up values in statistical tables. From here on out, we will assume that all statistical values will be calculated for us using a computer, either in Microsoft Excel or some specialized statistical software package. We will generally use the t distribution rather than the normal. But the same ideas we discussed above apply because as the sample size gets larger and larger, the t distribution turns into the normal distribution. The t statistic is calculated like the z statistic except that we use the sample standard deviation:

$$t = \frac{\bar{X} - \mu}{S / \sqrt{n}}$$

where $\bar{X}$ is the sample mean, μ is the assumed population mean, S is the sample standard deviation, and n is the sample size. In the situation where you are not comparing a sample mean with a population mean, but are comparing two sample means, the t statistic is calculated as:

$$t = \frac{\bar{X}_1 - \bar{X}_2}{S_P \sqrt{\dfrac{1}{n_1} + \dfrac{1}{n_2}}}$$

where $\overline{X}_1$ is the mean of one sample, $\overline{X}_2$ is the mean of the other sample, S_p is the pooled standard deviation, and n_1 and n_2 are the two sample sizes.

Confidence Intervals

The mean and standard deviation of a sample are called *point estimates*, which are just single-value guesses about the population parameters. As we saw above, repeated calculations of a statistic like the sample mean result in a distribution of values. Somewhere in that distribution will be the true value of the population mean. The problem is, we have only performed one experiment and calculated one sample mean. We don't know if the true population mean is above or below our sample mean, nor how far away it is (how much error is in our estimate).

We accept that point estimates have built-in error, so we need to decide how much confidence to place in them. In medicine the convention is to keep the error less than or equal to 5%. That means we would like a confidence level of 95%.

Thinking in terms of the sampling distribution, a confidence level of 95% means that we expect the true population parameter (the mean in this case) to be in an area that makes up 95% of the area under the curve. Since we do not know if our sample mean is above or below the true value, we assume that there is equal probability that it lies below it as above it. In other words, we assume that our mean value lies within a certain number of standard errors above or below the true value. If we were using the normal distribution, it would be two standard errors above and below the mean. But for the *t* distribution, the number of standard errors depends on the sample size. For now, let's just say the sample mean lies within *t* standard errors of the true value with 95% confidence.

If our sample mean is within *t* standard errors from the true value, it follows logically that the true value is within *t* standard errors from the sample mean. Written in equation form,

true value = sample mean $\pm$ *t* standard errors

Stated another way, we are 95% confident that the true value lies in the interval between the sample mean minus *t* standard errors and the sample mean plus *t* standard errors. Written as an equation, we have

$$\overline{X} - t\frac{S}{\sqrt{n}} \leq \mu \leq \overline{X} + t\frac{S}{\sqrt{n}}$$

The interval given in the above equation is called the *confidence interval*. Thus, a confidence interval is the range of values that are believed to contain the true parameter value. The value of *t* can be found in a statistical table or with a computer. **Table 10.4** combines the *t* value and the square root of the sample size into a *k* factor. This simplifies the above equation to

$$\overline{X} - kS \leq \mu \leq \overline{X} + kS$$

For example, suppose we perform an experiment that produced a set of 20 Pao$_2$ measurements with a mean value of 83 mm Hg and a standard deviation of 5 mm Hg. We wish to

Table 10.4

Factors for Determining 95% Confidence Interval for the Mean

n	*k*	*n*	*k*
2	8.98	16	0.53
3	2.48	17	0.51
4	1.59	18	0.50
5	1.24	19	0.48
6	1.05	20	0.47
7	0.92	21	0.46
8	0.84	22	0.44
9	0.77	23	0.43
10	0.72	24	0.42
11	0.67	25	0.41
12	0.64	26	0.40
13	0.60	27	0.40
14	0.58	28	0.39
15	0.55	29	0.38
		30	0.37

n = sample size

construct a 95% confidence interval (CI) that contains the true mean value of the population of Pao_2 values from which the sample was taken:

$$CI = \overline{X} \pm \left(\frac{t}{\sqrt{n}} \right) \times S$$

$$CI = 83 \pm 0.47 \times 5$$

$$CI = 83 \pm 2.35$$

$$CI = (80.6, 85.4)$$

The confidence interval is interpreted as follows: If the experiment was repeated 100 times and 100 confidence intervals were calculated, then 95 of those intervals would contain the true (but still unknown) population mean. Thus we are only 95% confident that the interval we calculated above contains the true value.

Confidence intervals can be calculated for many different statistics. For example, we could calculate the CI for the difference between two means, such as the Pao_2 before and after oscillating positive expiratory pressure therapy. In this case you would calculate the difference in Pao_2 (Pao_2 after therapy minus Pao_2 before therapy) for each patient. Then, you would calculate the mean difference and the standard deviation of the differences to use in the CI calculation.

Confidence intervals are sometimes used in place of hypothesis tests. If the confidence interval includes the hypothesized mean value under the null hypothesis, then we do not reject the null hypothesis. In the example above, if the CI for the difference in mean values contains zero as a value, then we would conclude that there was no difference in the mean Pao_2 before and after therapy (zero might be the true value of the mean difference).

Error Intervals

Clinical decisions are often based on single measurements or on a few consecutive measurements that show some consistency. We need to estimate the error of single measurements and judge how much confidence we can place in these estimates. Confidence intervals do not provide this information because they summarize groups of data rather than describe individual measurements. We need analogous intervals, which we will call *error intervals*, that describe the combined effects of systematic and random errors on individual measurements. We can also say something about how much confidence should be placed in the estimate. An error interval is the range of values that is expected to contain a given proportion of all future individual measurements at a given confidence level.[*] For example, we could specify a 95% error interval at the 99% confidence level. This specification means that 95 of the next 100 measurements are assumed to lie within this range. Further, if we repeated the experiment that generated the data 100 times, our assumption would be true for 99 of the error intervals we calculated.

Many studies involve the assessment of new devices or methods compared with existing standards, and many statistical concepts are involved. We will simplify the subject and discuss only three cases. The first case would be when a new batch of control solutions for a blood-gas analyzer is purchased. Laboratory standards require us to verify the manufacturer's specifications for the expected lower and upper limits of individual measured values for the analyte. If an individual measurement falls outside one of these limits, the analyzer may be malfunctioning.

A second case would be the evaluation of the performance of a new blood-gas analyzer by measuring control solutions with known Po_2 values.

The third case might be the comparison of Po_2 values from a new model of blood-gas analyzer with measurements from a currently used analyzer.

Although apparently similar, these three problems are actually different. In the first case, it is necessary to determine a range of values within which any given individual measurement should fall when measuring a known value. This range is known as a *tolerance interval*. In the second case, we wish to determine the range of values for the differences between the known (assumed true) value and the measured value. This range is called an *inaccuracy interval*. In the third case, the true value is not known, so we can assess only the range of values for the difference between one measurement system and another. This range is called an *agreement interval*. In each case, the error interval will have the form

$$\text{error interval} = \text{bias} \pm \text{imprecision}$$

as described in the section on inaccuracy, bias, and imprecision in Chapter 9. Error intervals will be wider than confidence intervals because the imprecision of individual measurements is larger than that of group statistics (the standard deviation is larger than the standard error by a factor of $\sqrt{n}$).

---

[*]A simplified version of error intervals, called "agreement intervals," was first described in Bland JM, Altman DG. Statistical methods for assessing agreement between two methods of clinical measurement. *Lancet*. 1986;1:307.

Tolerance Interval

Given a set of repeated measurements of the same quantity, we are interested in finding the range of values we might observe with a specified degree of confidence. If the true mean and standard deviation of an infinite number of repeated measurements were known, then a "two-sigma" (approximately two-standard-deviation) tolerance interval would be $\mu \pm 1.96\ \sigma$. This interval includes exactly 95% of the measurements, and we can say this with 100% confidence because we have just made an infinite number of measurements. Of course, μ and σ are really unknowable. Therefore, we must substitute the point estimates $\bar{X}$ and S. Because of the random error involved with estimating μ and σ using $\bar{X}$ and S, the proportion of the population of measured values covered by the tolerance interval is not exact. As a result, the confidence level must be based on the sample size.

The *tolerance interval* (TI) is expressed as

$$TI = \bar{X} \pm k_1 S$$

where $\bar{X}$ is the sample mean, S is the sample standard deviation from an experiment consisting of repeated measurements of a known quantity, and k_1 is a factor determined so that we can be 99% confident that the given interval will contain at least 95% of all future measurements (**Table 10.5**).

For example, if we made 20 repeated measurements of a blood gas control solution and found the average $Paco_2$ was 30 mm Hg with a standard deviation of 2 mm Hg, then the tolerance interval for the solution would be

$$TI = 30 \pm 3.18 \times 2$$

$$TI = 30 \pm 6.36$$

$$TI = (23.64, 36.36)$$

Now we could take these results into the blood gas lab and instruct the technicians to do a diagnostic procedure on the analyzer any time they observe a value below 23.6 or above 36.4 when that control solution level is analyzed.

Inaccuracy Interval

A tolerance interval gives only the imprecision (i.e., random error) of measurements. To assess the total error or inaccuracy of a measurement system, we need estimates of both bias and imprecision from experiments in which *known quantities* are repeatedly measured. Bias is estimated as the mean difference between measured and known (or assumed true) values. Imprecision is estimated as the standard deviation of the *differences* between measured and true values. Inaccuracy is expressed as the sum of the bias and imprecision estimates. Thus, we can construct an *inaccuracy interval* (II) similar to the tolerance interval:

$$II = \bar{\Delta} \pm k_1 S_\Delta$$

Table 10.5

Factors for Determining Two Sigma Error Intervals or Intervals Containing 95% of Observed Measurements at the 99% Confidence Level

n	*k₁*	*n*	*k₁*	*n*	*k₁*	*n*	*k₁*
6	6.37	30	2.85	54	2.55	120	2.32
7	5.52	31	2.83				
8	4.97	32	2.81	56	2.54	130	2.30
9	4.58	33	2.79				
10	4.29	34	2.77	58	2.52	140	2.28
11	4.07	35	2.76				
12	3.90	36	2.74	60	2.51	150	2.27
13	3.75	37	2.73				
14	3.63	38	2.71	65	2.48	160	2.26
15	3.53	39	2.70				
16	3.44	40	2.68	70	2.46	170	2.25
17	3.36	41	2.67				
18	3.30	42	2.66	75	2.44	180	2.24
19	3.24	43	2.65				
20	3.18	44	2.64	80	2.42	200	2.22
21	3.14	45	2.63				
22	3.09	46	2.62	85	2.40	300	2.17
23	3.05	47	2.61				
24	3.02	48	2.60	90	2.38	400	2.14
25	2.98	49	2.59				
26	2.95	50	2.58	100	2.36	500	2.12
27	2.93						
28	2.90	52	2.56	110	2.34	1000	2.07
29	2.87					infinity	1.96

n = sample size

where

- $\overline{\Delta}$ is the mean difference between measured and true values.
- S_Δ is the standard deviation of the differences. The standard deviation of the differences is the same as the difference between standard deviations. The standard deviation of the true value is zero because it is the same value each time. Therefore, we can substitute the standard deviation of the measured values, S, for S_Δ.
- k_1 is a factor determined so that we can be 99% confident that the given interval will contain at least 95% of all future measurements (refer to Table 10.5).

Agreement Interval

How do we know if some new measurement system will give results comparable to the one that is currently in use? Can the new system serve as a substitute for the old while preserving the quality of care? Assessing agreement between two measurement systems is similar to assessing inaccuracy, except that instead of repeatedly measuring on a level of a known quantity, several levels of the known quantity are selected and split samples are measured by both systems. For example, in assessing the agreement between old and new models of a blood-gas analyzer, several samples of patient blood would be split in half and analyzed with each device. Then an *agreement interval* (AI) is expressed as $AI = \bar{\Delta} \pm k_1 S_\Delta$, where $\bar{\Delta}$ is the mean difference between the pairs of split sample values. The difference for a pair is the result from new machine minus result from old machine; S_Δ is the standard deviation of the differences; and k_1 is a factor determined so that we can be 99% confident that the given interval will contain at least 95% of all future measurements (refer to Table 10.5).

For example, suppose we wish to compare a new point-of-care blood-gas analyzer with our standard bench model. We conduct an experiment in which we obtain samples of blood from 100 patients who have a wide range of Pao_2 values. Each sample is split in half, with one portion analyzed on the new blood-gas machine and the other half analyzed on the old machine. For each pair of results, we calculate the difference in Pao_2. Then we calculate the mean and standard deviation of the 100 differences. Suppose that $\bar{\Delta} = 5$ mm Hg and $S_\Delta = 9$ mm Hg. The agreement interval is then

$$AI = 5 \pm 2.36 \times 9$$

$$AI = 5 \pm 21.24$$

$$AI = (-16.2, 26.2)$$

Notice that we rounded the answer to one decimal place because that is the limit of the blood-gas machine resolution. We interpret the agreement interval as follows, keeping in mind that the differences were calculated by subtracting the value of the old machine from that of the new machine: Any individual measurement with the new machine can be expected to be anywhere from 16.2 mm Hg below to 26.2 mm Hg above the value you would have gotten if you had used the old machine. The next question is: Will this expected level of agreement change the quality of medical decision? In this case, you might conclude that the new point-of-care analyzer would lead you to make an unnecessary Fio_2 change on a patient: you would not have made the change if the sample were analyzed on the old machine. Assuming you had confidence in the accuracy of the old machine, you would conclude that adopting the new technology would degrade your standard of care.

Incorrect Methods to Evaluate Agreement

In the past, the most frequently used statistical analyses to assess the comparability of measurement devices were least-squares linear regression, the *t* test, the *F* test, and Pearson's product-moment correlation coefficient. However, these techniques are inappropriate for agreement studies.

As mentioned previously, least-squares regression minimizes the sum of squares of the vertical distances between the observed data and the regression line. The underlying assumption is that only the data plotted on the Y axis show variability. This assumption is inappropriate in the comparison of two measurement systems that both have variability. Also, regression is sensitive to nonlinearity of the data and will give misleading results if the range of data is too narrow.

Both the *t* test (for differences between means) and the *F* test (for differences between standard deviations) are sometimes used as indicators of agreement. But they are intended only to indicate whether the differences between the two methods are significant. If the calculated value for the statistic is larger than some critical value, the performance of the new system is judged not acceptable. If the statistic is smaller, the conclusion is usually that the methods agree and the new system is accepted. Such judgments may be erroneous for several reasons.

The F test is simply the ratio of the variances of the data from two measurement systems. It is a comparison of error levels, indicating the significance of any difference, and it is not an indicator of the acceptability of errors or their magnitude.

The t test is a ratio of systematic and random errors:

$$t = \frac{\text{bias} \times \sqrt{n}}{S_\Delta}$$

where bias is the difference between the true value and the mean value of the sample $(\bar{X} - \mu)$, S_Δ is the standard deviation of the differences between paired measurements, and n is the sample size. As a ratio of errors, t does not provide information about the total error or magnitude of disagreement. This situation is analogous to the determination of blood pH by the ratio of bicarbonate to carbon dioxide tension. A low pH does not make clear whether the bicarbonate is low or the carbon dioxide is high. Treatment of acidosis requires information about both metabolic and respiratory errors separately. In addition, there are at least four situations that can cause erroneous judgments when using the t value.

- The t value may be small when systematic error is small and random error is large. Thus, the farther apart the pairs of measurements are, the more likely we are to conclude that the methods agree.
- The t value may be small (and we conclude that the methods agree) even when both systematic and random errors are large.
- The t value may be large (and we conclude that the methods do not agree) even when both systematic and random errors are small.
- The t value gets smaller as the sample size gets larger. Thus, even if systematic and random errors are acceptable, we might erroneously conclude that the methods do not agree if the sample size is large and vice versa.

Perhaps the most widely misused indicator of agreement is the Pearson r. The fundamental problem with this statistic is that it is a measure of linear association, which is not the same as agreement. For example, suppose we plotted the data from two methods that gave exactly the same results. The data would all lie on the line of identity. The r value would be 1.0 (i.e., a perfect correlation) and we would naturally conclude that the methods had perfect agreement. However, if one method were out of calibration and gave exactly twice the value of the other, or say twice the value plus 3 units, the data would still lie on a straight line with $r = 1.0$. Obviously, the two methods do not agree, as the regression line would be displaced from the line of identity and would have a different slope (indicating both constant and proportional systematic error). The r value is an indicator of random error and is completely insensitive to systematic error.

Other problems are associated with the use of the *r* statistic. Correlation is sensitive to the range of measurements and will be greater for wide ranges than for small ones. Because you will usually compare methods over the whole range of values expected to be measured, a high correlation is almost guaranteed. Also, the test of significance (that *r* is significantly different from zero) will undoubtedly show that the two methods are related, as they are designed to measure the same quantity. The test of significance is therefore irrelevant to the question of agreement.

All of the above statistics share one additional weakness: they all describe characteristics of a group of data and say nothing about individual measurements. Recall that this is important because many clinical judgments are based on single measurements.

Data Analysis for Device Evaluation Studies

Establishing Standards

Measurement system performance studies are intended to show how close a single measurement value will be to the true value and how much confidence can be placed in it. Before any judgment can be made, we must have decided *beforehand* what level of inaccuracy is acceptable. This decision can be both elusive and confusing. Standards for allowable error may be generated in several ways:

- *On the basis of the intended application.* For example, a simple oxygen analyzer used in an adult ICU may have an allowable error of $\pm2\%$ of full scale because a small discrepancy will have little clinical effect. However, measurement of oxygen concentration for the purpose of calculating gas exchange parameters requires much better accuracy. For example, an error of 1% in the measurement of oxygen concentration leads to an error of 24% in the calculation of oxygen consumption and 32% in the calculation of respiratory exchange ratio. For this purpose, the allowable error would be about 0.1%.
- *On the basis of agreement with similar, commonly used measurement systems.* For example, the accuracy of pulse oximeters should be comparable to in-vitro oximeters.
- *On the basis of professional consensus.* For example, the American Thoracic Society has published accuracy and calibration standards for pulmonary function equipment.
- *On the basis of arbitrary statistical methods.* For example, if the standard deviation of the measurement method is one-fourth or less of the normal population standard deviation, then analytic imprecision may be judged negligible.

Note that even if the allowable error can be agreed upon, we must know the value, or range of values, of measured quantities that represent cutoff points for medical decisions. For example, an imprecision in transcutaneous Po_2 readings of ±15 torr might be reasonable for Po_2s above 100 torr but would not be adequate for lower values in the range that might indicate hypoxemia.

General Experimental Approach

In general, pairs of data (measured versus known values or values from two methods) should be gathered over a wide range of input levels (one data pair per level). These data will provide information about bias and some information about imprecision. Additional data pairs may be gathered from repeated measures at selected levels (critical levels corresponding to cutoff points for making decisions) to provide better estimates of imprecision. The sample size for a given experiment will be limited by many practical factors but should be no less than 20, with larger samples being preferable.

Experimental results should be planned with a consideration of the possible sources of bias and imprecision discussed above. For example, to estimate the inaccuracy expected in the normal daily operation of a measurement system, data should be collected over the entire range of measurements that will be used clinically (to account for errors due to the magnitude of measurements) and over a period of days (to account for environmental and operator factors and even calibration errors). In contrast, if the inaccuracy of the system alone is desired (to compare it with another system), repeated measures of the same quantity should be made within a short period, with the same operator, and with all other possible confounding factors held as constant as possible.

Data Analysis Procedure

Step 1. The first step in any data analysis should be to create a scatter plot of the raw data to get a subjective impression of their validity. The mean and standard deviation should be calculated and used to identify outliers (see below). In determining *tolerance intervals*, the data should be plotted along with the data mean and standard deviation. For *inaccuracy intervals*, the difference between the true (known or standard) values and the measured values should be plotted on the vertical axis against the true values on the horizontal axis. For *agreement intervals,* the differences between data pairs from the two measurement systems are plotted against the mean value for each pair. The mean values are used as the best estimate of the true values, which are not known. The purpose of these plots is not only to identify any outliers but also to make sure that the differences are not related to the measurement level. If they are, the standard deviation may be overstated at one point of the measurement range and understated at another. In other words, calculation of one value for standard deviation for all the data will not accurately describe the variability of the data over the entire range of measurements. You might be able to solve this problem by using a logarithmic transformation of the data. Alternatively, you could derive worst-case error specifications as a percentage of full scale. The hypothesis that the data points are correlated with the measurement level can be tested formally with Pearson's product-moment correlation coefficient (i.e., test the hypothesis that r is significantly different from zero).

Step 2. The next step is to make sure the data comply with the assumption of normality (that they are adequately described by the normal or Gaussian distribution). All of the statistical procedures described hereafter are based on this assumption. The data can be assessed for normality with the Kolmogorov-Smirnov test. It may be sufficient to simply plot the frequency distribution and make a subjective judgment as to whether or not it is bell-shaped.

Step 3. Once the data are judged to conform to the underlying assumptions, the mean and standard deviation are used to calculate error intervals as described above.

Step 4. Finally, the data should be presented in graphic form and labeled with the numerical values for the error intervals (**Figure 10.15**).

Figure 10.15

Suggested format for plotting data and error intervals for inaccuracy and agreement studies.

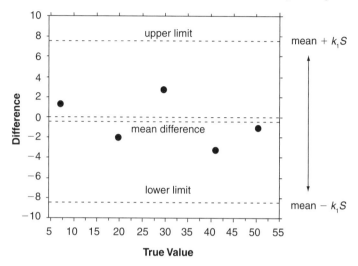

Each data point represents the difference between the measured value and the true value (inaccuracy study) or the difference between two measurements of the same specimen using two different devices (agreement study). For inaccuracy studies, the magnitude of the difference (vertical axis) is plotted against the true or known value (horizontal axis). For agreement studies, the true value is not known so it is estimated as the mean of the two measurements (horizontal axis). For example, S = sample standard deviation and k_1 is the factor for determining a two-sigma error interval (from Table 10.6). The product of k_1 times S is added to the sample mean to get the upper limit of the error interval. The product is subtracted from the mean to get the lower limit.

If the study is designed to compare the error intervals of several measurements, the data can be plotted as shown in **Figure 10.16**.

Treatment of Outliers

Spurious data may be caused by temporary or intermittent malfunctions of the measurement system or by operator errors. Such errors should not be included in the error analysis. The plot of the data should be inspected for outliers, values that depart from the expected distribution. Outliers at the upper and lower limits of the range will have a strong effect on the estimates of systematic error. Any of the sources of error mentioned previously can cause unusually large deviations from the desired linear relation and falsely increase the estimate of inaccuracy. Outliers are identified as any measurements that are more than k_2 standard deviations from the mean, where k_2 is based on the sample size (**Table 10.6**). Any occurrence of an outlier should be examined for evidence of a real source of nonlinearity rather than assuming it to be a spurious error. The occurrence of more than three unexplained outliers per 100 observations suggests the presence of a serious problem with the measurement system. Outliers are eliminated from

Figure 10.16

Suggested format for plotting error intervals when comparing several different devices (accuracy study).

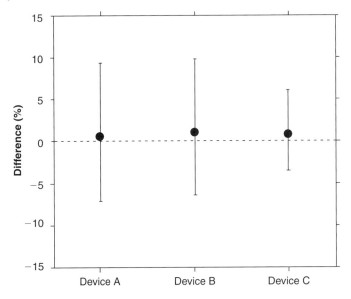

The dots represent the mean difference between measured and true values. The vertical lines through the mean values represent the error intervals calculated as the mean difference $\pm\, k_1 S$ as shown in Figure 10.15.

Table 10.6

Factors for Determining Outliers at the 95% Confidence Level

n	k_2	n	k_2
3	1.15	13	1.84
4	1.39	14	1.85
5	1.57	15	1.86
6	1.66	16	1.87
7	1.71	18	1.88
8	1.75	20	1.89
9	1.78	25	1.90
10	1.80	30	1.91
11	1.82	40	1.92
12	1.83		

Figure 10.17

Procedure for handling outliers in a set of measurements.

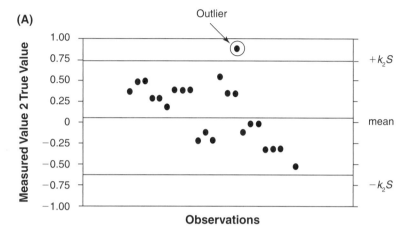

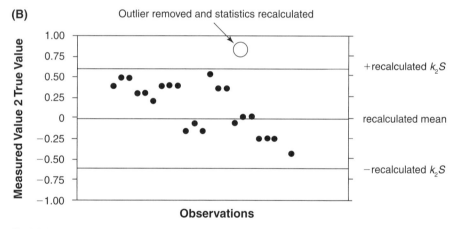

An outlier is identified in the original data set as a data point outside the limits calculated as ± k_2 standard deviations (refer to Table 10.5). It is removed and the outlier limits are recalculated. This time, no outliers are found.

the data one at a time until no more are identified. Each time an outlier is rejected, a new mean and standard deviation are calculated for the reduced sample (**Figure 10.17**).

Interpreting Manufacturers' Error Specifications

In evaluating a new device, our main concern is with how much error can be expected in normal use. Knowing that any specification of error is just an estimate, we want to know how much confidence to place in it. You would think this is a straightforward question with a simple answer, but manufacturers can be rather cryptic about their error specifications. For example, the operator's manual for a leading brand of pulse oximeter has a section titled "Specifications." There we find a specification for "accuracy" listed as "percent $SpO_2 \pm 1$ SD." From this specification we gather that the error in measured saturation is given as a "one-sigma" interval (one standard deviation). Next, we find that for saturations in the range of 70% to 100%, the accuracy is "± 2 digits." Given that the readout is digital and the units for SpO_2 are percent, we surmise that "digits" means percent. So what does this mean? First, we have to assume that the standard deviation (SD) referred to is that of the population of all future measurements made with the instrument, because we are not given a sample size. (Besides, we happen to know that error specifications for pulse oximeters are based on thousands of measurements, so the sample is a good estimate of the population.)

Second, as clinicians, we like to keep our risk of error below the 5% level for any kind of measurement. To achieve that level, we have to double the specified error to get a two-sigma interval (refer to Figure 10.12). Thus, we can expect 95% of measurements with this device to fall within $\pm 4\%$ of the true value. And because we have no further information, we just assume that we can have 100% confidence in this estimate.

Next, consider the operator's manual for a serum ionized calcium analyzer from a leading manufacturer. The manufacturer has defined inaccuracy as the mean difference between the measured value on a group of instruments and the estimated true value (what we have called bias). Imprecision is defined as the standard deviation of the measurements. You will recall that the standard deviation of the measurements is the same as the standard deviation of the differences between measured and true values, assuming the true value is constant. We are told that 100 samples were analyzed with a calculated bias of 0.04 mmol/L and imprecision of 0.02 mmol/L. We have enough information to create a two-sigma error interval at the 99% confidence level (an inaccuracy interval). From Table 10.4 we see that the k_l value for $n = 100$ is 2.36. The inaccuracy interval is thus $0.04 \pm 2.36 \times 0.02 = 0.04 \pm 0.05 = (-0.01, 0.09)$.

Note that the observed inaccuracy of a device may be different from the manufacturer's specifications, depending on how it is used. Instrument specifications do not, for example, include the various types of operator errors.

The user must be aware of the implications of error specifications. If a specification is given as a percentage of the full-scale reading, the device will be more accurate for measuring quantities at the upper end of the scale than on the lower end. For example, suppose the scale range is from 0 to 100 and the error is $\pm 2\%$ of full scale. If a known quantity having a value of 95 is measured, the instrument will probably give a value between 93 and 97, which is 98% to 102% of the true value. However, if a known quantity of 5 is measured, the reading will be between 3 and 7, or 60% to 140% of the true value. This represents an inaccuracy for that particular reading of $\pm 40\%$, which might be unacceptable, depending on the application. In contrast, if the specification is given as a percentage of reading, the instrument will have the same error at the upper and lower ends of the scale.

Inverse Estimation

In *creating* error specifications, the manufacturer's task is to describe the spread of measured values around the true value. But in *using* error specifications, the problem is reversed. For a given measured value, we want to know the range of values in which the true value will lie. If the mean (systematic error), standard deviation (random error), and sample size are given, we simply construct an inaccuracy interval, as described previously.

When the error specification is given as a percentage of full scale, the systematic and random errors have been lumped together into an equivalent constant systematic error. The lower and upper limits for the true value (true$_L$ and true$_U$) are given by:

$$\text{true}_U = \text{measured value} + \frac{\text{error} \times \text{full scale reading}}{100}$$

$$\text{true}_L = \text{measured value} - \frac{\text{error} \times \text{full scale reading}}{100}$$

For example, an instrument with a scale of 0 to 200 and an error of ±4% of full scale show a reading of 83. The true value will be in the interval

$$\text{true}_U = 83 + \frac{4 \times 200}{100} = 91$$

$$\text{true}_L = 83 - \frac{4 \times 200}{100} = 75$$

Notice that the true value is between 8 units below and 8 units above the measured value; the error band is symmetrical.

When the error specification is given as a percentage of reading, the systematic and random errors have been lumped together into an equivalent proportional systematic error. Because the error is proportional to the reading, the limits of the estimated true value are not symmetrical. The lower limit is closer to the measured value than the upper limit is. In this case, the limits are given by

$$\text{true}_U = \frac{\text{measured value} \times 100}{100 - \text{error}}$$

$$\text{true}_L = \frac{\text{measured value} \times 100}{100 + \text{error}}$$

Using the same example as before, but with an equivalent error of 10% of reading, we get

$$\text{true}_U = \frac{83 \times 100}{100 - 10} = 92$$

$$\text{true}_L = \frac{83 \times 100}{100 + 10} = 75$$

Now the true value is between 8 units below and 9 units above the measured value.

Hypothesis Testing

In hypothesis testing, we translate a research hypothesis into a formal mathematical statement, obtain a sample statistic, and find the probability of our sample statistic from the appropriate sampling distribution. Based on the probability we obtain, we either accept or reject our hypothesis.

Hypothesis testing is a technique for *quantifying* our guess about a hypothesis. We never know the "real" situation. Does drug X cause Y or not? We can figure the odds and quantify our probability of being right or wrong. Then, if we can decide what odds (or risk of being wrong) we can live with, we have a ready-made decision rule. If the probability that drug X causes result Y is high enough, then we decide that X does cause Y. We first give an illustrated example of a hypothesis test, and then summarize the steps in the procedure. You may have difficulty understanding the concepts of hypothesis testing until you actually work through a problem.

For example, let's say you are a staff therapist in a busy university hospital. Much of your day is devoted to delivering aerosol medications to patients on acute care floors. Thinking of yourself as a lone star in a world of "slackers," you wonder if you are actually working harder than your colleagues. For one week, you record the number of aerosol treatments you give each day. You find that you average 32 aerosols per day. Then you ask your supervisor what a fair aerosol treatment workload should be. She looks up some historical data and tells you that based on the total number of aerosol treatments done in a year and the number of therapists in the department, the average should be about 26 per day. Now the question is whether your average is significantly higher than the department average, or is your average due to a chance fluctuation? In other words, do you really work harder on average than the rest of the department, or were you just having a busy week?

The key concept to remember is that the value of a sample mean will fluctuate with different random samples, even if all samples come from the same population. This fluctuation is due to random sampling error. In other words, even though the population mean is 26, different samples will have different values for their means. A sample mean of 32 is possible even if the population that the sample comes from has a mean of 26. Of course, we don't know whether your sample represents an actual mean of 26 with a chance fluctuation, or if it represents a truly different population (your average assignment) with a mean greater than 26.

It is possible by chance to have a sample mean of 32 with a true population mean of 26 because of random error. Therefore, we calculate the probability of a sample mean of 32 to make our decision. If the probability is high, then we accept that the sample mean of 32 represents a population with a mean of 26. We conclude that there is no *actual* difference between 26 and 32, only a *chance* difference. This conclusion represents the *null* (no-difference) case or hypothesis. The symbol for the null hypothesis will be H_0. In contrast, if probability of a sample mean of 32 due to chance, given a population mean of 26, is low, then we will reject the no-difference hypothesis and accept the alternate hypothesis that your sample workload comes from a population with a mean that is greater than 26, and there is a difference between 26 and 32. The symbol for the alternate hypothesis is H_A. We must now decide what probability values we would consider to be "high" and "low."

If we set a cutoff value, below which all values are considered low, then we have set a *significance level.* The significance level is symbolized by the Greek letter alpha (α). For example, if alpha is set at 0.05, we are saying any probability of 0.05 or less is not likely. The value of 0.05 is commonly used by convention. In the methods section of most research articles you will find a statement like "The significance of our statistical tests was set at 0.05."

Let us summarize the information we have for our example:

- *Outcome variable:* Workload in units of aerosols delivered per person per day.
- *Research hypothesis:* My workload is higher than the departmental average.
- *Sample data:* (33, 49, 22, 27, 30).

Now let's review the procedure for testing the hypothesis.

Step 1. Formulate the statistical hypotheses.

$$H_0: \mu = 26 \text{ (null hypothesis)}$$

$$H_A: \mu \neq 26 \text{ (alternate hypothesis)}$$

The null hypothesis is that your sample came from a population with a mean of 26. The alternate hypothesis is that the sample comes from a population with a mean of greater than or less than 26, since we cannot foretell in which direction it might be. For example, your average workload may indeed be higher than the department's. Alternatively, your average workload may be less, but you were having a really busy week when you collected your sample. This type of hypothesis and is called "two-tailed" for reasons that will become clear later.

Step 2. Calculate the descriptive statistics for the sample data.

$$\overline{X} = \frac{33 + 49 + 22 + 27 + 30}{5} = 32.2$$

$$S = \sqrt{\frac{(33 - 32.2)^2 + (49 - 32.2)^2 + (22 - 32.2)^2 + (27 - 32.2)^2 + (30 - 32.2)^2}{5 - 1}} = 5.9$$

Of course, you would not do this calculation by hand as shown above but would use a spreadsheet or a calculator. Note that we are retaining one more significant digit in the answers than in the data to prevent round-off errors. The final answer will have the correct number of significant digits (no more than the fewest number in the data, in this case, two). You have to pay attention to little things like rounding error.

Step 3. Calculate the test statistic. In hypothesis testing, we assume that there is no difference (assume the null hypothesis is true) and find the probability of our sample mean value. To do that, we need to know what probability distribution to use. The appropriate distribution is our sampling distribution. Let us assume our sampling distribution is adequately described by the *t* distribution (because the sample size is small and we do not know the department's population standard deviation). Now, what is the probability of a sample mean of 32 or greater if the population mean is 26?

We calculate the t statistic for our data:

$$t = \frac{\overline{X} - \mu}{S / \sqrt{n}} = \frac{32 - 26}{5.9 / \sqrt{5}} = 2.374$$

Step 4. Determine the rejection region under the t distribution curve. We need the cutoff value of t associated with the desired significance level (0.05). This cutoff value of t allows us to rule off two areas under the t distribution curve that each represent half of the desired significance level (again, because we cannot say beforehand whether the population our sample came from has a mean higher or lower than the department mean). These areas represent unlikely values of t in the "tails" of the distribution. That is why the hypothesis test it is called a "two-tailed" test (**Figure 10.18**). The idea is that if the value of t from our sample data (Step 3) is larger than the critical value of t, then we conclude that our results are unlikely to occur by chance.

We can look up the cutoff value in a statistical table or we can use the Microsoft Excel spreadsheet equation =TINV(significance level, degrees of freedom) where the degrees of freedom equals $n - 1$. Thus, we type =TINV(0.05,4) in a cell, press the enter key, and get the value 2.776.

> *Figure 10.18 is the key to hypothesis testing and confidence intervals. If you can understand all the concepts it illustrates, then you will be prepared to read research articles and even do basic statistical testing.*

The graph in Figure 10.18 is somewhat simplified in that there is no vertical axis. The vertical axis is probability, as we discussed in an earlier section. The horizontal axis gives values of t from negative infinity to positive infinity. That is why the curve never touches the horizontal axis. The vertical line in the center of the curve marks the mean of the distribution.

Figure 10.18

Areas under a t distribution for a sample size of 5.

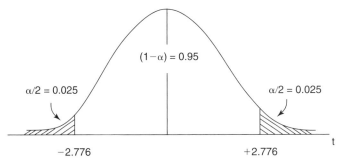

The cutoff value of ±2.776 represents the distance above and below the true population mean that encompasses a probability of 95%. The cutoff value will change for different samples sizes or significance levels. The shaded areas represent the "rejection regions".

As with the z distribution, the mean of the t distribution is zero. The vertical line also corresponds with the mean value of the population we are assuming under the null hypothesis, H_0, which in this example is 26.

The vertical line divides the distribution into two equal areas of 50% each. But we are more interested in the two shaded areas. The shaded areas, added together, make up a probability of 5%. That 5% corresponds to the significance level, α, that we set beforehand. Those areas represent occurrences that we consider rare. The unshaded area represents occurrences that are not rare. Occurrences of what? Well, we mean values of t, which represent occurrences of sample statistics (in this case mean values) from experiments. So, a sample mean that was close to the population mean would produce a t value close to zero and it would be in the unshaded region. A sample mean that was unusually far away from the mean would produce a t value that would be in the shaded region. We would consider the occurrence of such a sample mean (and corresponding t statistic) rare. So rare that if we observe one we would sooner conclude that it was from a different curve, a curve with a different mean. That is why the shaded regions are called "rejection" regions, because we would reject the null hypothesis. The unshaded regions are called acceptance or, more correctly, "do not reject" regions. (Remember, philosophically speaking, we never really accept that a hypothesis is true; we simply do not reject it until such time as more data are available.)

Step 5. Form a conclusion. If you have understood everything up to this point, making the conclusion is simple. Your value of t from the sample is 2.374. It is between 0 and the critical value of 2.776. That puts your t value within the "do not reject" region of the curve, so you do not reject the null hypothesis. Translated, that means you cannot conclude that your sample workload came from a population with a higher mean. So, despite the fact that for one week your average workload was higher than the departmental average, you cannot conclude that in general, your productivity is higher than your colleagues. What could have caused the mean to look higher but still not be a significant difference? Look again at the sample data. Notice that there is one day that sticks out at 49 treatments. This relatively large value had two effects. It increased the mean value a little but it increased the standard deviation substantially. For example, if that day had been 32 instead of 49, the mean would be 6% lower, but the standard deviation would be 59% lower. Now look at the equation for t again:

$$t = \frac{\overline{X} - \mu}{S / \sqrt{n}}$$

Notice that as the standard deviation, S, increases, t decreases. True, the mean also increases, which would tend to increase t, but we have just seen that the effect on the standard deviation is much larger. So data with a lot of variability are less likely to indicate a significant difference. Also notice that t is directly proportional to the square root of the sample size. That means our small sample size of only five days also tended to make the difference in the mean values insignificant. Consider what would have happened if we set the significance level at 0.10 or 0.01 instead of 0.05.

What would have happened if your sample had produced a t value larger than 2.776? That value of t would have been in the rejection region. Therefore, you would have concluded that your sample came from some population with a larger mean value than the population the

Figure 10.19

Values of the test statistic that lie in the rejection region under the null hypothesis, H_0, (top curve) are assumed to lie in the acceptance region of the distribution described by the alternative hypothesis (bottom curve).

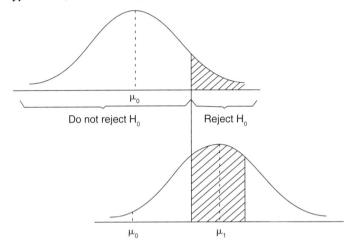

departmental data represented. What you are really saying is that if the sample mean of 32 is unlikely to have come from a population with a mean of 26, then it follows logically that the sample is more likely to have come from a population with a larger mean. We are not saying what that larger mean value is, just that it exists. **Figure 10.19** illustrates this reasoning: under the null hypothesis (population mean $= \mu_0$), observed values far from the mean are rare. If they are rare enough (occur less than 5% of the time) we consider them to be in the rejection region (shaded area in upper curve). If they are in the rejection region we conclude that they actually come from a different population (mean $= \mu_1$), where they have a higher probability of occurrence (shaded area in lower curve).

If Figure 10.19 does not make sense to you, consider this simple thought experiment: I place before you a container filled with marbles. I tell you that it contains either 1 white marble and 99 black marbles or 1 black marble and 99 white marbles. Let's say the null hypothesis is that the container is filled with mostly white marbles. You have to test this hypothesis by picking out a sample of five marbles. You do this by removing one marble, noting its color, replacing it, and repeating until you have observed five marbles. If you took an infinite number of samples of five marbles, the expected distribution of the ratio of black to white marbles under the null hypothesis would be represented by the top curve in Figure 10.19. A large percentage of the time you would observe mostly white marbles, represented by the unshaded portion of the curve. A small percentage of the time you would observe mostly black marbles, represented by the shaded portion of the curve.

Now for the experiment: You can't see into the container, just the marbles you take out. You take out one marble, note that it is black, replace it, and shake up the container.

You repeat the procedure and again it is a black marble. All five times you draw a marble it is black. What is your guess about the population of marbles? Do you think that you drew the same black marble five times in a row from a container filled mostly with white marbles? That could happen, but it would be very rare. (This corresponds to the shaded region in the top curve of the figure.) Or is it more likely that you were picking from a container with mostly black marbles? (This corresponds to the shaded region in the bottom curve of the figure.) Obviously, your choice would have to be the container of mostly black marbles. We reject the null hypothesis (H_0) and accept the alternative hypothesis. That is all we are doing in Figure 10.19, selecting the distribution that is most probable, knowing that we would make the wrong decision about 5 times in 100 identical experiments (5%) as determined by the significance level of the test.

The step-by-step procedure we have just used can be found in just about any statistical textbook along with tables for looking up t values. However, it is not very practical. Assuming you have statistical software or you have set up statistical calculations within a computer spreadsheet, then the procedure is simplified. For example, with your workload data you would do the following:

Step 1. Enter the data into a spreadsheet. In this case, you simply enter the daily number of aerosol treatments into a single column of the spreadsheet. Statistical software usually has a data entry screen that looks just like an accounting spreadsheet.

Step 2. Select and run the desired statistical analysis. Your problem requires a single sample t test. A statistical program like SigmaPlot (Systat Software, Inc.; www.sigmaplot.com) even has a "Wizard" that asks you a set of questions about your research problem and then suggests the correct statistical test.

Step 3. Interpret the results. SigmaPlot is very helpful in that it prints out a full report. The report not only summarizes the data but also checks the underlying assumptions of the chosen statistical test. For example, it will check to make sure the sample data are approximately normally distributed. If not, it will suggest an alternative nonparametric test. If the data pass the normality test, you get a calculated value for the statistic, which in our example would be a value for t. Then it gives the p value. The p value is the probability of observing values of t equal to or larger than the one for your sample data. In other words, the p value is the probability associated with the shaded areas in Figure 10.18. Remember, we set the significance level at 0.05. Therefore, if the p value is greater than 0.05, your t value does not lie in the rejection region, and you would conclude that there was no significant difference between your sample mean (32) and the population mean under the null hypothesis (the department mean of 26). This is the same thing as comparing the t to a critical value and deciding if it is in the rejection region or not. But statistical software and research articles usually give p values, not critical values for statistics. For example, using the Microsoft Excel spreadsheet equation =TDIST(t, degrees of freedom, tails), where t is the value that you calculated from your sample data (2.374), the degrees of freedom equals $n - 1$ or 4, and tails is 2 for a two-tailed test (and 1 for a single-tailed test, which is seldom seen in the medical literature because it gives less conservative results). Thus, we type =TDIST(2.374,4,2) in a cell, press the enter key, and get the p value of 0.08. This means that the probability of observing a sample mean of 32 from a population with a mean of 26 would happen 8 times out of 100 experiments, or 8% of the time. But our significance level of 0.5 says that only events occurring as rarely as 5 times or less out of 100 are significant. Because 0.08 is greater than 0.05, you conclude that your sample was not sufficiently rare. It probably does not come from a different population.

Let's review the important terms used in hypothesis testing.

- *Research hypothesis*: A statement of the proposed relationship between or among variables. Example: T-tube trials reduce weaning time compared with synchronized intermittent mandatory ventilation (SIMV).
- *Statistical hypothesis:* A precise statement about the parameters of a population. The two forms are the null hypothesis (H_0) and alternate hypothesis (H_A). The null hypothesis states "no difference" or "no association." The alternate hypothesis states that there is a difference or association. Example: H_0 (mean weaning time with T-tube is equal to the mean weaning time with SIMV) versus H_A (mean weaning time with T-tube is not equal to the mean weaning time with SIMV).
- *Test statistic*: The statistic such as a z or t score used to test the statistical hypothesis.
- *Statistical test*: A procedure allowing a decision to be made between two mutually exclusive statistical hypotheses, using the sample data. Also known as a hypothesis test.
- p *value*: The probability that the observed results or results more extreme would occur if the null hypothesis were true and the experiment were repeated many times.
- *Significance level (alpha):* The level of probability at which it is agreed that the null hypothesis will be rejected. This is the cutoff level for what is considered improbable.

Type I and II Errors

In hypothesis testing, we have a rule for deciding between the two mutually exclusive statistical hypotheses, the null and the alternate. Two decisions are possible: accept the null hypothesis (the treatment made no difference) or reject it (the treatment was effective). However, we never know for sure whether the treatment is effective.

Two situations are possible in actuality. Either the null hypothesis is true, or the null is not true. This gives four possible combinations between our decision and reality, as illustrated in **Figure 10.20**.

To simplify the discussion, let us suppose that the actual population mean is either 100 or 103. Both the distribution under the null hypothesis (H_0: mean $=100$) and the distribution under the alternative hypothesis (H_1: mean $= 103$) are shown in Figure 10.20. Alpha sets a cutoff point on the distribution under the null hypothesis. Suppose the mean is actually 100 (H_0 is true). Then we have a probability of $1 - \alpha$ of correctly accepting the null hypothesis. We also have a probability α of rejecting a true null hypothesis. This is called a *Type I error,* the error of rejecting the null hypothesis when it is true. In contrast, suppose the mean is actually 103, which could be the case as far as we know, and now H_0 is false. Unfortunately, because of random error in sampling, this distribution (right side of Figure 10.20) overlaps the distribution under the null hypothesis. The area of the two distributions that coincides to the *left* of alpha leads to acceptance of the null hypothesis, but the *null hypothesis* is *not true* now. The Greek letter beta (β) symbolizes the probability of a *Type II error*, which consists of accepting a false null hypothesis. Of course if the mean is really

Figure 10.20

Illustration of probabilities for Type I and Type II errors.

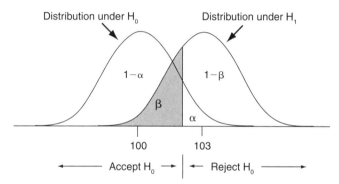

Actual Case

	H_0 true (μ=100)	H_0 false (μ=103)
Accept H_0	Correct prob = $1-\alpha$	Type II error prob = β
Reject H_0	Type I error prob = α	Correct prob = $1-\beta$

Decision

Distribution under H_0 Distribution under H_1

$1-\alpha$ $1-\beta$

β

α

100   103

⟵ Accept H_0 ⟶ | ⟵ Reject H_0 ⟶

H_0 = the null hypothesis (e.g., mean value = 100), H_1 = the alternate hypothesis (e.g., mean value = 103).

103, the area denoted by $1 - \beta$ gives the probability of correctly rejecting the null hypothesis. The term for $1 - \beta$ is *power*.

Now we can see that lowering alpha to 0.01 or to 0.001 involves a tradeoff. If we lower alpha, we reduce the risk of a Type I error, but concomitantly we increase the risk of a Type II error. In Figure 10.20, mentally slide the cutoff point designated by alpha to the right. Alpha is decreased, but the area of beta increases. One solution to keep alpha low *and* to lower beta is to decrease the variability, or spread, of the two distributions. These are sampling distributions, or distributions of the statistic $\bar{X}$. The standard deviation of the $\bar{X}$ values is given by the SEM. A smaller SEM indicates less variation, and we can decrease the size of the SEM by increasing sample size, $n\,(SEM = \sigma/\sqrt{n})$. This will decrease the size of beta and increase power $(1 - \beta)$.

Which type of error is more serious is relative to the research question. If a new drug is investigated, we would want a definite effect (a large difference) to conclude that the drug is effective. We would desire a small value for alpha, so we would rather accept a false null hypothesis (Type II error) than reject a true null hypothesis (Type 1 error). In other words, we would rather throw out a drug as ineffective when it is really effective than foist a truly ineffective drug on the public, thinking the drug is efficacious. Alpha is made small, although beta increases. In contrast, if we are testing for accuracy between two monitors, we want only a very small difference before we say the difference is significant. We desire a large alpha, so that a difference is more likely to be called significant. Here we would rather reject a true null hypothesis (Type I error) than accept a false, null hypothesis (Type II error). In this case, you would be better off to reject the conclusion of accuracy (even though the monitors are accurate) than say the monitors are accurate when they are not.

Power Analysis and Sample Size

Once the mechanism of hypothesis testing and basic statistical tests are understood, we can discuss the question of adequate sample size and the related concept of power analysis with statistical tests.

We have previously identified two types of errors that can occur, Type I and Type II (refer to Figure 10.20). If the null hypothesis represents reality, then α is our probability of rejecting the null hypothesis when it is true (a Type I error), and $1 - \alpha$ is the probability of accepting the null hypothesis when it is true, a correct decision.

But to be complete, we must consider the case where the null hypothesis is false—that is, the alternative hypothesis truly represents reality. Then we saw that there is a probability, β, of accepting the null hypothesis when the alternate hypothesis is really true. The probability of rejecting the null hypothesis—that is, accepting the alternate—is given by $1 - \beta$. The size of β and $1 - \beta$ are determined by the degree of overlap of the sampling distribution under the null and under the alternate hypotheses. This is shown in Figure 10.20.

For a given null and alternate distribution, *decreasing* the risk of a Type I error (lowering alpha) *increases* the risk of a Type II error (beta increases), as we can see in Figure 10.20. By making alpha too small, we can cause beta to become quite large, and thus we run the risk of incorrectly accepting the null. For example, suppose we lowered alpha to 0.001, causing beta to have a value of 0.60. Although we reduced our risk of rejecting a true null hypothesis to 1 in 1,000, we now have a risk of accepting a false null hypothesis that is greater than 1 out of 2. We could do better tossing a coin instead of doing an experiment! Novice researchers often make the mistake of ignoring power when their study results are negative, meaning that their data apparently showed no difference between outcome variables. If the power of their statistical tests was low, the results must be judged inconclusive.

How do we decrease *both* alpha and beta? Or to put the question another way, how can we have a large probability of accepting a the null hypothesis when it is true ($1 - \alpha$) and also have a large probability of accepting the alternate when *it* is true ($1 - \beta$)? The last probability, $1 - \beta$, is termed *power*, which is the probability of correctly rejecting the null hypothesis.

The most practical means to control power is to manipulate sample size. If we look at Figure 10.20 we can understand the rationale for this. Remember that the distributional curves in Figure 10.20 are distributions of possible sample means. The dispersion in the distributions is given by the standard error of the mean ($SEM = \sigma / \sqrt{n}$). If we make the SEM smaller, we could decrease the amount of overlap between the two distributions and still have each centered as seen on mean values of 100 and 103. This we can do by increasing sample size.

An example can make the effect of sample size on the SEM obvious. Let σ equal 9; then for an *n* of 9 and 81, respectively, the SEM is as follows:

$$SEM = 9 / \sqrt{9} = 3$$
$$SEM = 9 / \sqrt{81} = 1$$

The variance of the population, σ, will not change. Therefore, the SEM will decrease as sample size increases, and the distribution of the sample means will be less dispersed. If the two distributions in Figure 10.20 are each made narrower, then the area indicated by beta must become smaller with a given value for alpha. If beta is smaller, then power, or $1 - \beta$, will be increased.

To summarize, for a given population variance and alpha level, we can increase power, or the probability of correctly rejecting the null hypothesis, if we use a larger sample. But we may waste time and money by using too large a sample if a smaller sample achieves a desired power for a given population variance and alpha level.

The power of a statistical test, at any given significance level, is directly proportional to both the sample size and the treatment effect. The treatment effect, or *effect size*, is the expected magnitude of the effect caused by the treatment, or independent variable. Effect size is calculated differently depending on the sample statistic used. However, most often you will think of the effect in terms of a difference between two mean values (such as between two sample means or between a sample mean and a population mean). The difference in means is "standardized" (similar to the reasoning for a *z* score) by dividing it by the standard deviation. That allows us to use one table or nomogram for any effect size. For hypothesis tests where you will be comparing a single sample mean to the mean of a population, use:

$$\text{effect size} = \frac{\overline{X} - \mu}{S}$$

where $\overline{X}$ is the sample mean, μ is the population mean, and S is the sample standard deviation. For tests where you want to compare two sample means, use

$$\text{effect size} = \frac{\overline{X}_1 - \overline{X}_2}{S_P}$$

where $\overline{X}_1$ and $\overline{X}_2$ are the two sample means and S_P is the pooled standard deviation. Once you have the effect size, use the nomogram in **Figure 10.21** to estimate either the sample size or the power of the test.

Use the nomogram by connecting any two known values by a straight line and reading the unknown value where the line intersects the appropriate scale. For example, if the effect size is 1.0 and the desired power is 0.80, then the required sample size is 30. You can also evaluate the power of a test after the fact. For example, in the experiment we used in the discussion about hypothesis testing, you collected workload data for five days and found that the mean workload did not differ from the department's historical average. Because the *p* value from the

Figure 10.21

Nomogram relating effect size, total study size (sum of two equal sample sizes), and the power of a t test for the difference between mean values.

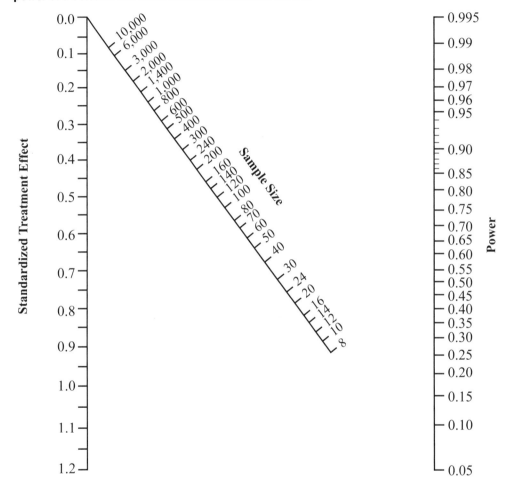

Connect any two known values by a straight line and read the unknown value where the line intersects the appropriate scale. For example, if the effect size is 1.0 and the desired power is 0.80, then the required sample size is 30. If the study requires only one sample, divide the sample size by 4 for a rough approximation.

hypothesis test was higher than 0.05, we did not reject the null hypothesis. In doing so, we run the risk of committing a Type II error, accepting the null hypothesis when it is really false. From our discussion about the power of a test, you should suspect that the negative results may be due to the small sample size.

To evaluate the power of the test, we first need to calculate the effect size. We can start with the actual mean values. You will recall that your sample mean from five days was 32.2 with a standard deviation of 5.9, while the population mean from departmental records was 26:

$$\text{effect size} = \frac{\overline{X} - \mu}{S} = \frac{32.2 - 26}{5.9} = 1.05$$

On the nomogram in Figure 10.21, we line up the effect size of 1.05 with the sample size of 8 (the smallest number on the scale and fairly close to 5) and extend the line through the power scale. Where the line intersects the scale we read a power of about 0.33. From Figure 10.20 we see that the probability that we made a correct decision was only 33%. Because power = $1 - \beta$, then the probability of a Type II error is $\beta = 1 - \text{power}$. Thus, the conclusion that your workload was no different from the departmental average had a probability of $1 - 0.33$ = 0.67, or a 67% chance of being wrong! That does not mean that you are great and the other workers are slackers; it means that you did not collect enough data to make a strong conclusion.

The selection of power is somewhat arbitrary, depending on which type of error is more serious in a given research situation. Usually, Type I error is more serious than Type II error: we would not want to conclude that there *is* a treatment effect if one does not exist because the subject is unnecessarily exposed to the risk of adverse reactions to treatment. Usually, a power of 0.80 (β of 0.20) is commonly used.

So how many days of data would you have to collect to be confident in your results? First decide on how big of an effect you want to show. Let's say that you would be content to show that you worked 20% harder than your coworkers. Twenty percent of 26 is 5.2. Now calculate the effect size:

$$\text{effect size} = \frac{5.2}{S} = \frac{5.2}{5.9} = 0.88$$

Second, decide how much power the hypothesis test should have. Again, this is an arbitrary decision, based on how much you want to avoid making a Type II error (low power means high probability of error). Concluding that your workload is no different from that of your coworkers will cause little more harm than hurting your ego, so you set the power at 0.75. Now, on the nomogram in Figure 10.21, use a ruler to line up the effect size of 0.88 with the power of 0.75, and you see the required sample size is about 35. Assuming you worked five days a week, you would have to collect data for seven weeks to make an accurate judgment about your workload compared with the average department workload.

There are some important lessons here. First, negative results are not always negative. Your confidence in a negative result depends on the power of the hypothesis test. Second, your efforts in collecting data for five days were not wasted just because you could not make conclusive results. What you did was conduct a *pilot study*, in which you learned something about how much effort is required to collect the data (giving you an idea of the feasibility of the study). More important, you were able to estimate the sample variability (the sample standard deviation) and use this to estimate the sample size needed for a larger study that would give more conclusive results.

Rules of Thumb for Estimating Sample Size

The following rules of thumb let you estimate approximate sample sizes under a variety of conditions without the use of nomograms, tables, or computers.[1] Assume a two-tailed hypothesis with significance level = 95% and power = 80%.

Estimates Based on Mean and Standard Deviation

These rules are useful when you have some data from a pilot study.

Difference Between Means (Single Sample)
Use this equation when a single sample mean is compared with a hypothesized population mean:

$$n = \frac{8}{\Delta^2}$$

where Δ is the standardized effect size:

$$\Delta = \frac{\overline{X} - \mu}{S}$$

in which n is the required sample size, $\overline{X}$ is the sample mean, μ is the hypothesized population mean, and S is the sample standard deviation. For example, if the standardized effect size is 0.5, then $n = 8/0.5^2 = 32$.

Difference Between Means (Two Samples)
Use this equation when comparing the difference between two sample means:

$$n = \frac{16}{\Delta^2}$$

where Δ is the standardized effect size:

$$\Delta = \frac{\overline{X} - \mu}{S}$$

in which n is the required sample size per group, $\overline{X}$ is the sample mean, μ is the hypothesized population mean, and S is the average of the two sample standard deviations (or just take the larger one for a conservative estimate of n). For example, if the standardized effect size is 0.5, then $n = 16/0.5^2 = 64$.

Estimates Based on Proportionate Change and Coefficient of Variation

These rules are useful when you do not have data from a pilot study but you can say, for example, that you want to detect a 20% change in the mean and the that sample data will probably have a 30% variability. You estimate the effect size in terms of a proportionate change of the mean (difference between means divided by population mean) and estimate the variability of the data in terms of the coefficient of variation (population standard deviation divided by the population mean).

Difference Between Means (Single Sample)
Use this equation when a single sample mean is compared with a hypothesized population mean:

$$n = \frac{4CV^2}{PC^2}[1+(1-PC)^2]$$

where n is the required sample size, CV is the estimated coefficient of variation (from the sample data), PC is the proportional change in the mean you want to detect, and S is the average of the two sample standard deviations (or just take the larger one for a conservative estimate of n). For example, if you would like to detect a 20% change in the mean value and you think the variability of the data should be about 30%, then

$$n = \frac{4(0.30)^2}{(0.20)^2}[1+(1-0.20)^2] \approx 15$$

If you have no idea of what the variability of the data may be, use

$$n \approx \frac{0.5}{PC^2}[1+(1-PC)^2]$$

Difference Between Means (Two Samples)
Use this equation when comparing the difference between two sample means

$$n = \frac{8CV^2}{PC^2}[1+(1-PC)^2]$$

where n is the required sample size per group, CV is the estimated coefficient of variation (from the sample data), PC is the proportional change in the mean you want to detect, and S is the average of the two sample standard deviations (or just take the larger one for a conservative estimate of n). For example, if you would like to detect a 20% change in the mean value and you think the variability of the data should be about 30%, then

$$n = \frac{8(0.30)^2}{(0.20)^2}[1+(1-0.20)^2] \approx 30$$

If you have no idea of what the variability of the data may be, use

$$n \approx \frac{1}{PC^2}[1+(1-PC)^2]$$

Estimates for Confidence Intervals

Frequently, we need to calculate a sample size for a fixed confidence interval width. We include the situation where the confidence interval is in the original measurement units (interval width = w) and where the interval is in units of the standard deviation (interval width/standard deviation = w^*).

Confidence Interval for the Mean

$$n = \frac{16\sigma^2}{w^2} = \frac{16}{(w^*)^2}$$

where σ is the population standard deviation (perhaps estimated from a pilot sample standard deviation).

Confidence Interval for the Difference Between Two Means

$$n = \frac{32\sigma^2}{w^2} = \frac{32}{(w^*)^2}$$

where σ is the population standard deviation (perhaps estimated from a pilot sample standard deviation).

Sample Size for Binomial Test

This rule of thumb is most accurate for sample sizes between 10 and 100.

Difference Between Proportions (Two Independent Samples)

$$n = \frac{4}{(p_1 - p_2)^2}$$

where p_1 and p_2 are the two proportions and n is the sample size per group. For example, if one sample proportion is 0.5 and the other sample proportion was 0.7, the sample size would have to be 100 for each sample group for the difference to be significant.

Unequal Sample Sizes

Case Control
Sometimes a study results in unequal sample sizes. For example, you may not be able to observe more cases of patients with a particular disease, but normal controls are plentiful. Suppose n subjects are required per group, but only m are available for one group ($m < n$). We need to know how much to increase n to maintain the power of the statistical test. We calculate the factor k such that km is the required larger sample size:

$$k = \frac{n}{2m - n}$$

For example, suppose that the sample size calculations indicate that $n = 16$ cases, and 16 controls are needed in a case-control study. However, only 12 cases are available ($m = 12$). How many controls will be needed to obtain the same precision? The answer is:

$$k = \frac{16}{2(12) - 16} = 2$$

So we need $km = 2 \times 12 = 24$ controls to obtain the same results as with 16 cases and 16 controls.

Cost Control

In some two-sample situations the cost per observation is not equal, and the challenge is to choose the sample sizes in such a way as to minimize cost and maximize precision. Suppose the cost per observation in the first sample is c_1 and in the second is c_2. How should the two sample sizes n_1 and n_2 be chosen?

$$\frac{n_2}{n_1} = \sqrt{\frac{c_1}{c_2}}$$

This equation is known as the square root rule: pick sample sizes inversely proportional to the square root of the cost of the observations. If costs are not too different, then equal sample sizes are suggested (because the square root of the ratio will be close to 1.0). For example, suppose the cost per observation for the first sample is 160 and the cost per observation for the second sample is 40. The rule of thumb states that you should take twice as many observations in the second group as compared with the first.

To calculate specific sample sizes, first calculate the required sample size on an equal sample size base using one of the previous equations. Now you know n and k ($k = n_2/n_1$) in the equation from the previous section on case control. Rearranging that equation and solving for m yields:

$$m = \frac{n(k + 1)}{2k}$$

Suppose that on an equal sample basis, $n = 16$ observations are needed. On the basis of cost, we calculate that we need twice as many of one sample as the other ($n_2/n_1 = 2$). Then the smaller sample, m, is:

$$m = \frac{n(k + 1)}{2k} = \frac{16(2 + 1)}{2 \times 2} = 12$$

So the sample sizes to minimize cost and maintain precision are 12 and $2 \times 12 = 24$.

Rule of Threes

The rule of threes can be used to address the following types of question, "I am told by my physician that I need a serious operation and have been informed that there has not been a fatal outcome in the 20 operations carried out by the physician. Does this information give me an estimate of the potential postoperative mortality?" The answer is yes!

Given no observed events in n trials, the maximum expected rate of occurrence of the event (at the 95% confidence level) is:

$$rate = \frac{3}{n}$$

In our example, the "observed event" is a fatal outcome. No fatal outcomes have been observed in the last 20 operations. Given no observed events in 20 trials, the rate of occurrence could be as high as $3/20 = 0.15$ or 15%. In other words, if the physician had performed 100 operations, we could expect to observe as many as 15 fatalities.

If we know the rate, we can solve for n. For example, if the rate of extubation failure is 0.15, how many patients will I extubate before I am 95% certain to see at least one fail? The answer is $n = 3/rate = 20$.

Clinical Importance Versus Statistical Significance

The statistical tests we have discussed have the general form:

$$test\ statistic = \frac{difference}{standard\ error}$$

The size of the test statistic for a given difference is determined by the standard error, which in turn is determined by the sample size. Therefore, statistical significance can be obtained simply by increasing the sample size, so that even a very small effect size is significant. However, we must interpret the results of the hypothesis test with a little common sense. If the difference between two mean values (treatment group vs. control group) is significant but so small that it does not have any practical effect, then we must conclude that the results are not clinically important. For example, when comparing weaning modes, a 20-minute average difference in duration of ventilation may be statistically significant, but is it clinically important?

There is admittedly no easy way to determine clinical importance. The sample size should not, however, be artificially increased beyond that needed for an acceptable power level.

Matched Versus Unmatched Data

When picking a statistical test to compare two groups, you must know the relationship (if any) between data points. Data are said to be *unmatched* (or unpaired or independent) if values in one group are unrelated in any way to the data values in the other group. In other words, the values obtained in one group do not affect the values obtained in the other group. The two sample groups are just selected randomly from (supposedly) the same population. In this case, the differences between the two groups are partly due to the effects of the different experimental treatments given and partly due to the natural variability among study subjects.

In contrast, *matched* (or paired or dependent) data are selected so that they will be as nearly identical as possible. Pairing decreases or eliminates the differences between the two groups due to variability among study subjects. Pairing usually results in the need for smaller sample sizes for any given statistical power. This decreased variability must be accounted for in the statistical procedures used to test hypotheses. Groups of data may be paired in three ways: natural pairing, artificial pairing, and self-pairing.

Natural Pairing

Naturally paired groups are obvious pairs such as twins (in humans) or litter mates (in animals).

Artificial Pairing

If you cannot get natural pairs, you can get close by selecting pairs of subjects who are matched on as many confounding variables as possible. For example, you could match subjects on age, weight, gender, race, severity of disease, and so on. Keep in mind that the more variables you try to match on, the harder it will be to find subjects that match.

Self-Pairing

Perhaps the best solution, when possible, is to have each experimental subject act as his or her own control. For example, you would select a subject, randomly select a treatment, give the treatment, wait until the effects wore off, then give the other treatment. In this way, a single subject generates a pair of data values. This procedure results in the smallest sample size you can get for the desired level of statistical power.

Questions

Definitions

Define the following terms:

- Qualitative variable
- Quantitative variable
- Discrete variable
- Confidence interval
- Error interval
- Null hypothesis
- Alternate hypothesis
- *p* value

- Alpha (level of significance)
- Type I error
- Type II error
- Power (statistical)

True or False

1. The number 170.0 has only three significant figures.
2. The answer to the calculation: 73.5 + 0.418 should be expressed as 73.9 rather than 73.918.
3. A pie chart is most useful for illustrating the difference between several mean values.
4. A percentiles plot helps you decide how often a certain range of values occurs.
5. The symbol Σ indicates that a set of numbers is to be added together (summed).
6. The bar above the X in the symbol represents the mean (average) value.
7. A correlation coefficient of –0.9 indicates that as one value increases, the correlated value has a strong tendency also to increase.
8. The equation for a straight line has the form $Y = a + bX$. The value of a tells you the value of Y when $X = 0$, and the value of b tells you how much Y changes for a unit change in X.
9. The value of r^2 is always larger than the value of r.
10. The power of a statistical test increases as sample size or treatment effect increases but decreases as the sample variability increases.

Multiple Choice

1. Data consisting of categories, such as gender and race, are measured on which level?
   a. Nominal
   b. Ordinal
   c. Continuous (interval)
   d. Continuous (ratio)
2. Data such as height and weight are measured on which level?
   a. Nominal
   b. Ordinal
   c. Continuous (interval)
   d. Continuous (ratio)
3. The Celsius temperature scale is an example of what level of measurement?
   a. Nominal
   b. Ordinal
   c. Continuous (interval)
   d. Continuous (ratio)
4. A pain scale such as None = 0, Moderate = 1, and Severe = 2 is an example of what level of measurement?
   a. Nominal
   b. Ordinal

    c. Continuous (interval)

    d. Continuous (ratio)

5. A measure of central tendency (i.e., average) appropriate for data measured on the continuous scale is the:

    a. Mean

    b. Median

    c. Mode

6. The ____ is the value below which 50% of the observations occur.

    a. Mean

    b. Median

    c. Mode

7. The ____ is most appropriate for data on the nominal level of measurement.

    a. Mean

    b. Median

    c. Mode

8. The statistic that gives you an idea of the average distance from the mean value is the:

    a. Range

    b. Standard deviation

    c. Coefficient of variation

    d. z score

9. The statistic that is calculated as the largest value in a data set minus the smallest value is the:

    a. Range

    b. Standard deviation

    c. Coefficient of variation

    d. z score

10. If you wanted to compare the variability of two different measurements, you would use the:

    a. Range

    b. Standard deviation

    c. Coefficient of variation

    d. z score

You record the number of aerosol treatments given to patients on a particular floor. The resulting data were:

    2, 3, 6, 2, 4, 4, 4, 1

Use this set of data for Questions 11–15.

11. What is the mean for this set of data?

    a. 3.3

    b. 3.5

    c. 4.0

    d. 5.0

    e. 1.6

12. What is the median?

    a. 3.3

    b. 3.5

    c. 4.0

    d. 5.0

    e. 1.6

13. What is the mode?

    a. 3.3

    b. 3.5

    c. 4.0

    d. 5.0

    e. 1.6

14. What is the range?

    a. 3.3

    b. 3.5

    c. 4.0

    d. 5.0

    e. 1.6

15. What is the standard deviation?

    a. 3.3

    b. 3.5

    c. 4.0

    d. 5.0

    e. 1.6

16. The mean $\pm$two standard deviations encompasses what percentage of observations?

    a. 68%

    b. 95%

    c. 99.7%

    d. 100%

17. The difference between a confidence interval and an error interval is:

    a. A confidence interval says something about a group of measurements, while an error interval says something about individual measurements.

    b. An error interval for a measurement is always smaller than its confidence interval.

    c. Confidence intervals are more useful for interpreting bedside measurements like blood gases.

    d. Error intervals are used to test the hypothesis that two mean values are equal.

18. Which error interval is used when the data are composed of the differences between measured and known values?

    a. Tolerance interval

    b. Inaccuracy interval

    c. Agreement interval

19. Which error interval is used to describe the range of values we might expect to find with repeated measurements of a blood gas control solution?
    a. Tolerance interval
    b. Inaccuracy interval
    c. Agreement interval
20. Which error interval is used to compare measurements from two devices when the true value is unknown?
    a. Tolerance interval
    b. Inaccuracy interval
    c. Agreement interval
21. A Type I error occurs when you:
    a. Accept the null hypothesis when it is true.
    b. Accept the null hypothesis when it is false.
    c. Reject the null hypothesis when it is true.
    d. Reject the null hypothesis when it is false.
22. A Type II error occurs when you:
    a. Accept the null hypothesis when it is true.
    b. Accept the null hypothesis when it is false.
    c. Reject the null hypothesis when it is true.
    d. Reject the null hypothesis when it is false.
23. You perform an experiment comparing the effects of two different modes of ventilation on the mean airway pressure. The mean of one group of patients was 12.1 cm H_2O, while that of the other was 12.4 cm H_2O. The p value was 0.04. You would most appropriately conclude:
    a. The mean difference in pressure was 0.1 cm H_2O.
    b. There is a statistically significant difference between the groups.
    c. There is no clinically important difference between the groups.
    d. All of the above.
24. Suppose in the example above the p value was 0.40 and the power to detect a difference of 2 cm H_2O was 0.50. Now what would you conclude?
    a. There is a 50% chance of making a Type I error.
    b. The p value indicates that there is no statistically significant difference, but the probability of being right in this conclusion is no better than tossing a coin.
    c. The difference is even more significant than before (Question 23).
    d. There is a clinically important difference.
25. In the example above (Question 24), what could you do to improve the power of the test?
    a. Increase the difference you want to detect to 4 cm H_2O.
    b. Increase the sample size.
    c. Both of the above.
    d. Neither of the above.
26. Matched groups, such as twins, are an example of:
    a. Natural pairing
    b. Artificial pairing
    c. Self-pairing

27. When each experimental subject acts as his or her own control, the matching is called:
   a. Natural pairing
   b. Artificial pairing
   c. Self-pairing
28. When pairs of experimental subjects are matched on as many confounding variables as possible, it is called:
   a. Natural pairing
   b. Artificial pairing
   c. Self-pairing
29. List all contraindications, adverse effects, unexpected results, and confounding variables.

Reference

1. Adapted from: van Belle G, Millard SP. 1998. *STRUTS: Statistical Rules of Thumb.* Seattle: University of Washington.

CHAPTER 11

Statistical Methods for Nominal Measures

D ata on the nominal level of measurement consist of named categories without any particular order to them. Numbers are used here to name or distinguish the categories and are purely arbitrary. Nominal measures are usually summarized in terms of percentages, proportions, ratios, and rates. Proportions and percentages are also applicable to ordinal data. Usually, the first step in describing the data is to create a contingency table.

Describing the Data

Contingency table: A contingency table is used to display counts or frequencies of two or more nominal variables. For example, a simple 3×2 (rows by columns) contingency table of treatment outcomes might look like **Table 11.1**.

Proportion: A proportion is the number of objects of a particular type (such as with a disease) divided by the total number of objects in the group:

$$proportion = \frac{number\ of\ objects\ of\ particular\ type}{total\ number\ of\ objects\ in\ group}$$

Table 11.1

Data Arranged in a Contingency Table

Outcome	Treated	Not Treated	Total
Improved	10	1	11
Worsened	2	15	17
No change	1	2	3
Total	13	18	

For example, if 10 people improved out of a group of 13 people treated, the proportion improved would be 10/13 = 0.77. Thus, a proportion is defined as a part divided by a whole. It is a special case of the mean, where objects are given values of 0 (e.g., for "death") and 1 (e.g., for "lived"). Then the numerator of the equation for the mean is the sum of the 1s and 0s, while the denominator is the count of all 1s and 0s.

Percentage: A percentage is a proportion multiplied by 100%:

$$percentage = \frac{number\ of\ objects\ of\ particular\ type}{total\ number\ of\ objects\ in\ group} \times 100\%$$

For example, if 15 people got worse out of a group of 18 people who were not treated, the percentage that got worse would be (15/18) × 100% = 83%.

Ratio: A ratio is the number of objects in a group with a particular characteristic of interest (e.g., died) divided by the number of objects in the same group without the characteristic (e.g., did not die):

$$ratio = \frac{number\ of\ objects\ with\ characteristic}{number\ of\ objects\ without\ characteristic}$$

For example, if a survey of 31 people with a particular disease showed that 13 were treated and 18 were not treated, the ratio would be 13/(31 − 13) = 13/18 = 0.72.

Odds: A ratio of the probabilities of the two possible states of a binary event.

$$odds = \frac{probability\ of\ event\ occurring}{probability\ of\ event\ not\ occurring}$$

For example, the odds of randomly selecting an ace out of a deck of cards is (number of aces)/(number of remaining cards) = 4/48 = 1/12.

Rate: Strictly speaking, a rate is the number of objects (or quantity of something) occurring per unit of time. However, in statistics, a rate is often defined as:

$$rate = \frac{number\ of\ events\ in\ a\ specified\ period}{total\ number\ of\ events\ in\ specified\ period} \times base$$

where the base is a number used to convert the rate to a conveniently large whole number. For example, if the proportion of deaths in a study was 10/50 and this result was to be related to the whole population, then an appropriate rate might be (10/50) × 1,000 = 200 deaths per 1,000 patients or, equivalently, 2,000 deaths per 10,000 patients.

Characteristics of a Diagnostic Test

Perhaps the most common source of nominal data is diagnostic testing. The underlying measurements are often at the continuous level of measurement (such as blood gases), but they are used to classify patients as having or not having a condition of interest (like respiratory failure). Given that the condition of interest is either present or absent, and the diagnostic test is either positive (condition is present) or negative (condition is absent), four distinct outcomes are possible (**Table 11.2**).

For example, consider a simple bedside screening procedure to predict a patient's ability to be weaned from mechanical ventilation. To date, the procedure most successful at prediction is based on the rapid/shallow breathing index (RSBI). This index is the ratio of a patient's breathing frequency divided by the tidal volume while breathing spontaneously during a short discontinuation of mechanical ventilation. A ratio of 0.64 has been shown to accurately predict successful continuation of spontaneous breathing without the ventilator for adults.

Suppose you wanted to repeat this study in children to determine if the same cutoff value applies. In addition, you also want to evaluate another index, the CROP index, which is composed of measures for lung compliance, inspiratory pressure, oxygenation, and respiratory rate. Ultimately, you want to know which index is more useful and what the cutoff value is.

The experimental data are given in **Table 11.3**. Notice how data on the continuous level of measurement (RSBI and CROP) have been simplified to the nominal level of

Table 11.2

Characteristics of a Predictive Test

Confirmed Condition

Test Result	Present	Absent
Positive	*a* True positive	*b* False positive
Negative	*c* False negative	*d* True negative

Note: True positive means test is positive and condition is present; *false positive* means test is positive but condition is absent; *false negative* means test is negative but condition is present; *true negative* means test is negative and condition is absent.

Table 11.3

Data for Experiment to Compare Weaning Indicators

Outcome	RSBI	CROP	Outcome	RSBI	CROP
Success	12.0	0.36	Failure	17.2	0.05
Success	10.1	0.50	Failure	16.7	0.06
Success	9.1	0.52	Failure	13.5	0.13
Success	7.2	0.43	Failure	12.4	0.07
Success	6.3	0.19	Failure	11.6	0.03
Success	5.8	0.48	Failure	9.1	0.04
Success	5.2	0.15	Failure	15.1	0.09
Success	2.4	0.08	Failure	15.0	0.06
Success	3.2	0.45	Failure	11.5	0.08

Abbreviations: RSBI, rapid/shallow breathing index; CROP, index using compliance, respiratory rate, oxygenation index, and inspiratory pressure.

measurement (success or failure) so that we can use the statistical techniques designed for diagnostic tests.

The next step is to look at the data graphically. We are trying to decide if there is a natural grouping of scores that would discriminate between weaning success and failure.

What we would like is a specific cutoff value for the RSBI such that any time we observe a patient with a higher value, we will conclude that weaning would fail and thus we will continue mechanical ventilation. We would like the same type of cutoff value for the CROP index, but here a high value indicates success. Unfortunately, the plots show that there are no values of RSBI or CROP that perfectly discriminate between success and failure. Therefore, we try to select cutoff values that minimize the false-positive and false-negative decisions. A false-positive decision means that we predict success but the patient fails. A false negative means we predict failure but the patient could really have succeeded if given the chance. We can select the cutoff values mathematically, but we will not go into that here. Assume that the dotted lines in **Figure 11.1** are the cutoff values for RSBI and CROP, either based on these data or obtained from some other set of data. Now we would like to know how accurate our predictions will be if we use these values to evaluate patients in the future. We evaluate this by converting the data in Table 11.3 into a table that looks like Table 11.2 using the cutoff values in Figure 11.1. This is shown in **Table 11.4**.

Figure 11.1

Graphic representation of data in Table 11.1.

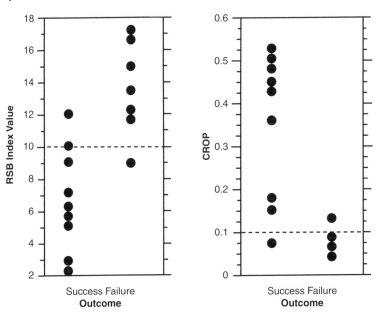

The dotted lines indicate cutoff values that maximize both sensitivity and specificity. For RSBI, values below 10 predict weaning success. For CROP, values above 0.10 predict weaning success.

Table 11.4

Calculating the Characteristics of the Rapid/Shallow Breathing Index (RSBI) Using the Data from Table 11.1 and the Cutoff Values from Figure 11.1

		Weaning Outcome	
		Success	**Failure**
Index Prediction	Success (positive)	7	1
	Failure (negative)	2	8

True- and False-Positive Rates

The true-positive rate is the probability that a test will be positive when the condition of interest (e.g., ability to wean successfully in our example, or for a lab test, disease) is present. The true-positive rate is the same as *sensitivity*. From Table 11.2:

$$\text{true-positive rate} = a/(a + c) = 7/9 = 0.78 = 78\%$$

Therefore, out of 100 patients who are weaned successfully, 78 will have an RSBI score predicting success.

The false-positive rate is the number of false-positive results expressed as a percentage of all positive results. From Table 11.4:

$$\text{false-positive rate} = b/(a + b) = 1/8 = 0.13 = 13\%$$

True- and False-Negative Rates

The true-negative rate is the probability that the test will be negative when the condition of interest is absent. The true-negative rate is the same as *specificity*. From Table 11.2:

$$\text{true-negative rate} = d/(b + d) = 8/9 = 0.89 = 89\%$$

This means that out of 100 patients who failed to wean, 89 will have an RSBI score predicting failure.

The false-negative rate is the number of false-negative results expressed as a percentage of all negative results. From Table 11.4:

$$\text{false-negative rate} = c/(c + d) = 2/10 = 0.20 = 20\%$$

Sensitivity and Specificity

Sensitivity is the ability of a test to correctly identify patients with the condition of interest (e.g., ability to breathe spontaneously in our example, or for a lab test, disease). Sensitivity answers the question "If the patient has the condition, how likely is she to have a positive test?" To remember this concept, think *sensitive to disease.* A highly sensitive test is a good *screening* test because it identifies most of the people who have the condition and only a few who do not. From Table 11.4:

$$\text{sensitivity} = a/(a + c) = 7/9 = 0.78 = 78\%$$

This means that out of 100 patients who are weaned successfully, 78 will have an RSBI score predicting success.

Specificity is the ability of a test to correctly identify patients who do not have the condition of interest. Specificity answers the question "If the patient does not have the condition, how likely is she to have a negative test?" To remember this concept, think *specific to health.* A highly specific test is a good *diagnostic* test because it identifies most of the people who do not have the condition and only a few who do. From Table 11.4:

$$\text{specificity} = d/(b + d) = 8/9 = 0.89 = 89\%$$

This means that out of 100 patients who failed to wean, 89 will have an RSBI score predicting failure.

Sensitivity and specificity are not affected by the *prevalence* of the condition of interest. Prevalence is the proportion of the population affected by the condition.

The selection of a cutoff value often involves a tradeoff between sensitivity and specificity, as seen in Figure 11.1. For example, suppose we decide that leaving a patient on the ventilator a little longer than necessary is better than having them fail weaning and be reintubated. We might adjust the cutoff value so that false positives are eliminated. For RSBI, we might select a cutoff value of 8 instead of 10. Now the sensitivity is lower (67%) but the specificity is higher (100%). We have just made the RSBI a less useful tool for screening patients who should undergo a weaning trial but a better instrument for predicting failure.

Positive and Negative Predictive Value

The positive predictive value of a test (or predictive value of a positive test) is the probability that the condition of interest is present when the test is positive. From Table 11.4:

$$\text{positive predictive value} = a/(a + b) = 7/8 = 0.88 = 88\%$$

Therefore, out of 100 patients who have an RSBI score predicting success, 88 will likely be weaned.

The negative predictive value of a test (or predictive value of a negative test) is the probability that the condition of interest is absent when the test is negative. From Table 11.4:

$$\text{negative predictive value} = d/(c + d) = 8/10 = 0.80 = 80\%$$

Out of 100 patients with an RSBI score predicting failure, 80 will likely fail the weaning attempt.

Unlike sensitivity and specificity, predictive values are affected by the prevalence of the condition of interest. For example, if the number of people who successfully weaned in Table 11.4 doubled, the positive predictive value would increase:

$$\text{positive predictive value} = a/(a + b) = 14/(14 + 1) = 0.93 = 93\%$$

and the negative predictive value would decrease:

$$\text{negative predictive value} = d/(c + d) = 8/(8 + 4) = 0.67 = 67\%$$

Diagnostic Accuracy

The diagnostic accuracy of a test is the proportion of correct results out of all results:

$$\text{diagnostic accuracy} = (\text{true positives} + \text{true negatives})/\text{all results}$$

From Table 11.4:

$$\text{diagnostic accuracy} = (a + d)/(a + b + c + d) = 15/18 = 0.83 = 83\%$$

Likelihood Ratio

The likelihood ratio for a positive test combines sensitivity and specificity into a single number expressing the odds (probability that an event occurs divided by the probability that it does not occur) that the test result occurs in patients with the condition versus those without the condition. A major advantage of the likelihood ratio is that you have to remember only one number, the ratio, instead of two numbers, sensitivity and specificity. From Table 11.4, the likelihood ratio for a positive test is:

$$\text{likelihood ratio} = \text{sensitivity}/\text{false positive rate} = 0.78/0.13 = 6.0$$

We conclude that a positive test result is six times more likely to occur in patients who successfully weaned than in patients who failed.

Receiver Operating Characteristic (ROC) Curve

As discussed earlier, there is usually a tradeoff between the sensitivity and specificity of a diagnostic or screening test, depending on what value we select for the cutoff. Therefore, a graph that illustrates this relationship would be helpful. Furthermore, we may want to compare two diagnostic tests to see which would be most useful. The receiver operating characteristic (ROC) curve is a device that fills these needs. ROC curves were developed in the communications field as a way to display signal-to-noise ratios (hence the term "receiver," as in radio receiver). For a diagnostic test, the true positives could be considered the "signal" and the false positives the "noise." The ROC is a plot of the true-positive rate against the false-positive rate for a test over a range of possible cutoff values (**Figure 11.2**). The line of identity (diagonal line) corresponds to a test that is either positive or negative by chance alone. That is, the probability of a true positive is equal to the probability of a false positive. In this case, a coin toss would be easier and just as accurate as the test in calculating the index. Plotted values that lie above the line of identity indicate a diagnostic test is whose predictive ability is better than tossing a coin, while values below the line indicate a test that is worse.

The closer the ROC curve is to the upper left-hand corner of the graph (true positive = 100%, false positive = 0%), the more accurate the diagnostic test is. As the cutoff value for the test becomes more stringent (more evidence is required for a positive test), the point on the curve corresponding to the sensitivity and specificity moves down and to the left (lower sensitivity, higher specificity). Note that the false positive rate equals one minus the specificity. If less evidence is required for a positive test, the point on the curve corresponding to sensitivity and specificity moves up and to the right (higher sensitivity, lower specificity). The cutoff value that results in the curve coming closest to the upper left-hand corner maximizes both sensitivity and specificity.

Plotting the ROC curves for two diagnostic tests together gives us an easy graphical method to decide which is better. The curve with the most area under it will lie closest to the

Figure 11.2

Receiver operating characteristic curves for two weaning tests, the RSBI and the CROP index.

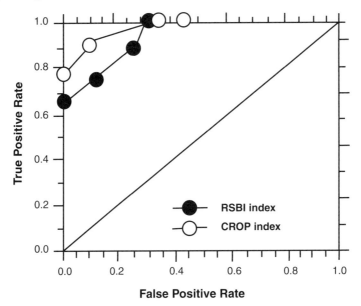

False Positive Rate

The CROP is a better test because there is more area under its curve compared with the RSBI curve.

upper left-hand corner over the range of cutoff values and indicates the more accurate test. The area under a the curve for a perfect test is 1.0, while the area for a test that is no better than tossing a coin is 0.5. In **Figure 11.3**, we see that the CROP index is a more accurate predictor of weaning success than the RSBI for our simulated experiment (see page 197).

Correlation

As discussed in Chapter 10, correlation means that the values of one variable go up or down with the values of another variable (for example, age is correlated with height). But nominal variables are not "higher" or "lower" when compared; they are just different. Therefore, the idea of association relates to frequencies in categories.

A common issue with diagnostic tests that generate nominal data is the need to establish the *reliability* of the test. If the test is repeated, we want to evaluate the agreement between results; high agreement means high reliability. If one person measures the same variable twice and the measurements are compared, an index of within-observer variability is called an *intra-rater reliability* index. When two or more people measure the same variable and their measurements are compared, an index of between-observer variability is called an *inter-rater reliability* index. Two examples of reliability indexes are the kappa and phi coefficients.

Kappa

Frequently in medicine, clinicians must interpret test results as indicating or not indicating disease or abnormality. The outcome is either yes or no, a nominal measure. Suppose we want to evaluate the inter-rater reliability of two physicians who have reviewed a set of 100 pulmonary function tests. From **Table 11.5**, we can begin to describe the agreement between physicians as:

$$\text{observed agreement} = \frac{a+d}{a+b+c+d} = \frac{75}{100} = 0.75 \ or \ 75\%$$

Table 11.5

Example Data Analysis for Assessing Agreement Between Two Observers

	Physician 2	
Physician 1	**Abnormal**	**Normal**
Abnormal	*a* 20	*b* 15	35
Normal	*c* 10	*d* 55	65
	30	70	

However, 75% is an overestimate because some agreement will occur by chance. The index corrected for chance is called kappa (κ):

$$\kappa = \frac{\text{observed agreement} - \text{chance agreement}}{1 - \text{chance agreement}}$$

where

$$\text{chance agreement} = \frac{(a+b)(a+c)}{a+b+c+d} + \frac{(c+d)(b+d)}{a+b+c+d}$$

Use **Table 11.6** as a guide to interpretation.

Although kappa is widely used in the literature, it has a limitation: as two observers classify an increasingly higher proportion of patients in one category or the other (such as normal or abnormal), the agreement by chance increases. Thus, kappa will increase even if the way raters interpret diagnostic tests does not change. One solution is to use another index, called *phi*.

Phi

Phi (Φ, rhymes with pie) is an index of agreement independent of chance. Thus, you will get similar values for phi whether the distribution of results is 50% positive and 50% negative or whether it is 90% positive and 10% negative, which is not true for kappa. Also, phi allows testing of significant differences between raters, which kappa does not. Again using the data from Table 11.5, phi is calculated as follows:

$$\Phi = \frac{ad - bc}{\sqrt{(a+b)(c+d)(a+c)(b+d)}}$$

Values for phi range from -1.0 (representing extreme disagreement) through 0.0 (chance agreement) to $+1.0$ (representing extreme agreement).

Table 11.6

Guide to Interpreting Values of Kappa

Value of Kappa (κ)	Strength of Agreement
< 0	Poor
0–0.20	Slight
0.21–0.40	Fair
0.41–0.60	Moderate
0.61–0.80	Substantial
0.81–1.0	Almost perfect

Comparing a Single Sample with a Population

Binomial Test

When comparing a proportion (or rate, or percentage) obtained from a single sample to a proportion from a known population, the problem is to decide if the sample proportion is unlikely to have occurred or not. As described in the chapter on basic statistics (in the discussion of hypothesis testing), we would get different outcomes every time we repeat the experiment. Some proportions may be higher, some lower, due to chance. Because our outcome variable is nominal, the possible proportions can only be whole numbers (2 out of 10, or 20%; we would never get a fractional outcome like 2.5 out of 10, or 20.5%). Because the outcomes are discrete numbers, the sampling distribution is discrete. For example, suppose you toss a coin 10 times as an experiment. After 10 tosses, you count the number of heads you got. If you repeat the experiment you will likely get a different number. If you repeated this experiment an infinite number of times and plotted the probability of each outcome, you would have a distribution similar to that shown in Figure 11.3. This distribution is called a binomial distribution because the outcome can be only one of two possible types (or numbers; head or tails, one or zero).

Let's apply this distribution to a clinical situation. Suppose that you wanted to test the hypothesis that patients with acute respiratory distress syndrome (ARDS) have a different survival rate in your ICU than the national average, say 50%. The null hypothesis is that an

Figure 11.3

Binomial distribution showing the probability of getting various numbers of heads in 10 coin tosses.

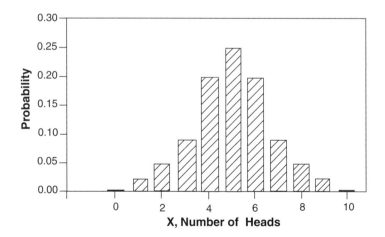

This assumes the probability of getting heads on a single toss is 0.50.

observed proportion from a sample of patients is equal to the assumed population proportion of 0.50. You obtain a sample of 10 patients, 9 of whom survived.

As we discussed in the section on hypothesis testing, you need to decide if your observed proportion of 9/10 falls within the rejection regions on the distribution. In other words, would sample proportions of equal or greater difference from 50% be unlikely (have probability less than α or 5%)? We do not know beforehand if the sample proportion will be higher or lower than the population proportion, so we have a two-tailed rejection region. This example happens to correspond to Figure 11.3. Thus, we want to know the combined probability of observed patient proportions of 9/10, 10/10 on the right tail plus proportions or 1/10 and 0/10 in the left tail. If this total probability is less than 0.05, we reject the null hypothesis and conclude that our sample came from a population with a true probability of survival different from 50%.

The probability in the left tail is calculated using the Microsoft Excel spreadsheet equation =BINOMDIST(successes, sample size, hypothesized proportion, true). This equation gives the cumulative probability for the distribution up to the proportion indicated by the number of successes in the sample (the value "true" tells the equation you want the cumulative probability). So, for our example we enter the equation

$$=BINOMDIST(1,10,0.5,true)$$

and receive the answer 0.011. The probability in the right tail is 1 minus the cumulative probability up to a proportion of 8/10. Thus we enter the equation

$$=1\text{-}BINOMDIST(8,10,0.5,true),$$

which gives the value of 0.011. Notice that because the distribution in this example is symmetrical, the area in the left tail is the same as the area in the right tail, and we could have simply done one spreadsheet calculation and multiplied by 2. But the distribution is symmetrical only when the hypothesized proportion is 0.50.

The total area in the rejection regions is $0.011 + 0.011 = 0.022$. This means that the probability of observing sample proportions as far away from the hypothesized population proportion as our sample is about 2.2%. Because we have set the significance level at $\alpha = 0.05$, or 5%, a p value from the hypothesis test ≤ 0.05 will indicate a significant difference. Therefore, we conclude that there is a significant difference between the survival rate in our ICU and that of the national average. In fact, we conclude that our survival rate is higher.

z Test

The binomial distribution approaches the normal distribution as the sample size gets larger. When the sample size is large enough, we can use a z test with the normal distribution to simplify the calculations. The statistic is calculated as:

$$z = \frac{p - p_0}{\sqrt{\dfrac{p_0(1 - p_0)}{n}}}$$

where p is the sample proportion, p_0 is the hypothesized population proportion, and n is the sample size. The sample size is considered large enough to use the normal approximation of the binomial distribution when

$$n \times p_0 > 5 \text{ and } n \times (1 - p_0) > 5$$

Using our previous example, $n = 10$ and $p_0 = 0.50$, so $n \times p_0 = 5$ and $n \times (1 - p_0) = 5$, so we could not use the normal distribution. You can see that the larger n is, the more appropriate the approximation. Let's say our sample size was 20. Then

$$z = \frac{p - p_0}{\sqrt{\dfrac{p_0(1 - p_0)}{n}}} = \frac{0.9 - 0.5}{\sqrt{\dfrac{0.5(0.5)}{20}}} = \frac{0.4}{\sqrt{0.0125}} = \frac{0.4}{0.11} = 3.58$$

The cutoff values of z for a two-tailed test are ± 1.96. Because 3.58 is larger than $+1.96$, we reject the null hypothesis and conclude that a significant difference between the proportions is present. If the sample proportion had been 0.10, then z would be -3.58, which is less than -1.96, and again we would reject the null hypothesis.

The cutoff values for various significance levels (i.e., different values of α) can be calculated with the Microsoft® Excel spreadsheet equation =NORMSINV(probability), where probability is $1 - \alpha$ for a one tailed test and $1 - \alpha/2$ for a two-tailed test. For example, if the significance level is 0.05, and we want a two-tailed test, then $1 - \alpha/2 = 1 - 0.025 = 0.975$. Then NORMSINV(0.975) yields the value 1.96. A 95% confidence interval (CI) for a sample proportion is constructed using:

$$CI = \text{sample proportion} \pm 1.96 \times \text{standard error of proportion}$$

$$CI = p \pm 1.96 \sqrt{\frac{p(1 - p)}{n}}$$

If the sample proportion was 0.45 and the sample size was 30

$$CI = 0.45 \pm 1.96 \sqrt{\frac{0.45(1 - 0.45)}{30}} = 0.45 \pm 1.96 \sqrt{\frac{0.45 \times 0.55}{30}} = 0.45 \pm 0.18 = (27, 063)$$

which means we can be 95% confident that the interval between 0.27 and 0.63 contains the true proportion of patients who survive ARDS in our ICU.

Comparing Two Samples, Unmatched Data

Having unpaired data means that there are data from two independent groups of experimental objects, such as two different groups of patients. For example, instead of comparing the survival rate of ARDS patients in our ICU with a benchmark value, suppose we wanted to compare survival rates in two ICUs. From now on, hypothesis tests will be more complicated, so we will use statistical software instead of manual calculations. For most examples, we use Sigma-Plot (Systat Software, Inc.; www.sigmaplot.com).

Fisher Exact Test

The Fisher exact test is used for 2×2 contingency tables (which have exactly two rows and two columns).

Example

The contingency table for comparing survival rates in two ICUs might look like **Table 11.7**.

Null Hypothesis
There is no significant difference between the proportion of patients that lived (or died) in ICU A compared with ICU B.

Most statistical programs will let you enter the data in columns and rows either as tabulated data (a contingency table like above) or as raw data as in **Table 11.8**.

This latter format might be more convenient if you are transferring data from a spreadsheet with the actual experimental results. If we enter this example, we get a p value and possibly an interpretation as follows.

Report from Statistics Program
The proportion of observations in the different categories, which define the contingency table, is not significantly different than is expected from random occurrence ($p = 1.000$). Thus, we conclude that the survival rates in the two ICUs are not different.

Table 11.7

Sample Data for the Fisher Exact Test

Outcome	ICU A	ICU B
Lived	10	13
Died	2	4

Table 11.8

Sample Computer Data Entry Scheme

ICU A	lived
ICU A	died
ICU B	lived
ICU B	died
ICU A	died
etc.	etc.

Comparing Two or More Samples, Matched Data

Paired data result when patients act as their own controls or when two groups of patients are carefully matched for confounding factors like age, weight, sex, race, etc. When you are experimenting on pieces of identical equipment, obviously they are very well-matched.

McNemar Test

A McNemar test is an analysis of contingency tables that have repeated observations of the same individuals. The test is appropriate for

- Determining whether or not individuals responded to treatment
- Comparing results of two different treatments on the same people

Example

Suppose we wanted to test the acceptance of a new airway clearance technique among patients at your hospital with cystic fibrosis. We record the patients' impressions before and after trying the new treatment. The raw data are shown in **Table 11.9**. These data can be organized in a contingency table (**Table 11.10**).

A similar table would have been created if we had compared one form of airway clearance with another, with all patients getting both treatments (acting as their own controls). Remember that the McNemar test requires that the contingency table have exactly the same number of rows as columns (such as 2×2, 3×3).

Null Hypothesis
There is no significant difference between the paired proportions before and after treatment.

Table 11.9

Sample Data for McNemar Test

Before Treatment	After Treatment
approve	approve
approve	approve
approve	approve
approve	disapprove
disapprove	disapprove
disapprove	disapprove
disapprove	disapprove
disapprove	disapprove
disapprove	disapprove
disapprove	don't know
don't know	approve
don't know	disapprove
don't know	don't know

Table 11.10

Contingency Table for Data in Table 11.9

	After Treatment		
Before Treatment	**Approve**	**Disapprove**	**Don't Know**
Approve	3	1	0
Disapprove	0	5	1
Don't know	1	1	1

Report from Statistics Program

The proportion of observations in the different categories that define the contingency table is not significantly different than is expected from random occurrence ($p = 0.572$).

Thus, we conclude that patients' opinions did not change after trying the new treatment. This is not too surprising. Looking at the contingency table, we see that almost 70% of the patients (9/13) did not change their opinion after trying the treatment (3 approved, 5 disapproved, and 1 did not know).

Comparing Three or More Samples, Unmatched Data

Chi-Squared Test

The chi-squared test can be used for analyzing contingency tables that are larger than 2×2.

Example

Suppose we wanted to test the effectiveness of three different drugs (or three dosages of one drug). The contingency table is shown in **Table 11.11**.

Null Hypothesis

The proportions (effective/total or not effective/total) are all equal (or equivalently, there is no association between drug and effectiveness).

Table 11.11

Contingency Table for a Chi-Squared Test

Outcome	Drug A	Drug B	Drug C
Effective	11	6	3
Not effective	2	6	7

Report from Statistics Program

Power of performed test with alpha = 0.05: 0.671.

The power of the performed test (0.671) is below the desired power of 0.800.

You should interpret the negative findings cautiously. The proportions of observations in different columns of the contingency table vary from row to row. The two characteristics that define the contingency table are outcome and drug type, and they are significantly related ($p = 0.026$). Thus, we reject the hypothesis that the drugs had equal effectiveness. The data suggest that there is an association between the type of drug and effectiveness.

Questions

Definitions

Define the following terms:

• Contingency table
• Proportion
• Percentage
• Ratio
• Odds
• Rate
• Sensitivity
• Specificity
• Positive predictive ability
• Negative predictive ability
• Receiver operating characteristic (ROC) curve

True or False

1. The kappa and phi statistics are used to evaluate the strength of agreement between two sets of data, such as the diagnoses of two physicians.
2. The choice of the cutoff value has no effect on a diagnostic test's sensitivity or specificity.
3. When two diagnostic tests are compared with ROC curves, the one with the most area under its curve is the most accurate test.

Multiple Choice

1. Which test is most appropriate for comparing the percentage of accidental extubations in your hospital with that of a known benchmark percentage?
   a. Binomial test
   b. Fisher exact test
   c. McNemar test
   d. Chi-square test

2. Suppose you were comparing the percentage of patients who changed their opinions of a treatment before and after trying it. What would be the best test?
   a. Binomial test
   b. Fisher exact test
   c. McNemar test
   d. Chi-square test
3. If you wanted to compare the survival rates of three ICUs, what would be the most appropriate test?
   a. Binomial test
   b. Fisher exact test
   c. McNemar test
   d. Chi-square test
4. You want to compare the percentage of positive responses to therapy in two different groups of patients. What test is most appropriate?
   a. Binomial test
   b. Fisher exact test
   c. McNemar test
   d. Chi-square test

CHAPTER 12

Statistical Methods for Ordinal Measures

D ata on the ordinal level of measurement have discrete categories with a particular order to them. Numbers are used to indicate relative high and low values of a variable (e.g., a Likert-type scale). Like nominal measurements, ordinal measurements are often summarized in terms of percentages, proportions, ratios, and rates. When continuous measurements have extreme values or outliers, converting the data to the ordinal level (by sorting individual values by rank) often makes inferential tests more reliable.

Describing the Data

Usually, the first step in describing the data is to create a *contingency table*. Such a table is used to display counts or frequencies of two or more ordinal variables. The contingency table in **Table 12.1** was used in a study of retinopathy in premature infants. The number and the percentage of patients can be given for each of the five stages of retinopathy.

Calculation of a mean or average is not appropriate for ordinal data. These data are often displayed with bar graphs or pie charts.

Table 12.1

A Contingency Table for Displaying Ordinal Data

Retinopathy Stage	Patients	Percent
0	6	30
I	6	30
II	2	10
III	3	15
IV	3	15
Total	20	100

Correlation

Because ordinal data can be ranked according to their relative values, we can compare two sets of ordinal data to see if an increase (or decrease) in one variable corresponds to an increase (or decrease) in the other.

Spearman Rank Order Correlation

The Spearman rank order correlation coefficient (also called *Spearman's rho* or *rank correlation*) is a nonparametric test that does not require the data points to be linearly related with a normal distribution about the regression line with constant variance. This statistic does not require that variables be assigned as independent and dependent.

The value of rho can take values from −1 through 0 to +1. A value of −1 indicates that high ranks of one variable occur with low ranks of the other variable. A value of 0 indicates there is no correlation between variables. A value of +1 indicates that high ranks of one variable occur with high ranks of the other variable.

Use the Spearman rank order correlation when:

- You want to measure the strength of association between pairs of ordinal variables or between an ordinal variable and a continuous variable.
- You want to reduce the effect of extreme values on the correlation of data on the continuous level of measurement. The Pearson product-moment correlation coefficient is markedly influenced by extreme values and does not provide a good description of data that are skewed or that contain outliers. The solution is to transform the data into ranks (i.e., convert from continuous to ordinal scale) and then calculate the correlation.

Example

You suspect that Apgar scores are correlated with infants' birth weight. You collect the data in **Table 12.2** on a group of newborns.

Null Hypothesis
Weight (when converted to an ordinal scale) is not associated with Apgar score.

Table 12.2

Example Data for Calculating Spearman Rank Order Correlation Coefficient

Weight (grams)	Weight (rank)	Apgar Score
1,023	3	6
850	1	3
1,540	5	10
1,150	4	8
900	2	5

Report from Statistics Program
Correlation coefficient $= 0.900$; $p = 0.0833$.

Pairs of variables with positive correlation coefficients and p values below 0.050 tend to increase together. For pairs with negative correlation coefficients and p values below 0.050, one variable tends to decrease while the other increases. For pairs with p values greater than 0.050, no significant relationship exists between the two variables.

We must conclude that for this set of data, weight and Apgar score are not correlated. Even though the correlation coefficient (0.9) appears quite high, the p value tells us that it can be expected to occur by chance at least 8 out of 100 times. However, the p value of 0.0833 is not too much above the significance cutoff value of $p \leq 0.05$. This result should tell us that our experiment was a good pilot study. We are justified in collecting a larger sample that might yield positive results.

Comparing Two Samples, Unmatched Data

Mann-Whitney Rank Sum Test

This test is also called the *Mann-Whitney U test* or the *Wilcoxon rank sum test*. It is the non-parametric alternative to the unpaired t test. It tests the hypothesis that the medians of two different samples are the same.

Example

Your department has just implemented a respiratory therapy consult service. Using standardized assessment procedures, therapists assign triage scores to patients according to disease type and severity. You want to test the performance of a new supervisor (A) by comparing her assessment skills with those of a more experienced supervisor (B). Each supervisor assesses the same eight patients on a scale of 1 to 5 (**Table 12.3**).

Table 12.3

Example Data for Calculating the Mann-Whitney U Test

Supervisor A	Supervisor B
1	1
3	4
2	3
4	4
5	5
2	3
4	4
2	2

Null Hypothesis
There is no difference between these groups of triage scores; the two sets of data were not drawn from populations with different medians.

Report from Statistics Program
The difference in the median values of the two groups is not great enough to exclude the possibility that the difference is due to random sampling variability; there is not a statistically significant difference ($p = 0.442$).

Therefore, we conclude that the new supervisor's assessment skills are equivalent to those of the more experienced supervisor.

Comparing Two Samples, Matched Data

Wilcoxon Signed Rank Test

The Wilcoxon signed rank test is the nonparametric alternative to a paired *t* test. This test is appropriate when comparing treatments on the same individual or matched individuals.

Example

Your department has just completed a training program for therapists who will participate in a respiratory therapy consult service. The consult service employs standardized assessment procedures to assign triage scores to patients according to their disease type and severity. To test the effectiveness of the training program, you select a new therapist and ask him to assign triage scores (1 through 5) to a set of seven simulated patients before and after training (**Table 12.4**).

Null Hypothesis
There is no difference in the two groups of data.

Table 12.4

Example Data for Calculating the Wilcoxon Signed Rank Test

Before	After
4	1
5	2
3	3
5	4
3	2
4	2
4	3

Report from Statistics Program

The change that occurred with the treatment is greater than would be expected by chance; there is a statistically significant difference ($p = 0.031$).

We conclude that the training program resulted in learning (assuming that the "after" scores were closer to the ideal scores for the simulated patients). In fact, we can see that before training, the therapist tended to score the patients higher (missing signs of illness severity) than after the training.

Comparing Three or More Samples, Unmatched Data

Kruskal-Wallis ANOVA

Kruskal-Wallis ANOVA is the nonparametric alternative to the one-way (or one factor) analysis of variance (ANOVA). You would use it when you want to see if the groups are affected by a single factor. It tests the hypothesis that the groups are the same versus the hypothesis that at least one of the groups is different from the others.

Example

Your department has been trying to decide on the appropriate length of a training program for therapists who will participate in a respiratory therapy consult service. The consult service employs standardized assessment procedures to assign triage scores to patients according to disease type and severity. To test the effectiveness of different training program lengths, you select three groups of seven new therapists and grade their assessment skills (grade 0 through 5) on simulated patients after each of three training sessions (**Table 12.5**).

Null Hypothesis

All three sets of data came from the same population; there are no differences among the groups.

Table 12.5

Example Data for Kruskal-Wallis ANOVA

One Hour	Six Hours	12 Hours
0	1	4
5	4	5
2	3	3
3	4	4
2	5	5
4	3	3
3	4	4

Report from Statistics Program
The differences in the median values among the treatment groups are not great enough to exclude the possibility that the difference is due to random sampling variability; the difference is not statistically significant ($p = 0.211$).

You conclude that training therapists longer than one hour is a waste of time. Note that if the p value had been less than 0.05, we would be able to do pairwise comparisons among the three groups to see which were different (see "Report from Statistics Program" in the next section).

Comparing Three or More Samples, Matched Data

Friedman Repeated Measures ANOVA

The Friedman repeated measures ANOVA is the nonparametric alternative to a one-way repeated measures analysis of variance (ANOVA). Use this test when you want to see if a single group of individuals was affected by a series of three or more different experimental treatments, in which each individual received all treatments.

Example

You would like to see if a certain brand of incentive spirometer has any affect on patient compliance. You select a group of six postoperative surgical patients and have them try each of three different incentive spirometers. The patients rank their opinion numerically (0 = don't like, 1 = neutral, 2 = like). The data are entered as in **Table 12.6**.

Null Hypothesis
All three sets of data came from the same population; there are no differences among the groups.

Report from Statistics Program
The differences in the median values among the treatment groups are greater than would be expected by chance; there is a statistically significant difference ($p = 0.027$).

Table 12.6

Example Data for Friedman Repeated Measures ANOVA

Spirometer A	Spirometer B	Spirometer C
0	1	2
1	1	1
0	2	2
0	1	2
1	0	2
1	1	2

To isolate the group or groups that differ from the others, use a multiple comparison procedure. All pairwise multiple comparison procedures (Student-Newman-Keuls Method):

Comparison	$p < 0.05$
C vs. A	Yes
C vs. B	Yes
B vs. A	No

We conclude that the spirometers are not all the same in terms of patient preference. To find how they rank, the statistics program performed pairwise comparisons among the three spirometers. From that, we see that patients prefer spirometer C over A and C over B, but they had equal preference for B compared with A.

Questions

Multiple Choice

1. If you wanted to test the hypothesis that birth weight is associated with Apgar score you would use which test?
   a. Spearman rank order correlation
   b. Mann-Whitney rank sum test
   c. Wilcoxon signed rank test
   d. Kruskal-Wallis ANOVA
   e. Friedman repeated measures ANOVA
2. Suppose you want to compare the assessment skills of two supervisors, by each of them assigning triage scores for a set of simulated patients. What test would you use?
   a. Spearman rank order correlation
   b. Mann-Whitney rank sum test
   c. Wilcoxon signed rank test
   d. Kruskal-Wallis ANOVA
   e. Friedman repeated measures ANOVA
3. Suppose you wanted to determine the improvement in assessment skill for a single person after a training session. What test would you use to see if the person's set of triage scores for simulated patients was different pre- and post-training?
   a. Spearman rank order correlation
   b. Mann-Whitney rank sum test
   c. Wilcoxon signed rank test
   d. Kruskal-Wallis ANOVA
   e. Friedman repeated measures ANOVA
4. You want to determine the most appropriate length of treatment based on a post-treatment assessment score. Three groups of patients are treated for 10, 20, and 30 minutes, respectively. What procedure would you use to test the hypothesis that there was no difference in assessment scores among the three groups?
   a. Spearman rank order correlation
   b. Mann-Whitney rank sum test

c. Wilcoxon signed rank test

d. Kruskal-Wallis ANOVA

e. Friedman repeated measures ANOVA

5. You would like to see if the brand of incentive spirometer has any affect on patient compliance. You select a group of six postoperative surgical patients and have them try each of three different incentive spirometers. The patients rank their opinion numerically (0 = don't like, 1 = neutral, 2 = like). What procedure would you use to test the hypothesis that there was no difference in opinion scores among the three brands?

a. Spearman rank order correlation

b. Mann-Whitney rank sum test

c. Wilcoxon signed rank test

d. Kruskal-Wallis ANOVA

e. Friedman repeated measures ANOVA

CHAPTER 13

Statistical Methods for Continuous Measures

D ata on the continuous level of measurement can take on any value and include measurements on the interval and ratio levels (see Chapter 10). Most of the data we are familiar with are measured at the continuous level (such as pressure, volume, flow, weight, drug dosages, lab values, etc.). Compared with nominal and ordinal levels, data at the continuous level contain more information and allow the widest range of statistical procedures.

Testing for Normality

A key assumption of the tests in this section is that the sample data come from a population that is normally distributed. If the sample data are not normally distributed, you will have to use one of the nonparametric tests described for data measured at the nominal or ordinal level.

Kolmogorov-Smirnov Test

The Kolmogorov-Smirnov procedure tests whether the distribution of a continuous variable is the same for two groups. That is, it tests the null hypothesis that two distributions are the same under the assumption that the observations from the two distributions are independent of each other. It is calculated by comparing the two distributions at a number of points and then considering the maximum difference between the two distributions. This test is heavily influenced by the maximum value in a set of numbers and should be used with caution if outliers are suspected.

Example

You want to test the effect of prone positioning on the Pao_2 of patients in the ICU. Data are collected before and after positioning the patient and you intend to use a paired t test.

However, the first step should be to make sure the PaO_2 data are normally distributed. A statistics program like SigmaPlot (Systat Software, Inc.; www.sigmaplot.com) will perform this test automatically.

Null Hypothesis
The two distributions are the same.

Report from Statistics Program
Figure 13.1 shows a histogram of the data superimposed on a normal curve for visual comparison.

If the result of the K-S test is significant (i.e., $p < 0.05$), then the actual and ideal variables are probably not from the same distribution. A significant difference implies that the actual variable is not normally distributed, because the ideal variable is. In the example shown in Figure 13.1, the p value is > 0.999, which is > 0.05, so we do not reject the null hypothesis. We assume the PaO_2 values are normally distributed and can use the t test.

Testing for Equal Variances

Another key assumption of the tests in this section is that the data in two or more samples have equal variances. If the data do not meet this assumption, you will have to use one of the nonparametric tests described for data measured at the nominal or ordinal level.

F Ratio Test

A comparison of the variances of groups of measurements can be useful to validate the assumptions of t tests and for other purposes. The F test is calculated as the ratio of two sample variances and shows whether the variance of one group is smaller, larger, or equal to the variance of the other group.

Example

One of the pulmonary physicians in your hospital has questioned the accuracy of your lab's pulmonary function test results. Specifically, she questions whether the new lab technician you have hired (Tech A) can produce as consistent results as the other technician, who has years of experience (Tech B). You gather two sets of FEV_1 measurements on the same patient by the two techs. Since you are using only one patient, most of the variance in measurements will be due to the two technicians. You do not know what the "true" FEV_1 is, so you cannot determine which technician produces the most "accurate" results. You could determine an agreement interval to see how far apart individual measurements by the two technicians might be (see "Error Intervals" in Chapter 10). However, you are really more concerned about how much the two technicians' results vary in general. Because variance (the average squared deviation from

Figure 13.1

Kolmogorov-Smirnoff test of normality.

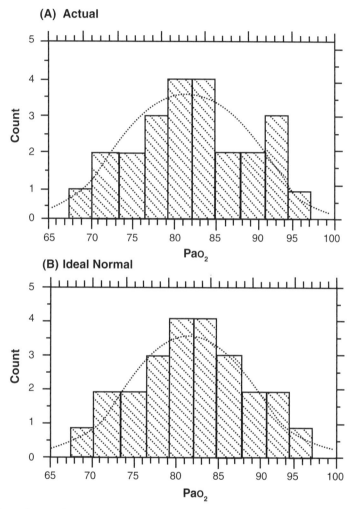

(A) Actual

(B) Ideal Normal

The top graph shows the actual sample data; the bottom graph shows ideal normal values from a normal distribution with the same mean and standard deviation as the sample. The normal curve is superimposed for visual comparison. The *p* value is > 0.999, which leads us to believe that there is no significant difference between the distributions. Therefore, the sample data are normally distributed.

the mean) represents random measurement error, you use the *F* test to compare the ability of the two techs to produce the same level of measurement accuracy. You enter the data into the statistics program as two columns of FEV_1 measurements (**Table 13.1**).

Table 13.1

Data Entry for an *F* Ratio Test

Tech A	Tech B
1.06	0.98
1.23	1.24
0.98	0.91
1.29	1.26
etc.	etc.

Null Hypothesis

The variances of the two groups of data are the same.

Report from the Statistics Program

The *p* value is less than 0.05, so we reject the null hypothesis and conclude that the variances are not equal.

From **Table 13.2** we can see that the variance of measurements made by Tech A (0.143) is much greater than the variance of measurements made by Tech B (0.033). We conclude that there may be something about the new technician's performance that is resulting in less consistent results than that of the more experienced technician.

Correlation and Regression

The concept of correlation implies that two variables co-vary; that is, a change in variable *x* is associated with a change in variable *y*. Another basic assumption of this section is that the association between the two variables is linear. Once we have established that there is an association, we can use a given value of one to predict the associated value of the other. For example, we can predict normal breathing frequency based on a person's age. This type of

Table 13.2

Results of *F* Ratio Test

	Variance Ratio	*F* Value	*p* Value	95% Lower	95% Upper
Tech A	0.232	0.232	0.0002	0.110	0.488
Tech B					

	Count	Mean	Variance	Standard Deviation	Standard Error
Tech A	30	1.206	0.143	0.378	0.069
Tech B	30	1.173	0.033	0.182	0.033

prediction can be extended to more than two variables, such as the prediction of pulmonary function values based on height, weight, and age. Correlation and regression are also described in Chapter 10.

Pearson Product-Moment Correlation Coefficient

The most common correlation coefficient with a continuous variable measurable on an interval level is the Pearson product-moment correlation coefficient (Pearson r). The Pearson r statistic ranges in value from -1.0 (perfect negative correlation) through 0 (no correlation) to $+1.0$ (perfect positive correlation).

Example

You decide to evaluate a device called the EzPAP for lung expansion therapy. It generates a continuous airway pressure proportional to the flow introduced at its inlet port. However, the user's manual does not say how the set flow is related to resultant airway pressure, and we generally use the device without a pressure gauge attached. You connect a flowmeter and pressure gauge to the device and record the pressures (in cm H_2O) as you adjust the gas flow (in L/min) over a wide range. You enter the data into a statistics program (see **Table 13.3**) and calculate the Pearson r.

Null Hypothesis
The two variables have no significant linear association.

Report from Statistics Program
Correlation coefficient: 0.942.

The p value is less than 0.001. The p value is from a test of the null hypothesis to see if the correlation coefficient is significantly different from 0. The p value is the probability of being wrong in concluding that there is a true association between the variables.

Pairs of variables with positive correlation coefficients and p values below 0.050 tend to increase together. For the pairs with negative correlation coefficients and p values below 0.050,

Table 13.3

Data Entry for Calculating the Correlation Coefficient

Flow	Pressure
3	5
4	5
5	6
6	7
etc.	etc.

one variable tends to decrease while the other increases. For pairs with p values greater than 0.050, no significant relationship exists between the two variables.

We conclude that a high degree of linear correlation exists between pressure and flow. This finding will allow us to predict how much flow we must set to get a desired level of airway pressure. To do that, we perform a simple linear regression.

Simple Linear Regression

A simple regression uses the values of one independent variable (x) to predict the value of a dependent variable (y). Regression analysis fits a straight line to a plot of the data. The equation for the line has the form $y = b_0 + b_1 x$, where y is the dependent variable, x is the independent variable, b_0 is the y-intercept (point where the line crosses the Y-axis on the plot), and b_1 is the slope of the line ($\Delta y / \Delta x$).

Example

Using the data table from the EzPAP experiment above, we perform a simple linear regression. The purpose of the experiment is to allow us to predict the amount of flow required for a desired level of pressure. Therefore, we designate pressure as the (known) independent variable and flow as the dependent variable. In other words, the amount of flow we will set on the flowmeter connected to the EzPAP will depend on how much airway pressure we want the patient to receive.

Report from Statistics Program
Refer to **Figure 13.2**.

Normality test: Passed ($p = 0.511$)
Constant variance test: Passed ($p = 0.214$)

	Coefficient	**p**
Y-intercept	1.045	0.021
Pressure	0.653	<0.001
R^2: 0.89		

Standard error of estimate: 1.482

The statistics program tested the two underlying hypotheses that (1) the data are normally distributed and (2) the two samples have equal variances. Both tests passed as indicated. The p values for the y-intercept and the slope indicate that they are both significantly different from 0. In other words, a significant correlation exists between pressure and flow.

The r^2 value (symbolized in Figure 13.2) is called the coefficient of determination (the square of the correlation coefficient; see Chapter 10). The value of 0.89 means that 89% of the variation in flow is due to the variation in pressure, as we would guess from the obvious linear association and the high correlation coefficient. Only 11% of the variation in flow is due to

Figure 13.2

Results of linear regression analysis.

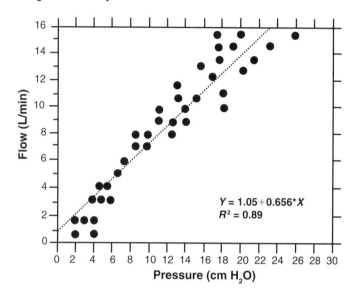

$Y = 1.05 + 0.656 * X$
$R^2 = 0.89$

random measurement error or nonlinearity in the relationship. Consequently, we can have a high degree of confidence in the accuracy of our predictions.

The differences between the measured values of *y* (in this case, flow) and those predicted by the regression equation are called *residuals*. Because the value predicted by the regression equation is the estimated mean value of repeated measurements and hence the best estimate of the true value of *x*, the residuals represent the random errors of measurement. The standard deviation of the residuals is called the *standard error of the estimate*. It is an estimate of the standard deviation of repeated measurements of *y* at any specific value of *x* and is thus an estimate of the imprecision of the measured values.

The regression equation says that the required flow (*y*) can be predicted by multiplying the desired pressure (*x*) by 0.65 (liters per minute per centimeter of water pressure) and adding 1.05 (liters per minute). To simplify the calculation, you round the numbers and inform the other therapists that they can get the required flow by multiplying the desired pressure by 0.7 and adding 1.

Multiple Linear Regression

Simple linear regression can be extended to cases where more than one independent (predictor) variable is present. When the independent variables are varied, they produce a corresponding value for the dependent (response) variable. If you are not sure if all independent variables should be used in the model, use *stepwise multiple linear regression* to identify the important independent variables from the set of possible variables. If the relationship does not fit a straight line or plane, use *polynomial* or *nonlinear* regression.

Multiple linear regression assumes an association between one dependent variable and an arbitrary number (symbolized by k) of independent variables. The general equation is:

$$y = b_0 + b_1x_1 + b_2x_2 + b_3x_3 + \ldots + b_kx_k$$

where y is the dependent variable, x_1, x_2, x_3,. . . x_k are the k independent variables, and b_0, b_1, b_2,. . . bk are the k regression coefficients. As the values of x vary, the value of y either increases or decreases depending on the sign of the associated regression coefficient b. An example of this would be the use of an equation to predict a pulmonary function value, like functional residual capacity, based on the patient's height and age.

Logistic Regression

Logistic regression is designed for predicting a qualitative dependent variable, such as presence or absence of disease, from observations of one or more independent variables. The qualitative dependent variable must be nominal and dichotomous (take only two possible values such as lived or died, presence or absence, etc.), represented by values of 0 and 1. The independent variables can be continuous, ordinal, or nominal. Independent ordinal variables can have names or be coded as 0 = absence, 1 = level 1, 2 = level 2, etc. (this coding is helpful when calculating P; see below). Like linear regression, logistic regression can be simple (one independent variable) or multiple (many independent variables). The general logistic regression model is as follows:

$$P = \frac{e^y}{1+e^y}$$

where $y = b_0 + b_1x_1 + b_2x_2 + b_3x_3 + \ldots + b_kx_k$. P is interpreted to mean the probability of the dependent event happening given the specific values of the independent variables (not to be confused with the p from hypothesis testing). The predictors, x_1, x_2, x_3,. . . x_k are the k independent variables, b_0, b_1, b_2,. . . b_k are the k regression coefficients, and e is the base of the natural logarithms (approximately equal to 2.718).

We can use the regression coefficients in two ways. One way is to use them with specific values for the independent variables in the above equation to calculate a value of P. The other way is to use the coefficients to calculate odds ratios. When P is small for all values of x, the *odds ratio* is approximately equal to the *relative risk*. For example, the relative risk of 10 in a smoking/lung cancer study would indicate that subjects who smoke are 10 times more likely to develop lung cancer than subjects who do not smoke.

Example

You conduct a study comparing two types of continuous positive airway pressure (CPAP) in premature infants. The dependent variable is the occurrence of complications such as nasal septum breakdown, deformation of the nares, or bleeding. The independent variables you think may influence the occurrence of complications include the type of CPAP delivery system, the CPAP fixation cap size, the duration of treatment, the infant's gestational age, and its birth weight. You enter the data into the statistics program as shown in **Table 13.4**.

Table 13.4

Data Entry for Multiple Linear Regression Analysis

Complication Present	CPAP Type	Wrong Cap	Duration (Days)	Age (Wks)	Weight (gms)
0	conv	yes	0.84	28	1084
0	fluidic	yes	0.52	28	1287
1	conv	no	1.30	32	1749
0	conv	yes	5.20	28	1002
1	fluidic	no	5.40	28	713
etc.	etc.	etc.	etc.	etc.	etc.

In Table 13.4, a value of 1 for *Complication Present* means that a complication was observed, while a value of 0 means there were no complications observed (remember that the dependent variable must be dichotomous). The types of CPAP compared were conventional and fluidic. The CPAP nasal prongs are secured by ties to a cotton cap on the infant's head. These caps come in several sizes; this variable could have been coded such that 1 means the wrong cap size was selected, 0 means the right size was selected. The wrong-size cap leads to incorrect fit of the nasal prongs and may lead to complications. *Duration* is the number of days of CPAP treatment. *Age* is gestational age of the infant in weeks, and *Weight* is birth weight in grams. It is important to pay attention to how the data are named. Each statistics program has its own way of determining what level of nominal variable to use as the level against which other levels are compared. In our example, *Complication Present* was associated with fluidic CPAP compared with conventional because "conv" appeared first in an alphabetized list of CPAP types.

Report from Statistics Program
The first column of **Table 13.5** gives the coefficients of the logistic regression. The second column shows the p values associated with the null hypothesis that each independent variable is unrelated to the incidence of complications.

The p values indicate that only CPAP type and duration are significantly related to complications. The odds ratio gives us the approximate increase in risk of using fluidic CPAP: about 3.5 times more likely to result in complications. Similarly, a unit increase in duration (1.0 day) leads to a 41% increase in risk of complications. The odds ratio for a unit increase in the independent variable is given by the equation *odds ratio* $= e^b$, where b is the coefficient of the independent variable of interest. Thus, if we want to calculate the odds ratio for two days (2 units), we would have

$$odds\ ratio = e^{2 \times 0.35} = 2.718^{0.70} = 2.01$$

Table 13.5

Results of Multiple Linear Regression Analysis

	Coefficient	p Value	Odds Ratio
CPAP type (b_1)	1.265	0.559	3.5
Wrong hat (b_2)	−0.033	0.9448	1.0
Duration (b_3)	0.350	0.0023	1.4
Gestational age (b_4)	−0.077	0.4459	0.9
Birth (b_2) weight (b_5)	0.0002	0.6724	1.0
Constant (b_0)	−0.991		

We can use the coefficients to calculate a specific probability of occurrence of complications. First, we calculate *y* using the equation given previously, the coefficients from the results table, and specific values of the independent variables. For example, suppose we want the probability of occurrence when *CPAP type* is fluidic (value of 1 versus 0 for conventional), *Wrong Hat* is yes (value of 1 versus 0 for right hat), *Duration* is 2 on day 2, *Gestational Age* is 30 weeks, and *Birth Weight* is 1000 grams. The value of *y* is:

$$y = -0.991 + 1.265(1) - 0.033(1) + 0.350(2) - 0.077(30) + 0.0002(1000)$$
$$y = -1.17$$

Next, the value of *y* is substituted into the equation for *P*:

$$P = \frac{e^y}{1+e^y} = \frac{e-1.17}{1+e^{-1.17}} = \frac{0.31}{1.31} = 0.24$$

Thus, on the basis of this study, an infant with the listed characteristics would have a 24% chance of having complications due to CPAP using the fluidic system.

Comparing One Sample to a Known Value

One-Sample *t* Test

The one-sample *t* test compares a sample mean to a hypothesized population mean and determines the probability that the observed difference between sample and hypothesized mean occurred by chance. The probability of chance occurrence is the *p* value. A *p* value close to 1.0 implies that the hypothesized and sample means are the same: the observed sample would probably not come from a population with the hypothesized mean. A small *p* value (less than 0.05) suggests that such a difference is unlikely (only 1 in 20) to occur by chance if the sample came from a population with the hypothesized mean. We would say that the sample mean is significantly different from the hypothesized value.

Example

You are considering the purchase of a new disposable ventilator circuit. The manufacturer claims that the tubing compliance is 1.5 cm H_2O. You take a sample circuit and connect it to a ventilator and lung simulator. A sample of 17 different tidal volume and airway pressure measurements yields a sample of 17 compliance values. You enter these values into a statistics program and request a one-sample t test comparing your sample mean compliance to the manufacturer's stated value of 1.5 cm H_2O.

Null Hypothesis
No difference exists between the sample mean and the hypothesized population mean for the tubing.

Report from Statistics Program
Table 13.6 shows the results. The sample mean is 1.7 cm H_2O, which is greater than the hypothesized value of 1.5 cm H_2O. However, the p value is greater than 0.05, so we do not reject the null hypothesis.

We conclude that the sample tubing compliance is not different from the manufacturer's specification. The program gives the 95% confidence interval for the true mean value as being between 1.348 and 1.958 cm H_2O.

Table 13.6

Results from a Sample t Test

	Mean	t **Value**	p **Value**	**95% Lower**	**95% Upper**
Compliance	1.653	1.062	0.304	1.348	1.958

Note: Hypothesized mean $= 1.5$.

Comparing Two Samples, Unmatched Data

Unpaired t Test

The unpaired t test compares the means of two groups and determines the probability that the observed difference occurred by chance. The chance is reported as the p value. A p value close to 1.0 implies that the two sample means are the same, because the observed sample would probably not come from a population with the hypothesized mean. A small p value (less than 0.05) suggests that such a difference is unlikely (only 1 in 20) to occur by chance if the sample came from a population with the hypothesized mean. We would say that the sample mean is significantly different from the hypothesized value. We could also say that the hypothesized difference between the means is zero.

If your data fail the normality or equal variance tests, use the Mann-Whitney rank sum test.

Example

Suppose we want to change vendors for our disposable ventilator tubing. We want to be sure that the new brand (Brand A) has the same performance as the one we currently use (Brand B) in terms of volume lost due to compliance. We connect samples of both kinds of tubing to a ventilator and lung simulator and measure the lost volume over a wide range of set tidal volumes. We enter the two sets of lost volume data into the statistics program as shown in **Table 13.7**.

Null Hypothesis
The average lost volume for Brand A is the same as for Brand B.

Report from Statistics Program
Refer to **Table 13.8**.

Normality test: Passed ($p = 0.298$)
Equal variance test: Passed ($p = 0.096$)
Hypothesized mean difference: 0
Power of performed test with alpha: 0.050; 0.878

Table 13.7

Data for Two-Sample *t* Test

Brand A	Brand B
33	28
30	25
25	27
etc.	etc.

Table 13.8

Results for a Two-Sample *t* Test

	Mean Difference	*t* Value	*p* Value	95% Lower	95% Upper
Brand A – Brand B	−1.8	−0.684	0.4991	−7.0	3.5

	Count	Mean	Variance	Std. Dev.	Std. Error
Brand A	17	33.3	50.1	7.078	1.717
Brand B	17	35.1	49.3	7.021	1.702

The difference in the mean values of the two groups is not great enough to reject the possibility that the difference is due to random sampling variability. There is not a statistically significant difference between the input groups ($p = 0.4991$).

Power of performed test with alpha: 0.050; 0.070
The power of the performed test (0.070) is below the desired power of 0.800.

You should interpret the negative findings cautiously. The results of two sample tests are often illustrated graphically, as in **Figure 13.3**. The dots in the graph represent the mean values for each sample. The lines above and below the dots represent one standard deviation. The lines through the mean values are called error bars. Sometimes you see graphs where the error bars represent standard errors or possibly 95% confidence limits. Remember that error bars representing the *standard deviation* refer to the random error of individual measurements, while bars that represent *standard error* refer to the random error of estimating the mean value.

Table 13.8 shows that the mean lost volume with Brand A is about 1.8 mL less than the volume lost with Brand B (because the mean difference is negative and was calculated as A minus B). However, this difference is due to chance and does not represent either a statistically significant or a clinically important difference ($p > 0.05$). We can be fairly confident that if we switch to Brand A, we will maintain the same standard of care. Although the power of the test was not very great, the consequences of making a Type II error are also not very great.

Figure 13.3

Plot of results for comparison of two means.

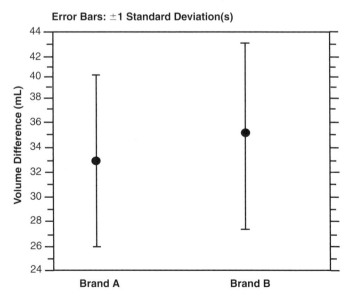

Dots represent the mean values and the error bars span ± standard deviation.

Comparing Two Samples, Matched Data

Paired *t* Test

The most common use of a paired *t* test is the comparison of two measurements from the same individual or experimental unit. The two measurements can be made at different times or under different conditions. The paired *t* test is used to evaluate the hypothesis that the mean of the differences between pairs of experimental units is equal to some hypothesized value, usually zero. A hypothesized value of zero is equivalent to the hypothesis that there is no difference between the two samples. The paired *t* test compares the two samples and determines the probability of the observed difference occurring by chance. The chance is reported as the *p* value. A small *p* value (less than 0.05) suggests that such a difference is unlikely (only 1 in 20) to occur by chance if the sample came from a population with the hypothesized mean. We would say that the sample mean is significantly different from the hypothesized value. We could also say that the hypothesized difference between the means is zero.

The paired *t* test is more powerful than the unpaired *t* test, because it takes into account the fact that measurements from the same unit tend to be more similar than measurements from different units. For example, in a test administered before and after a therapeutic treatment, the unpaired *t* test may not detect small (but consistent) increases in each individual's outcome measurements. The paired *t* test is more sensitive to the fact that one measurement of each pair essentially serves as a control for the others.

A subject acting as his or her own control is called self-pairing. The paired *t* test is also used for cases of natural pairing (such as identical twins or identical pieces of equipment) and artificial pairing (matching pairs of subjects on as many characteristics as possible). See the section on "Matched Versus Unmatched Data" in Chapter 10.

If your data fail the normality or equal variance tests, use the Wilcoxon signed rank test.

Example

Two groups of asthmatic patients treated in the emergency department are entered into a study of aerosolized bronchodilators comparing the effects of standard racemic albuterol with levalbuterol. The two groups are matched for age, gender, race, and severity of illness. The outcome variable is length of stay (in hours) in the emergency department. The data are entered in the statistics program as shown in **Table 13.9**.

Table 13.9

Data Entry for a Paired *t* Test

Racemic	Levalbuterol
33	28
30	25
25	27
etc.	etc.

Null Hypothesis
There is no difference in the mean length of stay between the two groups.

Report from Statistics Program
The data are often displayed as shown in **Table 13.10** for the unpaired *t* test.

Normality test: Passed ($p = 0.281$)
Hypothesized mean difference: 0
Power of performed test with alpha: 0.050; 0.050

The change that occurred with the treatment is not great enough to exclude the possibility that the difference is due to chance ($p = 0.690$). The power of the performed test (0.050) is below the desired power of 0.800.
You should interpret the negative findings cautiously.
We conclude that this study should be considered an encouraging pilot study. A larger study will be needed to be confident that the length of stay in the emergency room is not different between the two drugs.

Comparing Three or More Samples, Unmatched Data

When a statistical test is performed at a given level of significance, such as 0.05, then the risk of a Type I error is controlled at the 5% level. However, when multiple tests are run at the 0.05 level, then the risk of a Type I error begins to increase. With several independent comparisons, the probability of getting at least one falsely significant comparison when there are actually no significant differences is given by the equation:

$$probability\ of\ at\ least\ one\ false\ result = 1-(1-\alpha)^C$$

where α is the significance level and c is the number of independent comparisons. For example, suppose you want to know if patients treated with practice guidelines have better outcomes

Table 13.10

Results of Paired *t* Test

	Mean Difference	*t* Value	*p* Value	95% Lower	95% Upper
Racemic – Levalbuterol	0.120	0.405	0.690	–0.501	0.741

	Count	Mean	Variance	Std. Dev.	Std. Error
Racemic	20	2.3	1.073	1.036	0.232
Levalbuterol	20	2.2	0.721	0.849	0.190

than those treated without guidelines. You want to compare two groups of patients on three variables: length of stay, number of complications, and patient satisfaction score. If you perform three t tests and at least one of them shows a significant difference, you will be tempted to conclude that a difference exists among the groups (especially if this conclusion agrees with your preconceived notions). However, if you report a significant difference and your significance level was 0.05, then you would be underestimating your risk of a Type I error. In fact, the real Type I error with three comparisons is $1 - (10 - 0.05)^3 = 0.14$, which is considerably higher than the 0.05 that you assumed. Your real probability of making a Type I error in concluding there is a difference is 14%, not 5%. This mistake appears in published studies surprisingly often.

The proper way to compare more than two mean values is to use the analysis of variance (ANOVA) procedure.

One-Way ANOVA

A one-way (or one-factor) analysis of variance looks at values collected at one point in time for more than two different groups of subjects. It is used when you want to determine if the means of two or more different groups are affected by a single experimental factor. ANOVA tests the null hypothesis that the mean values of all the groups are the same versus the hypothesis that at least one of the mean values is different. If the test suggests that you reject the null hypothesis, other tests can be used to find which means are different. These are called post hoc (unplanned or after-the-fact) tests and are usually conducted as pairwise comparisons among all the possible pairs of groups. One common example is the Tukey test.

If your data fail the normality or equal variance tests, you should use the Kruskal-Wallis ANOVA on ranks.

Example

Suppose you want to compare the noise levels produced by four different brands of mechanical ventilators. You collect sound intensity (in decibels, dB) measurements from several ventilators in of each type. You enter the data into the statistics program as shown in **Table 13.11**.

Table 13.11

Data Entry for One-Way ANOVA

Brand A	Brand B	Brand C	Brand D
58.18	50.68	51.83	57.72
58.53	49.95	52.13	56.46
57.36	50.21	51.56	56.82
58.68	49.61	52.83	56.98

Null Hypothesis
There are no differences in mean sound intensity between any two of the four groups of measurements.

Report from Statistics Program
The data from this type of analysis are often illustrated with a table similar to the one shown for the unpaired *t* test, except that more than two groups would be shown (see **Table 13.12** and **Table 13.13**).

Normality test passed: ($p = 0.742$)
Equal variance test passed: ($p = 0.984$)
Power of performed test with alpha: 0.050; 1.000

   The differences in the mean values among the treatment groups are greater than would be expected by chance. The *p* value is < 0.001, indicating a statistically significant difference.

We conclude that none of the ventilators produce the same noise level. They are ranked from loudest to quietest in Table 13.12.

Table 13.12

Results for One-Way ANOVA

	Mean	Std. Dev.	Std. Error
Brand A	58.188	0.592	0.296
Brand B	50.111	0.452	0.226
Brand C	52.088	0.546	0.273
Brand D	56.994	0.531	0.265

Table 13.13

Pairwise Multiple Comparisons Using the Tukey Test

	Difference of Means	$p < 0.05$
Brand A vs. Brand B	8.077	Yes
Brand A vs. Brand C	6.100	Yes
Brand A vs. Brand D	1.194	Yes
Brand D vs. Brand B	6.883	Yes
Brand D vs. Brand C	4.906	Yes
Brand C vs. Brand B	1.977	Yes

Two-Way ANOVA

In a one-way ANOVA we were comparing values *between groups*. In a two-way (or two-factor) ANOVA, we are comparing values *within groups as well as between groups*. This analysis would be appropriate for looking at comparisons of groups at different times as well as the differences within each group over the course of the study.

In a two-factor ANOVA, there are two experimental *factors*, which are varied for each experimental group. The two or more different values of each factor are called *levels*. The test is for differences between samples grouped according to the levels of each factor and for *interactions* between the factors (**Table 13.14**).

Table 13.14

Data Structure for Two-Way ANOVA

	Factor 1	
Factor 2	**Level 1**	**Level 2**
Level 1	Subject A	Subject H
	Subject B	Subject I
	Subject C	Subject J
Level 2	Subject D	Subject K
	Subject E	Subject L
	Subject F	Subject M

A two-factor ANOVA tests three hypotheses:

1. There is no difference among the levels of the first factor.
2. There is no difference among the levels of the second factor.
3. There is no interaction between factors. That is, if there is any difference among levels of one factor, the differences are the same regardless of the second factor level.

Example

Suppose you want to test the effect of gender on ventilator weaning time (in hours) using two modes of ventilation, synchronized intermittent mandatory ventilation (SIMV) and pressure support (PS). One factor is gender, with two levels (male and female). The other factor is mode of ventilation, with two levels (SIMV and PS). **Table 13.15** shows how the data from a study including 12 patients might look. The data are entered into the statistics program as shown in **Table 13.16**.

Null Hypotheses
1. There is no difference between SIMV and PS.
2. There is no difference between males and females.
3. There is no interaction between gender and mode.

Table 13.15

Sample Data for Two-Way ANOVA

	Mode of Ventilation	
Gender	**SIMV**	**PS**
Male	38	15
Weaning time	32	18
(hours)	35	22
Female	51	59
Weaning time	49	61
(hours)	55	66

Table 13.16

Data Entry for Two-Way ANOVA

Gender	**Mode**	**Hours**
male	SIMV	38
male	SIMV	32
male	SIMV	35
male	PS	15
male	PS	18
male	PS	22
female	SIMV	51
female	SIMV	49
female	SIMV	55
female	PS	59
female	PS	61
female	PS	66

This type of data is often graphed using either points or bars (**Figure 13.4**). Make sure you specify what the error bars represent (either standard deviation or standard error).

Notice that the fill pattern for the dots or the bars is selected so that it will reproduce accurately on a black-and-white copier. Authors sometimes use only color to distinguish

Figure 13.4

Two different ways of displaying results for two-way ANOVA.

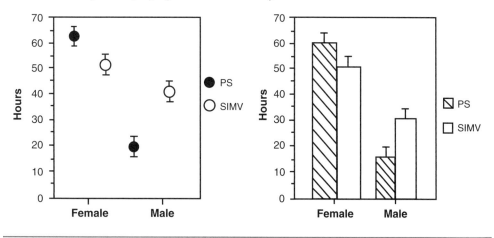

between groups on a graph, and this detail is lost when readers make black-and-white copies.

Report from Statistics Program
Refer to **Table 13.17** and **Table 13.18**.

Normality test: Passed ($p = 0.435$)
Equal variance test: Passed ($p = 0.959$)
Power of performed test with alpha: 0.0500; for Gender: 1.000
Power of performed test with alpha: 0.0500; for Mode: 0.207
Power of performed test with alpha: 0.0500; for Gender $\times$ Mode: 1.000

The difference in the mean values between the two genders is greater than would be expected by chance after allowing for effects of differences in mode. There is a statistically

Table 13.17

Results of Two-Way ANOVA

Factor 1	Mean	Std. Error
SIMV	43.333	1.349
PS	40.167	1.349

Factor 2	Mean	Std. Error
Male	26.667	1.349
Female	56.833	1.349

	p Value
Gender	<0.001
Mode	0.135
Gender $\times$ mode	<0.001

Table 13.18

Pairwise Multiple Comparison Procedure (Tukey Test)

	Mean	Std. Error
Female $\times$ PS	62.000	1.908
Female $\times$ SIMV	51.667	1.908
Male $\times$ SIMV	35.000	1.908
Male $\times$ PS	18.333	1.908

significant difference ($p < 0.001$). To isolate which group or groups differ from the others, use a multiple comparison procedure.

The difference in the mean values between the modes is not great enough to exclude the possibility that the difference is due just to random sampling variability after allowing for the effects of differences in gender. There is not a statistically significant difference ($p = 0.135$).

The effect of gender depends on which mode is present. There is a statistically significant interaction between gender and mode ($p < 0.001$).

Based on these results, we conclude that males wean faster than females but there is no difference between the modes. Furthermore, females take longer when they are on PS and males take longer when they are on SIMV.

Comparing Three or More Samples, Matched Data

One-Way Repeated Measures ANOVA

A one-way (or one-factor) analysis of variance looks at values collected at more than one point in time for a single group of subjects. It is used when you want to determine if a single group of individuals was affected by a series of experimental treatments or conditions. ANOVA tests the null hypothesis that all the mean values of all the groups are the same versus the hypothesis that at least one of the mean values is different. If the test suggests that you reject the null hypothesis, other tests can be used to find which means are different. These are called post hoc (unplanned or after-the-fact) tests and are usually conducted as pairwise comparisons among all the possible pairs of groups. One common example is the Tukey test.

If your data fail the normality or equal variance tests, use the Friedman repeated measures ANOVA on ranks.

Example

You have a care path for pediatric asthmatic patients that requires therapists to perform assessments at specified intervals of 2, 3, and 4 hours from the start of treatments. One of these assessments is forced expiratory volume in one second (FEV_1), which requires both time and equipment to perform bedside spirometry. You suspect that FEV_1 does not change that much over 4 hours and may thus be eliminated as an assessment procedure. For a group of 10 patients treated with the care path, you record FEV_1 values after 2, 3, and 4 hours of bronchodilator treatment (**Table 13.19**).

Null Hypothesis
There are no differences in mean FEV_1 between any two of the three groups of measurements.

Table 13.19

Sample Data for One-Way Repeated Measures ANOVA

2 Hours	3 Hours	4 Hours
1.23	1.81	1.81
1.38	1.38	1.77
1.01	1.46	1.56
0.96	1.41	1.60
1.31	1.44	1.77
1.12	1.26	1.28
1.09	1.48	1.72
1.19	1.46	1.80
1.27	1.00	1.63
1.17	1.23	1.80

Report from Statistics Program
The data from this type of analysis are often illustrated with a graph similar to the one shown for the unpaired *t* test, (Table 13.9) except that there would be more than two groups shown (see **Table 13.20** and **Table 13.21**).

Normality test passed: ($p = 0.405$)
Equal variance test passed: ($p = 0.204$)
Power of performed test with alpha: 0.050; 1.000

Table 13.20

Results for One-Way Repeated Measures ANOVA

	Mean	Std. Dev.	Std. Error
2 hours	1.173	0.132	0.0419
3 hours	1.392	0.207	0.0656
4 hours	1.676	0.166	0.0524

Table 13.21

Pairwise Multiple Comparisons Using the Tukey Test

	Difference of Means	$p < 0.05$
4 hours vs. 2 hours	0.503	Yes
4 hours vs. 3 hours	0.284	Yes
3 hours vs. 2 hours	0.219	Yes

The differences in the mean values among the treatment groups are greater than would be expected by chance; the difference is statistically significant ($p < 0.001$).

We conclude that FEV_1 does indeed increase at each assessment period. Although the difference between any two periods is statistically significant, we may conclude that there is not enough clinically important difference to justify the time and effort to collect the FEV_1 data.

Two-Way Repeated Measures ANOVA

In a one-way ANOVA we were comparing values *between groups.* In a two-way (or two-factor) ANOVA, we are comparing values *within groups as well as between groups.* This analysis would be appropriate for looking at comparisons of groups at different times as well as the differences within each group over the course of the study.

In a two-factor ANOVA, there are two experimental *factors*, which are varied for each experimental group (**Table 13.22**, **Table 13.23**, and **Table 13.24**). Either or both of these factors are repeated treatments on the same group of individuals. The two or more different values of each factor are called *levels.* The test is for differences between the different levels of each factor and for *interactions* between the factors.

A two-factor ANOVA tests three hypotheses:

1. There is no difference among the levels of the first factor.
2. There is no difference among the levels of the second factor.
3. There is no interaction between factors. That is, if there is any difference among levels of one factor, the differences are the same regardless of the second factor level.

If experimental subjects are divided into two groups, with each group treated with one factor, we say there is one repeated measure, and the data structure is as shown in Table 13.22.

Table 13.23 shows how data would be entered into SigmaPlot.

If all experimental subjects are treated with both factors, we say there are two repeated measures, and the data structure is as shown in Table 13.24.

Table 13.22

Data Structure for Two-Way Repeated Measures ANOVA with One Repeated Measure (Factor)

	Factor 1	
Factor 2	**Level 1**	**Level 2**
Level 1	Subject A	Subject A
	Subject B	Subject B
	Subject C	Subject C
Level 2	Subject D	Subject D
	Subject E	Subject E
	Subject F	Subject F

Table 13.23

Data Entry for Two-Way Repeated Measures ANOVA with One Repeated Measure (Factor)

Subject	Factor 1	Factor 2	Measurement
A	Level 1	Level 1	Value 1
A	Level 2	Level 1	Value 2
B	Level 1	Level 1	Value 3
B	Level 2	Level 1	Value 4
C	Level 1	Level 1	Value 5
C	Level 2	Level 1	Value 6
D	Level 1	Level 2	Value 7
D	Level 2	Level 2	Value 8
E	Level 1	Level 2	Value 9
E	Level 2	Level 2	Value 10
F	Level 1	Level 2	Value 11
F	Level 2	Level 2	Value 12

Note: Data entry format shown is for SigmaPlot; other programs require different formats.

Table 13.24

Design for Two-Way Repeated Measures ANOVA with Two Repeated Measures (Factors)

	Factor 1	
Factor 2	**Level 1**	**Level 2**
Level 1	Subject A	Subject A
	Subject B	Subject B
	Subject C	Subject C
Level 2	Subject A	Subject A
	Subject B	Subject B
	Subject C	Subject C

Data may be entered into SigmaPlot as shown in **Table 13.25**.

Example

Suppose you want to assess the effects on oxygenation of a mode of mechanical ventilation called automatic tube compensation (ATC) using two different ventilators, the Brand A and the Brand B. The outcome variable is PaO_2. You select three patients on the Dräger and three on the Bennett 840. For each patient, you select two different levels of tube compensation.

Table 13.25

Data Entry for Two-Way Repeated Measures ANOVA with Two Repeated Measures (Factors)

Subject	Factor 1	Factor 2	Measurement
A	Level 1	Level 1	Value 1
A	Level 2	Level 1	Value 2
B	Level 1	Level 1	Value 3
B	Level 2	Level 1	Value 4
C	Level 1	Level 1	Value 5
C	Level 2	Level 1	Value 6
A	Level 1	Level 2	Value 7
A	Level 2	Level 2	Value 8
B	Level 1	Level 2	Value 9
B	Level 2	Level 2	Value 10
C	Level 1	Level 2	Value 11
C	Level 2	Level 2	Value 12

Note: Data entry format shown for SigmaPlot; other programs require different formats.

This experiment uses a repeated measures design with one factor (tube compensation) repeated (**Table 13.26**). **Table 13.27** shows the data entry format for the SigmaPlot program.

Null Hypotheses
1. There is no difference between Brand A and Brand B.
2. There is no difference between 0% ATC and 100% ATC.
3. There is no interaction between ventilator and ATC level.

Report from Statistics Program
This type of data is often graphed using either points or bars as shown for the two-way ANOVA without repeated measures (Figure 13.4). Make sure you specify what the error bars represent (either standard deviation or standard error). Refer to **Table 13.28** and **Table 13.29**.

Table 13.26

Example Data for Two-Way Repeated Measures ANOVA with One Repeated Measure (Factor)

	Tube Compensation Setting	
	0%	100%
Brand A	85	130
	90	105
Brand B	55	55
	75	80
	70	75

Table 13.27

Sample Data for Two-Way Repeated Measures ANOVA with Two Repeated Measures (Factors)

Subject	Tube Comp. (%)	Ventilator	Pao_2 (mm Hg)
A	0	Brand A	90.8
A	100	Brand A	110.0
B	0	Brand A	84.2
B	100	Brand A	92.0
C	0	Brand A	79.6
C	100	Brand A	84.7
D	0	Brand B	87.9
D	100	Brand B	106.0
E	0	Brand B	77.5
E	100	Brand B	91.4
F	0	Brand B	73.8
F	100	Brand B	90.4

Note: Data entry format shown is for SigmaPlot; other programs require different formats.

Table 13.28

Results for Two-Way Repeated Measures ANOVA with Two Repeated Measures (Factors)

Factor 1	Mean	Std. Error		*p* Value
Brand A	90.252	5.003	Ventilator	0.751
Brand B	87.845	5.003	ATC level	0.004

Factor 2	Mean	Std. Error	Ventilator $\times$ ATC	0.285
0% ATC	82.338	3.712		
100% ATC	95.759	3.712		

Table 13.29

Pairwise Multiple Comparison Procedure (Tukey Test)

	Mean	Std. Error
Brand A $\times$ 0.000	84.928	5.249
Brand A $\times$ 100.000	95.576	5.249
Brand B $\times$ 0% ATC	79.748	5.249
Brand B $\times$ 100% ATC	95.942	5.249

Normality test: Passed ($p = 0.\ 0.272$)
Equal variance test: Passed ($p = 0.\ 0.060$)
Power of performed test with alpha: 0.0500; for Ventilator: 0.0503
Power of performed test with alpha: 0.0500; for ATC: 0.990
Power of performed test with alpha: 0.0500; for Ventilator $\times$ ATC: 0.0865

The difference in the mean values between the different ventilators is not great enough to exclude the possibility that the difference is due just to random sampling variability after allowing for the effects of differences in ATC. There is not a statistically significant difference ($p = 0.751$).

The difference in the mean values between the different levels of ATC is greater than would be expected by chance after allowing for effects of differences in type of ventilator. There is a statistically significant difference ($p = 0.004$). To isolate which group or groups differ from the others, use a multiple comparison procedure.

The effect of different ventilators does not depend on the level of ATC present. There is not a statistically significant interaction between ventilator and ATC ($p = 0.285$).

Based on these results, we conclude that there is no difference in the way ACT works on the two ventilators in terms of oxygenation. However, using ATC does improve oxygenation.

Questions

Multiple Choice

1. One of the assumptions of the t test is that the data you are analyzing are normally distributed. Before using this test, you should confirm this assumption using:
   a. Kolomogorov-Smirnov test
   b. F ratio test
   c. Pearson product-moment correlation coefficient
   d. Regression analysis
2. You have a set of data showing patients' room air PaO_2 at sea level and at a simulated altitude of 8,000 feet. If you wanted to use this data to predict PaO_2 at altitude from PaO_2 at sea level, you would use:
   a. Kolomogorov-Smirnov test
   b. F ratio test
   c. Pearson product-moment correlation coefficient
   d. Regression analysis
3. You have a new blood-gas machine that seems to be producing inconsistent results. In order to test the hypothesis that the variance of this machine's measurements is different from your old machine, you would use:
   a. Kolomogorov-Smirnov test
   b. F ratio test
   c. Pearson product-moment correlation coefficient
   d. Regression analysis
4. Suppose you want to determine whether or not training time is associated with competency scores. What would you use?
   a. Kolomogorov-Smirnov test
   b. F ratio test

    c. Pearson product-moment correlation coefficient

    d. Regression analysis

5. The procedure that uses one independent variable to predict the value of one dependent variable is:

    a. Simple linear regression

    b. Multiple linear regression

    c. Logistic regression

6. If you have more than one independent (predictor) variables, you would use:

    a. Simple linear regression

    b. Multiple linear regression

    c. Logistic regression

7. If you want to predict the presence or absence of a disease based on one or more independent variables, you must use:

    a. Simple linear regression

    b. Multiple linear regression

    c. Logistic regression

8. If you want to use the regression coefficients to calculate odds ratios, you need:

    a. Simple linear regression

    b. Multiple linear regression

    c. Logistic regression

9. A study suggests that the average length of stay reported by pediatric ICUs in the United States is 8.5 days. To test the hypothesis that your pediatric ICU has a shorter length of stay, you would use:

    a. One-sample t test

    b. Unpaired t test

    c. Paired t test

    d. ANOVA

10. You have been giving the same final exam year after year to a class of health care students. You have a set of six scores representing the average class performance. What would you use to test the hypothesis that the average class score has been decreasing over time?

    a. One-sample t test

    b. Unpaired t test

    c. Paired t test

    d. ANOVA

11. Two sets of patients are entered into a study. One set is treated with a new fast-acting bronchodilator and the other a placebo. What test would you use to make sure the two groups of patients had similar FEV_1 values at the start of the study?

    a. One-sample t test

    b. Unpaired t test

    c. Paired t test

    d. ANOVA

12. In the study above, what test would you use to compare the mean FEV_1 values before and after treatment?

    a. One-sample t test

    b. Unpaired t test

    c. Paired t test

Section IV

Publishing the Findings

CHAPTER 14

The Paper

Any research project that is important enough to require careful thought in design and sustained effort in data gathering merits a written report at its conclusion. Such a report serves at least two purposes. First, it forces the researcher to review the entire thought process involved, from the initial recognition of a clinical problem through the formation of a conceptual model relating the associated variables, to the comparison of this model with reality using actual measurements. Any flaws or ambiguities in this train of thought will become evident once the events are recreated in a written report. Someone once said that to understand a subject, one should teach it. A research report is a teaching instrument in the sense that it provides a concise review of the background and current perspective on a specific topic. A second, more obvious function of a research report is to expand the scientific community's knowledge base. Published reports become immortal pieces of the ever-changing puzzle we call scientific knowledge.

Publication of an article in a scientific journal can also result in personal benefits for the author. It is a measure of professional success and may lead to tenure and status. In the extreme case, one may find oneself in a "publish or perish" situation if employed as a faculty member of a university.

In this chapter we will review the basic procedures for publishing a full-length manuscript. In the next two chapters we will discuss more specialized aspects of publication, including how to submit an abstract and how to prepare a poster presentation based on the abstract.

Selecting an Appropriate Journal

In order for research to be accepted by the scientific community, it must "fit in." A journal with the appropriate readership must be selected. A topic that may seem original and interesting to one audience may be insulting to another. For this reason, you should select the journal in which you hope to publish the study findings before writing the paper. Several considerations in choosing an appropriate journal will now be reviewed.

Writing Style

Reading journals will give you a feel for the subject matter and level of complexity of articles selected by the editors. Some journals deal primarily with the more abstract topics of basic research (e.g., *Journal of Applied Physiology*), whereas others emphasize more clinically relevant matters (e.g., *Critical Care Medicine* or *Respiratory Care*). Also, some journals presume a high level of mathematical sophistication on the part of the reader, as indicated by frequent articles containing calculus or complex statistical procedures. An article based on a rather simplistic algebraic model is likely to be rejected by such a journal. Some journals will publish only clinical research and will reject device evaluations.

Before beginning to write, look for an "Instruction for Authors" page included in the print journal or on the journal's Web site. This page will provide detailed instructions concerning writing style, reference format, and preparation of illustrations. It will also indicate whether or not the journal charges a fee to publish the manuscript.

Types of Authors

Respiratory therapists sometimes have difficulty publishing a manuscript in a journal whose authors are almost exclusively MDs or PhDs. Review past issues to determine whether or not professionals with your credentials have published in the journal in question. An original investigation that would be of interest mainly to respiratory therapists is more likely to be accepted by a journal in which other therapists contribute articles. When published in such a journal, your article will get the greatest exposure to the most appropriate audience.

Types of Readers

Health care professions have become highly diversified, with journals catering to each specialty and subspecialty. In addition to journals of interest to specific professionals, such as nurses or cardiopulmonary technologists, there are journals that are read by a variety of medical personnel (e.g., *Critical Care Medicine*). Selecting an appropriate journal will depend somewhat on the research topic's degree of specialization, as well as the intended audience.

Indexing

One of the factors that determines how widely read an article will be is how easily it can be found by other investigators. Select a journal that is indexed in a major reference source such as Index Medicus or CINAHL (Cumulative Index to Nursing and Allied Health Literature). Services such as Current Contents Connect provide reviews of current published titles. Not all journals are covered by these sources, so you'll want to be sure to choose one that is.

Peer Review

Most respectable scientific journals are peer reviewed. Peer review means that the editor will send copies of a prospective manuscript to consultants who are familiar with the subject area of the paper. A biostatistician may also be asked to review the study design and data analysis. These consultants will provide the editor and the author with detailed criticisms of the manuscript. Such criticisms are beneficial to the author, who obtains a better idea of contemporary professional standards; to the journal, by establishing credibility; and to the reader, who can be more confident of the validity of the report. Having a paper accepted by a peer-reviewed journal is more difficult than gaining acceptance from a so-called throwaway journal. Subscriptions to this latter type are generally offered free because they are primarily vehicles for the advertisements of medical equipment manufacturers. Obviously, an article published in a journal with strict editorial policies means more to the author and the reader than one published in a less sophisticated periodical.

Getting Started

Authorship

All persons listed as authors must have participated in the reported work and in the shaping of the manuscript. All must have proofread the submitted manuscript. All should be able to publicly discuss and defend the paper's content. Authorship is not based solely on solicitation of funding, collection or analysis of data, provision of advice, or similar services. Persons who provide such ancillary services may be recognized in an acknowledgments section, but written permission is required from the person acknowledged (see also "Who Should Write It?" in Chapter 16).

The Rough Draft

Writing a high-quality manuscript is hard work, but the exertion of writing and rewriting a paper results in something that is worth reading. A good paper is generally rewritten at least three times (and as many as 10 times) before the final draft is completed. In light of this, you should minimize the time between each redaction so that enthusiasm for the project is not drained by having to "come up to speed" each time you begin. However, I recommend that you let the first or second draft sit for a week or so in order to achieve what Zen masters call "beginner's mind." This means that you can look at the manuscript with a fresh outlook. In this way you will see areas where you previously did not explain things with enough detail because you were too close to the project—you had assumed knowledge that the average reader cannot be expected to have simply because everything was so familiar to *you*.

Always start with an outline of the paper. Never just start writing off the top of your head. I believe you should start by writing the introduction, but only in abbreviated form—perhaps just a paragraph explaining the context of the study and why it is important. Next, write a very clear statement of the study purpose and hypotheses. If you have written an adequate study protocol, the introduction can simply be copied from that. Next write the results section, because that is what is uppermost in your mind and the writing is fairly simple. Starting with this can help you get over any "writer's block." Next write the methods section, making sure that the methods correspond with the results and, more important, with the study purpose and hypotheses stated in the introduction. Then write the discussion section and conclusions. After that, you should be well prepared to go back and expand the introduction, making it interesting, brief, and informative. Finally, write the abstract, using actual sentences from the body of the paper. Then, as I said before, leave the manuscript alone for a week or two. After a "cooling off" period, go back and read the manuscript again. Now that the project is not so fresh in your mind you will be better able to read it with the eyes of your audience, who is totally new to it. This process will help you to explain things in enough detail so that someone else can follow your train of thought rather than expecting your audience to read between the lines.

Have copies of all reference articles on hand before you begin writing. The format for listing references in the text may vary with each journal. For example, some journals require references to be numbered consecutively with superscripts. No matter what the specific requirements are, however, for the first few drafts you should simply list the last name of the article's first author and the year of publication. Each time you add a reference to the text, note it in complete bibliographical form on a separate sheet of paper. This format minimizes the work of changing the order and placement of references as you revise the manuscript. As the paper nears completion, you can change the manner in which the references are listed to conform to the style of a particular journal (e.g., consecutive numbering). Even better, purchase and learn how to use a bibliographic management program like EndNote (www.endnote.com) or RefWorks (www.refworks.com). Such programs greatly facilitate both acquiring reference citations from the Internet and placing them into your documents.

Before the writing begins, establish how the responsibility for writing will be allocated and in what order the authors will be listed. Actual writing of the manuscript usually proceeds most smoothly if one person is designated as the primary author. This person is responsible for writing the first draft. Contributing authors edit the first few drafts and provide input. The primary author then coordinates subsequent revisions and prepares the final manuscript for submission to a journal. I have found that the best way to manage this process is for the primary author to create a Microsoft Word file with the date or version number in the file name. Then the current version is distributed to the co-authors as an e-mail attachment. The co-authors add their comments and changes using the "Track Changes" feature in Word and send it back to the primary author. The primary author then uses the first version she receives, and using the Reviewing toolbar in Word, either accepts or rejects the changes in the manuscript, addresses the comments, and then deletes them. This manuscript is modified until all the reviews are in. Then, the new revision is renamed and sent out for another round of reviews. This process is repeated until all authors are satisfied with the work. In practice, there are two ways to do this. If you have plenty of time and you are fairly sure your reviewers are relatively prompt, send the manuscript to one reviewer at a time. That way you can always be working with one document and there is less chance for confusion. You simply accept or reject each edit from each author sequentially. If you are in a hurry, do it in parallel and send each version to all reviewers, but this way you will have to re-do the edits of the other reviewers on one master document.

If you are a primary author who has not published a manuscript before, find an experienced colleague to act as a mentor. Ideally, consult someone who has knowledge of or interest in your research topic and who has published several papers. If you are fortunate enough to find such an adviser, consider offering to include his or her name as a co-author. In this way both parties, and ultimately the manuscript, will benefit.

Finally, make sure you read Appendix I, Basic Science Writing, for some excellent tips on how to improve your technical writing skills.

The Structure of a Paper

Every scientific manuscript has five main sections, excluding the title. We review each section in the order in which they appear, which is usually not the order in which they are written. Refer to the model manuscript in Appendix V for specific examples.

Title

There is a certain art to wording a title. It should not be too vague, and all acronyms should be spelled out. For example, "An investigation of CPAP" is a poor title. A better title would be "The effects of early continuous positive airway pressure on length of stay in the neonatal intensive care unit." The title should serve to introduce the topic and catch the reader's attention, while avoiding any sense of drama or marketing of conclusions. The best way to learn the art of crafting a title is to look at how informative titles are worded in respected medical journals.

Abstract

An abstract is required by many journals and usually appears after the title in the published article. As a practical matter, it is generally written after the main body of the manuscript is finished. The purpose of the abstract is to provide a short, concise summary of the study for the reader who may not have the time to read the whole article. The abstract is essentially a miniature, condensed version of the paper containing the same format: introduction, methods, results, and conclusion. However, the results and methods are more important than the introduction and conclusion, and since space is limited, no more than one or two sentences should be devoted to a problem statement or discussion of conclusions.

In writing the abstract, avoid simply listing or describing the contents of the paper. The abstract should be informative and complete as a stand-alone piece of communication. Avoid phrases such as "Results will be given. . . " that force the reader to consult the text and defeat the purpose of a summary. However, the abstract should not contain information that is not presented in the text. Do not include opinions or conclusions without providing the evidence on which they were based.

Most journals specify a maximum length for the abstract. Requirements vary, but an appropriate length is approximately 300 words or less. In striving for brevity, remember to provide the same quality of grammar as the main body of the article. Do not eliminate essential prepositions, adjectives, and conjunctions such as "of," "the," and "a," but do try to eliminate words and "flowery language" that add nothing to the informative content of the summary. You will find the task easier if you write the abstract first without regard to the word count, making sure all the important data and concepts are included. Then use the "Word Count" tool in Microsoft Word to total the words. Now go through each sentence, word by word, and consider how to rephrase it to make it shorter but still convey the message. After going through every sentence, perform a word count again. Repeat.

Introduction

The introduction consists of two or three paragraphs that explain the purpose of the paper. It should contain a brief description of the background and significance of the research topic and include a few key references. The introduction should provide the reader with an awareness of the context and scope of the study.

A statement of the research problem or hypothesis should be included. Not including the hypothesis is a common mistake among beginners; not stating a *clear* hypothesis that relates to the measurable variables in the methods section is a frequent mistake even among experienced authors. Describing the hypothesis, or at least the research problem, in the introduction sets the stage for the methods (which must describe how the hypothesis was tested), the results (which must correspond to all the methods described), and the discussion (which tells how the results addressed the hypothesis).

The references cited in the introduction should support the theoretical framework of the hypothesis, although an in-depth explanation should be saved for the discussion section. The introduction should also contain definitions of the general concepts treated in the manuscript. Frequently used terms can be abbreviated after first being spelled out in the opening paragraphs.

Methods

The purpose of this section is to explain to the reader exactly what was done to answer the research question and/or test the hypotheses described in the introduction. It should be brief, but it must contain enough information to allow other researchers to duplicate the study. The ability to reproduce study results is the hallmark of the scientific method.

The methods section may contain several subdivisions. The experimental subjects and the criteria for including them in the study should be clearly explained. If patients are included in the study, a table of distinguishing characteristics may be helpful in summarizing demographic data. Such a table might include age, sex, diagnosis, mode of therapy, and so on. The sample selection procedure and the rationale for the study design must be clearly presented. This type of information is necessary if the results of the study are to be generalized to a broader population of similar patients.

An essential component of the methods section is a complete description of the equipment used to gather the data. The description should include the model number of the particular device and the manufacturer's name and address (city and state). For example, if airway pressure was measured, the text might read, "Patient response was simulated with a lung model (ASL 5000, IngMar Medical, Inc., Pittsburgh, PA)." The calibration procedure for each measuring device should be described along with any pertinent validation procedures. Validation procedures might include comparison of a measurement device with a laboratory standard (e.g., using a U-tube manometer to validate measurements made with a calibrated pressure sensor) or testing the dynamic response of a device to ensure accuracy at various frequencies (e.g., analysis of the frequency response of pressure- and flow-measuring systems).

Describe the procedure used to gather the data. This description might include an outline of the experimental protocol that was approved by the institutional review board. State whether informed consent was obtained from the patient. A description of the experimental procedure should include the actual steps involved in gathering the data and the time elapsed during each phase of the experiment. Be sure to mention any problems or unforeseen events that occurred during the study. The information in this section should be detailed enough to guide other researchers who might wish to verify the results. The methods section will also help the reader to evaluate the quality of the data gathered during the study.

Finally, include a brief description of how the data were analyzed. Provide a short discussion of the statistical procedures used and why they were appropriate for the experimental design. Unless the procedures were unusual, do not give the statistical equations used. However, many statistical procedures are based on certain assumptions about how the data were gathered (e.g., independence of data points used in a linear regression). Thus, you should provide enough information for the reader to evaluate the validity of any underlying assumptions and, hence, the adequacy of the analysis.

Results

This section of the paper presents the data gathered from the experiments. The order in which the information is given should correspond to the organization of the methods section. In that section, the reader was introduced to the step-by-step procedure used to study a particular problem. An expectation has been created in the reader's mind for the result of each step of the procedure. Therefore, the results should be presented in a logical progression from the beginning to the end of the experiment. This progression helps to assure the reader of the thoroughness of the experimental technique.

The actual presentation of the data can take many forms. Use tables to summarize large amounts of raw data. Tables avoid the drudgery of long, redundant verbiage in the text of the paper. Each table should be constructed so that its meaning is clear without having to refer to the text. The idea is to summarize and guide the interpretation of large amounts of data and to reduce the time necessary to read the article. If the table appears to be too large, use figures or graphs. Specific examples of data summary techniques can be found in Chapters 10–13.

The information presented in the results section is usually in the form of "bare facts" with little or no explanation of its significance. The data are interpreted in the discussion section. Of course, this is a general rule and may be suspended at times if it is felt that elaboration of some point in the results section would help the reader's understanding. However, the overall train of thought created by a research paper should proceed from the presentation of the problem, to an explanation of the methods used to examine the problem, to the results of the experimental methods, and finally to an interpretation of the results.

From a philosophical standpoint, the results of a study do not "prove" anything. They simply add supportive evidence to the stated hypothesis. Thus, you must avoid any claims that a hypothesis was proven, confirmed, or verified in the results section. Remember that conclusions are described in the discussion and conclusions sections, not in the results section.

The results of statistical analyses should be reported in the past tense. This is a subtle point. Consider, for example, the statement, "Airway pressures during high frequency ventilation *are* significantly lower than those during conventional ventilation." This implies that not only were the pressures analyzed during the study significantly different, but the author, by using the present tense, assumes that the results are unquestionably generalizable to all instances of high-frequency ventilation. Using the past tense (changing "are" to "was") emphasizes that the results pertain to a limited sample under the conditions of one particular study. The responsibility for interpreting the generalizability of the results ultimately rests with the reader. The significance of a statistical test is usually reported in terms of a p value. Differences associated with p values less than 0.05 are considered significant by convention in medical studies.

Discussion

The discussion shows how the results answered the research question first described in the introduction. The results of statistical hypothesis tests must be translated into conclusions about the research hypotheses. This section describes the implications and practical meaning of the study results. In addition, the discussion should describe the limitations of the study design, any problems encountered, and any recommendations for future studies. The process of interpreting the results not only concerns the data generated by the study but also relates that data to other studies and theoretical frameworks. The discussion is the appropriate place to include detailed reviews of other related research—including references—that would help to develop the reader's perspective and appreciation for the significance of the study.

Conclusion

Some journals require a separate conclusion statement at the end of the paper. The conclusions made should be thoroughly explained, including reasons for rejecting alternate interpretations. In addition, there should be a statement regarding the population to which the results can be generalized. Because the implications of a given study are usually speculative, it is appropriate to use words that are somewhat tentative in nature. For example, "The results of this study suggest that. . ." or "Because of the significant differences found, it may be possible to. . . ." Such language emphasizes the fact that your interpretation is itself a hypothesis that may be tested by further research.

Illustrations

The inclusion of a few well-composed illustrations can vastly improve the quality and readability of any manuscript. If drawings and photographs are to be included, it is usually best to consult a professional medical illustrator. However, with a few simple tools and a little practice, even a novice can achieve good results with graphs and simple charts. Simple line drawing can be done on a computer with a word processing program. I like to use an inexpensive drawing program called Zoner Draw (about $50). You can download a free trial version at http://www.zoner.com/draw. The beauty of this program, besides being easy to learn, is that you can export your drawings in a variety of file formats with adjustable resolution (i.e., dots per inch) so that you can meet any manuscript submission requirements. A good statistics program like SigmaPlot (www.sigmaplot.com/home.php) can also export graphs in a variety of formats. If you find that the file size of such an export is too large, and you are unable to change it in the statistics program, simply import it into your drawing program and re-export with the appropriate compression settings.

Formal training is not necessary to create professional-looking graphs and charts. Simply look at illustrations that appear in other manuscripts in various medical journals. Study the details and then carefully copy that style using your data. Having a manuscript published with original illustrations introduces a new dimension of satisfaction and economy.

Submission for Publication

First Steps

Read and follow the instructions to authors supplied by the journal to which you will send your manuscript. The instructions will tell you things like how many copies to submit, how to format the references, and how to submit electronically (if applicable).

Peer Review

After a manuscript has been submitted, the journal editor will look it over. The editor may return the manuscript with an explanation of why it is not acceptable. Sometimes the manuscript simply does not fit in with the typical subject matter of the journal, and the editor may suggest more appropriate journals. If it passes this initial screening, it is sent to two or three peer reviewers.

Peer reviewers are carefully selected content experts who have a thorough knowledge of the type of research being evaluated. Such experts have usually published extensively themselves. Ideally, the reviewers are not told the authors' names to help prevent bias. Most assuredly, you will not be given the names of the reviewers.

Reviewing is hard work. Editors have a responsibility to assemble knowledgeable reviewers and to protest when reviewers return an obviously biased or self-serving review. The reviewers have a responsibility to maintain their own integrity by looking beyond personal biases, to educate themselves about aspects of the study that may be unfamiliar to them, to weigh the quality of the paper with its potential value to the readership, and to deal fairly with the author.

As an author, you can expect the reviewers to provide detailed and clearly written explanations of the strengths and weaknesses of your paper and support for any criticisms. Your paper will be judged (1) acceptable for publication as submitted (rare); (2) in need of revision before a decision can be made; or (3) so flawed that adequate revision appears unlikely. An editor then gives consideration to the critiques of the two or three reviewers and informs the author.

Revision

Having a paper rejected is like being told your child is ugly and stupid. Most people react with negative emotions and give up. But if you can get past that phase, you have several options. First, examine whether the reviewers' comments are justified. Sometimes they have just misunderstood what you wrote (or failed to explain adequately). If the comments are justified, see what you can do to make the required changes. Keep two things in mind: (1) the time spent in revision is generally only a small fraction of the time already invested; (2) most manuscripts require revision and you are not being singled out. When the revision is complete, resubmit the manuscript with a cover letter listing each of the reviewers' comments and how you addressed them. Authors always have the right to overrule a reviewer's objection, but they must adequately support their point of view. Please see Appendix V for an example of a good manuscript that was peer reviewed and Appendix VI for the actual reviewer's comments and the authors' responses.

Production

After a manuscript is accepted for publication, it is first copyedited. Copyediting is the stage at which editors make the manuscript consistent with the journal's style. They may ask you to clarify some wording or supply missing information (e.g., incomplete reference data). When copyediting is complete, the manuscript is sent to be typeset. After it has been typeset, "proofs" or final page layouts are sent to the author for inspection and approval. These will most often be electronic files (e.g., PDF) rather than actual paper documents. Because of the costs involved, only minor changes can be made at this stage. When the author approves the proofs, he or she also grants the journal permission to publish the paper and assigns the copyright to the journal. The final stage of production involves careful proofreading (for typographical errors), pagination, transmission to the press, and the actual printing and binding.

Mistakes to Avoid

Here are some common reasons why manuscripts are rejected for publication:

- The paper did not describe the research question or it did not clearly explain the hypothesis.
- The study did not actually test the research hypothesis.
- The wrong measurement methods were used or measurement errors were made.
- The sample size was too small and the results were inconclusive.
- The study used the wrong design and did not adequately control for confounding factors.
- The statistical analysis was incorrect. (Surprisingly, some papers do get published with the wrong analyses.)
- The authors drew unjustified conclusions from their data.
- There is a significant conflict of interest (the authors might benefit from the publication of the paper and insufficient safeguards were seen to be in place to avoid bias).
- The paper is so badly written that it is incomprehensible.

Chapter 16, on writing the case report, goes into much more detail regarding common mistakes first-time authors make. Here are some things to keep in mind:

- The single most important principle to remember is this: *There must be a logical continuity throughout the different sections of the paper.* The title should hint at the hypothesis; the introduction should state the hypothesis; the hypothesis should dictate the experimental procedures in the methods section; there should be data for all the methods in the results section, and the discussion should refer back to, and make conclusions, about the original hypothesis. Neophytes usually make the mistake of breaking this chain of continuity, leaving the reader wondering what the paper is really about.
- Conduct the study without preconceived notions about the outcome. If you set out "to prove that. . ." instead of "to find out whether. . ." you will probably introduce personal bias.
- Always create an outline first and then follow the outline as you write.
- Supply all the detail necessary for other researchers to replicate your study. New authors sometimes keep all the necessary records but fail to include them in the paper.
- Repeat your measurements and report the number of repetitions. "Operator error" is a real concern and often can be detected by repeating measurements.
- Make sure your measuring devices are properly calibrated and document the calibration procedures.
- Report only the data collected, and draw conclusions based only on those data. Opinion can be included (sparingly) in the discussion but must be identified as such.
- Do a final proofreading of the manuscript after you have had a week or two (or even longer if possible) to forget about it. A fresh mind does the best proofreading.
- Submit a carefully prepared manuscript. Failing to consult the journal's instructions to authors and carelessness in preparation suggests that maybe the study was careless.

Writing for publication requires discipline, time, and energy, but it completes the work of the investigator. It makes your work part of medical history. It is worth the effort!

Questions

True or False

1. Peer review means manuscripts submitted for possible publication in a medical journal are first reviewed by a panel of experts on the topic of the paper.
2. Authorship is based entirely on who collected the data.
3. You should always start writing your paper with an outline.
4. The basic format of a scientific paper is title, abstract, introduction, methods, results, discussion, in that order.
5. The single most important thing to remember about writing a research paper is that there must be a logical continuity throughout the title, introduction, methods, results, and discussion sections.
6. Describing the calibration of measurement instruments is really not an important issue because readers assume your devices work properly.
7. Journals do not usually publish instructions for authors.

CHAPTER 15

The Abstract

A s we learned in the previous chapter, the abstract is a condensed version of a research paper that appears at the beginning of the publication. Many readers skim the abstract to see if they are interested enough to read the whole paper. Some readers don't have enough time to read anything more than abstracts. For these reasons, the abstract is an important element of a published paper. In fact, it is so important that sometimes it is published without the paper!

Background

Many medical associations (including Respiratory Care) hold annual scientific conventions during which researchers give presentations of their work. The presentations are of two basic types: lectures and poster presentations. During the time leading up to the convention, the medical association will send out a "call for abstracts" requesting that researchers submit the results of their unpublished studies in abstract form. These abstracts are then subjected to peer review. Accepted abstracts are published together in one issue of the medical association's professional journal. Authors of accepted abstracts are then invited to present their work at the convention in the form of either a lecture or a poster presentation. For the annual international Respiratory Care Congress, all accepted abstracts are presented as posters. I will describe poster presentations in Chapter 17. In this chapter, I will describe the type of abstract that is published in *Respiratory Care*, which is very similar to other medical journals.

Specifications

An abstract may report (1) an original study, (2) the evaluation of a method, device, or protocol, or (3) a case or case series. Topics may be aspects of adult acute care, continuing care/rehabilitation, perinatology/pediatrics, cardiopulmonary technology, or health care delivery. The abstract may have been presented previously at a local or regional (but not national) meeting and should not have been published previously in a national journal. The abstract will be the only evidence by which the reviewers can decide whether the author should be invited to present a poster at the annual meeting. Therefore, *the abstract must provide all important data, findings, and conclusions.* Give specific information. Do not write general statements like "Results will be presented . . ." or "Significance will be discussed . . . ."

Content Elements

Original Study

Abstracts *must* include: (1) background (statement of research problem, question, or hypothesis); (2) method (description of research design and conduct in sufficient detail to permit judgment of validity); (3) results (statement of research findings with quantitative data and statistical analysis); and (4) conclusions (interpretation of the meaning of the results).

Method, Device, or Protocol Evaluation

Abstracts *must* include: (1) background (identification of the method, device, or protocol and its intended function); (2) method (description of the evaluation in sufficient detail to permit judgment of its objectivity and validity); (3) results (findings of the evaluation); (4) experience (summary of the author's practical experience or a lack of experience with the method, device, or protocol); and (5) conclusion (interpretation of the evaluation and experience). Cost comparisons should be included where possible and appropriate.

Case Report

Abstracts *must* report a case that is uncommon or of exceptional educational value and must include: (1) introduction (relevant basic information important to understanding the case); (2) case summary (patient data and response, details of interventions); and (3) discussion. Content should reflect results of literature review. The author(s) should have been actively involved in the case, and a case-managing physician must be a co-author or must approve the report.

Format

Most, if not all, major medical journals require you to submit your abstract using the Internet. Thus, you will have to check with the journal's Web site for specific formatting instructions and things like the maximum number of words or characters permitted in the abstract.

In some ways, writing this type of abstract is more difficult than writing a whole paper. You must think carefully about what you must include and what you would like to include if space permits. The best way to write this type of abstract is to first read some published abstracts and study the ones that look neat and are easy to read and understand. Some good examples are included at the end of the chapter. Then create a rough draft of your own abstract. Don't worry about the size of the abstract, but keep it to one page. Start, as always, with an outline (and one with more detail than just introduction, methods, results, and discussion).

When the first draft is finished, go back and consider how you might reorganize the outline to make it shorter. Start thinking about the final size. Rewrite the abstract so that it is about the right length. Next, proofread each sentence. Try to think of ways to reword sentences to make them shorter. Use shorter words and abbreviations where possible. This should get you to the required size. Make sure you use boldface for the major headings (e.g., Background, Methods) so they stand out (assuming this is carried through to the final product—some submission processes may block formatting). Make sure your title is brief and correctly formatted (e.g., all bold, capital letters) so that it stands out too. Finally, make sure you submit the abstract following all the instructions to authors provided by the journal. *And, don't miss the deadline!*

Model Abstract

Following are two examples of well-written abstracts that were submitted, reviewed, accepted, and published in *Respiratory Care*. Study them carefully and note that they have all the elements required of a good abstract.

Model Abstract #1: Mid-Frequency Ventilation: Optimum Settings for ARDS[1]

Background: Studies support the use of small tidal volumes (6-8 mL/kg) during mechanical ventilation to reduce ventilator induced lung injury. The extreme of this philosophy is high frequency ventilation (HFV), which requires specialized ventilators. Conventional adult ventilation, even with low volumes, is applied with relatively low frequencies (<35/min). No studies have described a method of determining an optimum frequency using conventional ventilators. The purpose of this study was to develop a mathematical model that predicts a patient-dependent frequency that minimizes tidal volume while maximizing alveolar minute ventilation (AMV) during conventional pressure-controlled continuous mandatory ventilation (PC-CMV). ***Methods:*** We modified the Marini et al. model of PC-CMV (*J Appl Physiol* 1989, 67:1081-92) to include variable dead space fraction (DSF). The new model allows input of patient data including height, compliance, resistance, DSF, inspiratory pressure (IP), PEEP, and duty cycle (%I) and outputs AMV, tidal volume, mean airway, and autoPEEP as functions of frequency. If IP is adjusted until peak AMV equals physiologically required AMV, then optimum frequency and volume are those that produce peak AMV. The model simulated ARDS using resistance = 10 cm H_2O/L/s and compliance = 0.025 L/H_2O, DSF = 0.45, height = 170 cm. We varied model parameters to identify the effects of lung mechanics and DSF on output variables. ***Results:*** At nominal ARDS parameters the optimum frequency was 45/min delivering 4.3 mL/kg with autoPEEP = 1 cm H_2O (**Figure 15.1**). Changing resistance and compliance to double the time constant yielded optimum values at 28/min, 5.4 mL/kg. Increasing DSF to 0.60 yielded 46/min and 5.9 mL/kg. The lowest optimum tidal volume was always at

[1] Chatburn RL. Mireles-cabodevila E. Mid-frequency ventilation: optimum settings for ARDS. *Resp Care* 2008;*53* (11):1588.

Figure 15.1

Mid-frequency ventilation abstract.

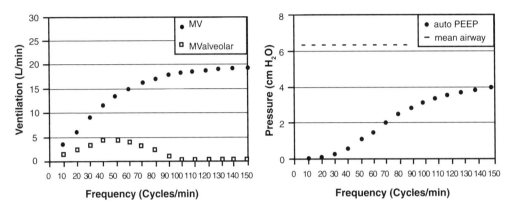

Source: Courtesy of RESPIRATORY CARE and the American Association for Respiratory Care.

%I = 50%; other values for %I yielded higher lower frequencies and higher tidal volumes. **Conclusion:** Measured lung mechanics and deadspace can predict optimum settings with this model. PC-CMV optimized for minimum tidal volume and maximum alveolar ventilation results in lower tidal volumes and higher ventilatory frequencies than conventionally used but below that requiring specialized ventilators.

Model Abstract #2: Laboratory Evaluation of Three Stockpiled Portable Ventilators[2]

Background: Several portable ventilators with different operational characteristics are stockpiled and designated for emergency use. **Objective:** The objective of this study was to evaluate the trigger characteristics during pressure support ventilation and effects of changing load (decreasing lung compliance and increasing airways resistance) on tidal volume delivery during volume controlled ventilation. We hypothesize that there would be performance differences among ventilator brands. **Methods:** The Impact Univent 750, Viasys LTV 1000, and Newport HT-50 ventilators were connected to an ASL 5000 lung simulator (IngMar

[2] Volsko TA, Chatburn RL, Coniglio N. Laboratory evaluation of three stockpiled portable ventilators. *Resp Care* 2008;*53*(11):1550.

Medical Inc). A passive model was used to test stability of tidal volume delivery. Each ventilator was set to volume controlled continuous mandatory ventilation (VC-CMV) at a frequency of 15/min with a 1.0 second inspiratory time and a PEEP of 5 cm H_2O. Set tidal volume was 500 mL or 1000 mL with normal load (compliance 75 mL/cm H_2O, resistance 6 H_2O/L/sec) and high load (compliance 40 mL/cm H_2O, resistance 15.0 cm H_2O/L/sec). Tidal volume delivery error was defined as 100% × (delivered volume – set volume)/set volume. To determine trigger performance during continuous spontaneous ventilation, we used an active lung model with a normal load and frequency of 15 breaths/min, PEEP of 5 cm H_2O and a pressure support of 15 cm H_2O above baseline. Differences in mean values were evaluated using one-way ANOVA. Statistical significance was set at $p < 0.05$. **Results:** The results are shown in **Table 15.1**. Tidal volume delivery was different among brands for the same pressure support settings. There were no differences in trigger variables, but expiratory resistance was higher in the LTV 1000. There were no differences in tidal volume delivery error. **Conclusion:** Stockpiled portable ventilators vary in some of their performance characteristics. Therapists must be aware of these differences in order to initiate and manage patients on portable mechanical ventilators.

Table 15.1

Performance Characteristics of Portable Ventilators

Ventilator	Insp. T_{90} (ms)	PIP (cm H_2O)	Trig Delay (ms)	Trigger Work (mJ)	Tidal Volume (mL)	T_I (ms)	Cycle Synchrony (ΔT_I)	Exp. T_{90} (ms)	R_E (cm H_2O/L/s)	$Load_{Lo}$ V_T Error (mL)	$Load_{Hi}$ V_T Error (mL)
			Pressure Support							*VC-CMV*	
LTV-1000	0	19	429	1.1	949	1440	44	1596	4.8	–7%	–6%
HT-50	537	21	435	1.9	1155	1330	33	838	0.3	–8%	–6%
Impact Eagle 750	NA	NA	164	6.4	NA	NA	NA	NA	NA	–10%	–2%
p value			*0.285*	*0.9*	*0.005*	*0.1*	*0.096*	*<0.001*	*<0.001*	*0.602*	*0.616*

Abbreviations: Insp T_{90} = inspiratory pressure at 90%, PIP = peak inspiratory pressure, Trig Delay = trigger delay, T_I = inspiratory time, Exp T_{90} = expiratory pressure at 90% of expiratory time, R_E = Median Expiratory Resistance, $Load_{Lo}$ V_T error = the percent error in tidal volume with normal resistance and compliance, $Load_{Hi}$ V_T error = the percent error in tidal volume with high resistance and low compliance.

What Not to Do (Analysis of Rejected Abstracts)

The following pages show sample abstracts similar to some I have seen as a reviewer and rejected for a variety of reasons. They are perfect examples of what not to do. Read each one through as if you were a reviewer and try to spot the problems. In Appendix III, you will find checklists that reviewers for *Respiratory Care* use to appraise papers and manuscripts. Use the appropriate checklist (original study, device evaluation, or case study) to judge the quality of the abstracts in this section. After each abstract, we will discuss the issues.

Abstract #1: Quality Improvement Using Therapist-Driven Protocols

One of our quality monitors is the oxygen saturation (Spo_2) of patients receiving O_2. We found that patients received prolonged administration of O_2 with inefficient weaning taking place. The criteria for "excessive O_2" was a consistent $Spo_2 > 96\%$. The quality committee felt that this situation was due to a lack of structure in our weaning process and proposed the development and implementation of a therapist-driven O_2 weaning protocol. We then conducted a literature search on weaning pediatric patients from oxygen. Also, we surveyed attending physicians about how they would like to see their patients weaned. Twelve of 22 physicians responded. They indicated they would like to see their patients checked at least every 3 hours and weaned for saturations $>95\%$ in approximately 5% decrements. An O_2 weaning protocol for the general care areas was written using this information. The goals of the protocol were to improve patient care, to allow for a more efficient use of O_2, and to reduce patient cost. The weaning protocol was approved by the Medical Executive Committee and the Respiratory Therapy medical director. In November the protocol was implemented. Following a random selection of patients with diagnoses that precluded the necessity of chronic O_2 administration, (e.g., as BPD and cystic fibrosis) 17 patients were selected for chart review from 2 years prior to the protocol to 1 year after. Diagnoses reviewed were asthma, croup, bronchiolitis, pneumonia, and post-op patients. For these patients, the average period on O_2 prior to the protocol was 2.6 days. After the protocol, the average period was 1.6 days. These preliminary findings, although not statistically significant ($p > 0.05$), indicate the protocol may be effective in decreasing O_2 use in these patients. The quality-improvement process, when appropriately used, can result in patient cost savings and improved patient care.

Review of Abstract #1

What is the very first thing you notice about this abstract? It is not in the standard format with subheads for background, methods, results, and conclusion sections. The first impression you get is that the authors were careless in preparation. They were probably inexperienced and lacking a good mentor. You can see this from the way the sentences were constructed. For example, they say, "Diagnoses reviewed were asthma, croup, bronchiolitis, pneumonia, and post-op patients." An experienced mentor would have pointed out that *diagnoses* were not reviewed but rather *data* (i.e., patient records) were reviewed for patients with specific diagnoses. Let's ask some basic questions:

- *Is the background information adequate?* In fact it reads like it is all background information—just a narrative and not a study at all. We can't even tell if this is an original study or a device/protocol evaluation.
- *Is there a hypothesis or explanation of device?* We can't really tell what the study question is, and there certainly is no hypothesis statement. It just rambles on without any real focus.
- *Is there enough detail in the methods?* Well, there was a literature search but we don't know why. There was some kind of survey but no detail of questions asked. Based on the survey a protocol was written and implemented. Patients were randomly selected, but selection criteria are not clear and we don't know why they were reviewed until we see results on oxygen usage (i.e., no prior hypothesis). Methods and results are scrambled together. A *p* value is given, but we don't know what statistical test was performed.
- *Are results complete?* We have to hunt for results and guess at their validity.
- *Are conclusions appropriate?* The only outcome variable seems to be period of oxygen use, and there was no difference before and after implementation of the protocol. There are no data on cost or quality of patient care, so no conclusions can be made on cost or quality.
- *Other problems:* The authors use the acronym BPD without defining it. Remember, the journal may be read by people outside the U.S. hospital environment, who would not know what this means. The number of physicians who responded to the survey was noted but not how many were asked to respond. What if the respondents represented a very small minority of the physicians? How can we generalize the results to the whole hospital?
- *Verdict:* This abstract needs major revision!

Abstract #2: Comparison of Whole-Body Plethysmography (WBP) with In-Line Pneumotachography (ILP) for Neonatal Pulmonary Function Measurements

ILP has long been the standard device for air-flow measurements in newborn pulmonary function. This device is known to be affected by barometric pressure Fio_2, temperature, airway pressure, and humidity.

Two ILP volume-monitoring devices (Bear NVM1 and Bicore 100) and a WBP device (Vitaltrends VT1000) were compared to understand the effects of changing gas conditions under typical clinical settings. Tidal volume (VT), inspiratory time (TI), and resistance (R) were compared.

Without BTPS and Fio_2 correction, the effect on volume measurement was found to be large for pneumotachography.

$(VT_{VT1000} = 1.24*VT_{Bicore} + 0.28, R^2 = 0.999, VT_{VT1000} = 1.18*VT_{NVM} + 0.31, R^2 = 0.993$ at $Fio_2 = 100)$. When corrected for Fio_2 and BTPS, the Bear NVM1 and the VT1000 show the same volumes ($VT_{VT1000} = 1.09*VT_{Bicore} + 0.29$, $R^2 = 0.993$ at $Fio_2 = 100$, $VT_{VT1000} = 0.93*VT_{NVM}$, $R^2 = 1$ at $Fio_2 = 21$). The VT1000 calibrates itself for Fio_2 and BTPS. The Bear NVM1 provides a lookup table for correction to BTPS conditions. When not taking into account the difference in mean level, the interclass correlation coefficient (ICC) in all cases was found to be significant (ICC = 0.98, 0.97, and 0.98 for VT1000 vs NVM1, VT1000 vs Bicore, and the Bear vs Bicore, respectively). Pulmonary mechanics measurements were similar between the VT1000 and the Bicore (ICC = 0.99) for TI, ICC = 0.99 for R). Although resistance trended similarly there was a large offset.

When uncorrected (as is typically the case in clinical settings), the ILP method can over- or underestimate minute volume by as much as 24% in our study. We concluded that WBP measurement is convenient for monitoring critically ill neonates and provides a more accurate bedside readout of minute volumes under conditions of varying Fio_2, RH, temperature, and atmospheric pressure.

Review of Abstract #2

Again, the first thing you notice about this abstract is that it is not in the standard format with subheads for background, methods, results, and conclusion sections, so they are not clearly identifiable. And again, an experienced mentor would have pointed out minor errors in wording. For example, the first sentence says "ILP has long been the standard device for air-flow measurements in newborn pulmonary function." But in the title, ILP is defined as inline pneumotachography, which is a procedure, not a device.

- *Is the background information adequate?* Maybe too brief, but it is there.
- *Is there a hypothesis or explanation of device?* There is no definite hypothesis statement, but we can piece together the idea that the authors wanted to evaluate the effects of gas condition on the accuracy of tidal volume, inspiratory time, and resistance measurements. You wonder why those particular measurements were chosen.
- *Is there enough detail in the methods?* What methods? The authors jump right into results. Are the measurements made on patients or a lung simulator? What were the gas conditions (e.g., temperature, barometric pressure, Fio_2)? A correlation coefficient is the wrong statistic to compare agreement among measurements (see Chapter 10). Regression may be all right in this case, but we only know the method was used if we are familiar with the format of the equations presented as results. The authors use the acronym BTPS without explanation, assuming readers will know it means body temperature and pressure saturated. Keep in mind that many medical journals have international readership, so readers may not be familiar with common abbreviations, acronyms, or jargon used in the United States.
- *Are results complete?* There are plenty of numbers, but we are not sure how they were obtained. It hurts my head to try to read, let alone interpret, all those equations bunched together. Also, the authors suddenly switch from using the term NVM1-to-Bear, to represent the Bear NVM1 device. This is confusing, especially since it occurs in the same sentence.
- *Are conclusions appropriate?* The authors assume the VT1000 is the standard (again we have to guess this from the format of the regression equations). Why should we believe that assumption? They conclude that WBP is accurate, but it was not compared with any type of

gold standard to make that conclusion. Indeed, it was compared only with devices expected to be inaccurate due to lack of correction factors.

- *Verdict:* This abstract was a little better than the last but still needs work.

Abstract #3: Effect of PEEP in Patients with Congenital Diaphragmatic Hernia

Introduction

Infants with congenital diaphragmatic hernia (CDH) continue to be a challenge to ventilate. Little data have been published on the use of PEEP in these infants post ECMO. We evaluated the effects of PEEP on lung compliance (Cdyn), physiologic deadspace (V_D/V_T), $Paco_2$, and Pao_2, during trials off of ECMO in infants with CDH.

Methods

Patients were sedated, paralyzed, and ventilated in the pressure control mode on the Servo 900C. Standard ventilator settings were a rate of 30 breaths/min and a PIP/PEEP of 30/5 cm H_2O. Cdyn, V_T/V_D ratios, and arterial blood gases were recorded during routine separations from the ECMO circuit. PEEP levels were lowered to 2 cm H_2O while maintaining the same peak inspiratory pressure. Measurements were then repeated. Decreasing the PEEP from 5 cm H_2O to 2 cm H_2O was associated with a significant improvement in Cdyn ($p = 0.006$), V_D/V_T ($p = 0.011$), and V_T/kg ($p < 0.001$). The $Paco_2$ also significantly improved on a lower PEEP ($p = 0.02$). However, there was no significant difference in the Pao_2.

Discussion

We conclude that both Cdyn and V_D/V_T in the CDH infant significantly improves on low levels of PEEP. The concurrent lowering of the mean airway pressure does not adversely affect the Pao_2. These findings suggest that PEEP levels greater than 2 cm H_2O worsen physiologic deadspace and compliance during trials off of ECMO, potentially altering the clinical assessment. Further studies are needed to determine whether it is the anatomic and/or alveolar deadspace that increases with higher PEEP levels.

Review of Abstract #3

At last we have an abstract with the correct format: Background, Methods, Results, Conclusion.

- *Is the background information adequate?* Yes, short, relevant, and to the point.
- *Is there a hypothesis or explanation of device?* Study purpose is stated, but it would have been clearer if a specific hypothesis was given.
- *Is there enough detail in the methods?* No description of study entry criteria for patients (although some info is in the results section). How many times were measurements repeated? How were deadspace and dynamic compliance assessed? The mode of ventilation is not clear. There is no description of statistical procedures.

- *Are results complete?* No actual data are given. We need summary data at least, like mean and standard deviation values for measured variables.
- *Are conclusions appropriate?* Assuming the statistical procedures were done correctly, the conclusions are justified.
- *Verdict:* Without more detail in the methods and some actual data, we cannot judge the value of this study. The authors ask us to take too much on faith. Close, but still not there.

This last example is very interesting. Read it carefully.

Abstract #4: Simulation of Closed-Chest Compression Using a Mechanical Test Lung

Background

Closed-chest compression during cardiopulmonary resuscitation (CPR) is recognized as an important lifesaving procedure. The function of breathing assistance devices, such as manual bag-valve and automatic resuscitators, is affected by chest compression because they are pressure sensitive. As breathing assistance devices evolve, the need exists to test these devices, techniques, and equipment to ensure safety and efficacy. Such a system is described below.

Equipment

The lung was simulated by a commercially available lung model (SMS, England). An external compression simulator was attached to the model as well as a pressure tap for data acquisition. The lung compression device was composed of an air cylinder with bidirectional flow adjustments to control compression speed, a pressure-adjustable air supply to control maximum force, and control circuits and a solenoid valve for actuation. The cylinder mount directed the cylinder rod against the mechanical test lung, and a stop was mounted to the frame to simulate the maximum depth of an external compression. The simulator was equipped with controls to regulate cycle rate, speed, force, and distance. A fine adjustment scale on the speed and pressure control ensured repeatability.

Methods

A breathing device, such as a manual bag-valve or automatic resuscitator, was used to simulate artificial ventilation. The chest compression simulator was activated to simulate CPR. This was helpful in evaluating synchronous and nonsynchronous compressions with breathing cycles at various compression rates.

Results

The compression rate was set at 80 times per minute with a ratio of 5 compressions per breath. The proximal airway pressure waveform was recorded utilizing a computer data acquisition system (see **Figure 15.2**). The pressure waveform represented external chest compressions during resuscitation.

Figure 15.2

Simulation abstract.

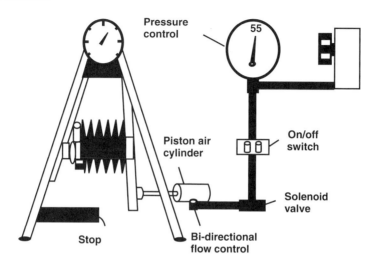

Labels: Pressure control, Piston air cylinder, On/off switch, Solenoid valve, Stop, Bi-directional flow control, 55

Conclusion

Because this lung compression system is so versatile, it can be used to evaluate different types of respiratory devices. In this study, closed-chest compressions were simulated under controlled conditions. This system can be effectively used to test the safety and efficacy of other breathing assistance devices.

Review of Abstract #4

So what do you think? It's beautiful, isn't it? Great layout, easy to read, good introductory sentence. It even has a nice line drawing. There is only one problem: this is not a device evaluation. It is just a narrative description. The equipment, methods, and results sections are all essentially the same thing, a description of a test setup. A nice little story, but not even close to being a scientific study.

Summary

By now, you should be familiar with what an abstract is and how to create one the proper way. The mistakes that novices make have been illustrated, and you have seen what good abstracts look like. Abstracts are important because for many people, they are the first (sometimes only) involvement in research publication. And of course, once the abstract is written and published, most of the work for a full-length paper has been done.

Keep in mind that even though most journals subject abstracts to peer review, abstracts still do not have the same credibility as papers. This lack of credibility is because the methods are necessarily abbreviated and readers cannot properly judge the study's validity. Many bad-quality abstracts slip by the reviewers due to the sheer numbers submitted. Always interpret any abstracts you read with a healthy skepticism.

Questions

True or False

1. You may publish only an abstract of a study and not write a whole paper.
2. Usual topics for an abstract are (1) an original study, (2) a device or method evaluation, and (3) a case study.
3. The abstract should give a brief overview of the study and not include any data.
4. A published abstract is just as credible as a published paper.
5. Abstracts are never peer reviewed like papers are.

The Case Report

Inclusion of a chapter on writing case reports might at first seem out of place in a text on clinical research. Properly selected and prepared, however, the report of a single case not only qualifies as legitimate clinical research but also presents an opportunity for health care practitioners to participate in the research and publication process when circumstances render other forms of research publication unfeasible. One need not have research funding, a laboratory, or a "sabbatical" from one's patient-care-based hospital position in order to prepare and publish an excellent case report. In addition, experience with a case report can help to create, in someone without previous research experience, the critical frame of mind that can be the crucial ingredient missing in unsuccessful attempts at formal research endeavors.

Virtually everyone participating in the assessment and care of patients encounters findings or outcomes, or solves clinical problems, in ways that could be "reportable" if they thought about them in the right way and then were able to follow through with "writing them up" correctly. The purpose of this chapter is to stimulate health care practitioners to think about the possibilities of investigating, learning from, and sharing with others in their field their experiences with patients, and to provide guidelines for turning those experiences into publications in the scientific literature. Case reports seldom make medical history. In general they are less significant scientifically than original investigations. However, there are some kinds of scientific information that cannot conveniently be communicated in any other way. The case report can be an important link in the larger chain of scientific progress and communication. Certainly, a case report must have the same sophistication, honesty, authoritativeness, and professionalism as a prospective study or comprehensive literature review. Thus, although it is one of the lesser players on the scientific stage, the case report requires no less care and must meet the same standards as its more celebrated colleagues in print.

Most case reports consist of a description of an individual illness, disease course, or treatment, followed by a discussion of the unique or particularly instructive features it demonstrates. In the majority of instances such a report is a few pages long at most and contains perhaps one figure or table and half a dozen references. Other formats, however, may occasionally be acceptable. Two cases may be reported, or even four or six, using the same basic outline, with discussion of the primary feature being reported coming after the last case description. The difference between such a multi-case report and a clinical series is mainly that the former is anecdotal, and thus less scientifically rigorous. Another format is the "case report and review of the literature," which consists of an extensive review of all the important published experience with a subject that is introduced by an illustrative individual case. In comparison with the usual, shorter type of case report, these have fewer opportunities for publication, since most medical journals today do not have the space to publish them.

A last variant of the basic case report is the case study, which is often a lengthy description of detailed laboratory investigation and represents highly original research, even though the research may be directed to elucidation of the disorders of a single patient. Detailed investigation of a single case is no substitute for a carefully designed clinical trial; instead, the instructive value of an individual case can sometimes be increased by careful modification of the circumstances under which the observation in question was made.

This chapter first discusses the qualifications for authorship of case reports and then summarizes the types of cases or observations that might be appropriate subjects for a published case report. Next comes a step-by-step discussion of the process of preparing and writing such a report, and a summary of its usual components. Finally, a dozen mistakes are described that authors of case reports, especially first-time authors, most frequently make. Ways are suggested to avoid these mistakes.

Who Should Write It?

The case report can be an ideal "first paper." Most reports of original investigation require expertise in several areas of scientific endeavor not ordinarily within the experience of the health care practitioner. But the case report can be written by anyone in the field, so long as he or she is prepared to work hard at it and obtain the right kinds of help. Writing a case report requires that the author thoroughly understand the case being reported and the disease or entity it is intended to illustrate; these requirements in turn imply access to reference materials and other facilities necessary to substantiate them.

A report of a new clinical finding or disease manifestation may well require expertise beyond your own, and simply reading about the conditions involved may not be sufficient for the task of writing the paper. In most circumstances, help will be required from someone with clinical experience in the relevant area, and the source of such assistance may not be immediately apparent. The medical director of health care services, another attending physician, or an instructor would be logical persons with whom to start, as would anyone else with personal experience with the condition in question.

Of course, a paper written for publication and the eyes of one's peers must be written in clear, correct English, and expertise in English composition is not necessarily a requirement for clinical work. Thus, the writing aspect of the case report may require help from someone more experienced, especially if English is not one's strong suit. This mundane aspect of the publication process is nonetheless vitally important, and medical journals often reject poorly written manuscripts irrespective of their scientific interest or accuracy.

There is no reason that one person cannot recognize, research, prepare, and submit a case report for publication. To do so requires expertise in the clinical practice, in literature review, and in scientific writing. Thus, most case reports, and especially those of first-time authors, have several contributors whose skills in different areas make the end product better than it would be with a single author. In most clinical cases, quite a number of individuals have been involved in various aspects. These may include the attending physician, consultants, nurses, respiratory therapists, laboratory personnel, statisticians, librarians, and secretaries. Who should and should not be listed as an author of the paper? This will vary depending on the complexity of the case, but as a rule most case reports should not require more than three or four authors. If more than four names appear on the title page, it is likely that one or two individuals really did the lion's share of the work; listing the others in effect detracts from the credit they deserve. Whoever had the original idea and actually wrote the paper should be first on the author list. The first listed author was usually responsible for the project and did more work than anyone else. Other individuals who made major contributions to the conception, background work, and writing should be co-authors. But do not include persons whose involvement was limited to taking care of the patient, running laboratory tests (unless these are experimental or special research procedures), interpreting x-rays, and so forth. Some department supervisors and medical directors insist that their names be on any paper to come out of their departments. This practice is unprofessional unless these individuals also made major contributions. Deciding early on who is and is not to be an author will save the project from later misunderstandings and unpleasantness.

Attributes of a Reportable Case

Case reports are generally seen as being less important contributions than papers describing prospective, controlled clinical trials and other kinds of research. This is true—case reports seldom make large impacts on medical progress. Several medical journals, in fact, no longer publish case reports at all. However, most editors recognize the distinct value of an appropriately prepared and targeted case report, and most clinical journals publish at least some.

What cases are appropriate varies with the journal and with its editorial policy. Here are three examples:

- The unique (or nearly unique) case, unreported previously
- The unexpected association of two or more known conditions or diseases in a single patient
- The unexpected outcome or event that suggests response to therapy or an adverse drug effect

In a broader sense, cases may be worthy of publication if their description and discussion presents either something new, or something already known, but in a particularly instructive example. To be something new does not necessarily require uniqueness in all the world's literature. Rather, such "news" should be previously unknown, or readily available within the health care setting. Also, a particularly instructive example may be defined differently in different situations.

Table 16.1 lists six settings in which publication of a case report may be justified. We discuss each of these settings below.

A New Disease or Condition

In recent history, acquired immune deficiency syndrome (AIDS) has reminded everyone connected with health care that medicine is not static. New diseases and disease-causing agents continue to appear. Still, a truly unique syndrome or entirely new disease is pretty rare. However, "new" need not mean "previously unreported anywhere," but rather a condition

Table 16.1

Possible Reportable Cases

- A new disease or condition
- A previously unreported clinical feature or complication of a known disease or condition
- A particularly instructive case of a previously known disease or condition
- A new diagnostic test or other assessment as illustrated by an individual case
- A new treatment modality
- A new outcome or complication of treatment

pertinent to the field that has not previously been described in the journals most likely to be read by one's peers.

A Previously Unreported Feature or Complication

Unreported features might include situations documented previously but not in the usual literature of the health care practitioner. There is, however, a burden of proof on the author to be certain that the disease or situation described has not in fact been similarly reported in the past. Thus, you must make as reasonably thorough a search of the literature as possible. Even when no prior description has been located, it is still unwise to make statements like "this is the first reported case." Few editors will allow such proclamations to be printed.

A Particularly Instructive Example of a Known Condition

A well-studied or unusually well-documented example of a known or even common condition can be a valuable teaching tool. Most medical journals do not publish formal case reports of such cases. Many journals have regular features that serve the same purpose—for example, "Case Records of the Massachusetts General Hospital" in *New England Journal of Medicine*, which provides a weekly clinico-pathological forum. Other journals (including *Respiratory Care*), however, may accept well-documented examples of known diseases or outcomes as case reports if they are authoritative and do not duplicate recently covered material.

A Case Illustrating a New Diagnostic Test or Monitoring Technique

Case reports in this category are exceptional. However, some methods of patient assessment cannot be initially evaluated with more rigorous trials involving large numbers of patients. A case report or small series of individual, anecdotal cases can be a reasonable alternative. For example, suppose persistent bronchopleural air leak during mechanical ventilation is an unusual occurrence at your institution. You have devised and documented a new, accurate way of quantitating the leak. A case report may constitute the only means readily available to disseminate information about it to your peers.

A New Treatment Modality

A management technique applied to an infrequently seen condition may have to be reported by means of a single case. The practitioner either sees too few of them or does not have the resources to perform a formal trial in a larger number of cases. This circumstance has admittedly been abused. The health care literature contains too many single-case reports of new treatments that appeared to work but have never subsequently been validated with appropriately designed investigations.

A New Outcome of Treatment

An unusual result or complication of treatment can form the basis of a case report, particularly if the events reported constitute a dramatic departure from the usual or expected. Cases in which a patient survives a previously uniformly fatal condition or dies from something that is not supposed to be serious should be documented. Documentation of adverse outcomes and complications is an important step in the eventual establishment of optimal patient care.

Steps in Preparing a Case Report

The principles of research design are applicable in many respects to the preparation of a single case report. In general, however, the process is less complex and some phases may be unnecessary. Preparing a case report is a project of much less complexity and magnitude than most formal research projects, mainly because only a single patient or event is being described and the topic is intentionally a narrower one. **Table 16.2** lists the stages through which most case reports pass, from initial conception to ultimate publication.

Identification of an Appropriate Case

Health care is a dynamic, rapidly evolving field that deals with diseases and treatments that were unheard of a generation or two ago. In this setting, the clinician inevitably encounters clinical presentations, complications, or outcomes that he or she has not previously seen. It is safe to predict that during a career in clinical health care, each of us will encounter cases or events that could be "reportable." We thus have the opportunity to contribute to the state of our knowledge in our field. In the great majority of instances, however, the unique or innovative will be overlooked. The cases reported in *Respiratory Care*, *Chest*, and *Anesthesiology* are not the only ones that happen; they are the ones that are recognized and pursued in the spirit of

Table 16.2

Steps in Writing a Case Report
- Identification of an appropriate case
- Review of the pertinent literature
- Consultation and discussion
- Planning the paper; assignment of roles and authorship
- Further investigation of the patient, institution of new therapy, or other original research
- Preparation of the first draft
- Preparation of tables and illustrations
- Consultation and discussion
- Revision of the manuscript
- Preparation and submission of final draft

scientific investigation. Thus, the vital ingredient enabling you to make the first step toward publishing a case report is a continual watchfulness for the interesting, the stimulating, and the different from what one usually sees. In most instances, cases so identified turn out to be instructive but already known to others in the profession. To find that one in five or one in twenty that could and should be pursued and published, however, it is important to establish an attitude of intellectual inquiry in your work. You should be thinking constantly of how one might learn more from everyday experience.

Review of the Pertinent Literature

Once you encounter a potentially new situation, you must learn more about the subject area in which it falls. Even "experts" who have performed research on the subject cannot say for certain that a particular circumstance has not been reported before. A literature search is always necessary. Start with textbooks or journals so that undue effort is not expended on expensive computerized searches. If you do not find any previous reference to a similar case, conduct a thorough literature search.

Consultation and Discussion

Before putting too much energy into a project, you should consult advisers whose experience is more extensive than your own. A therapist or technician might well discuss the case with the medical director of the department, or with a specialist in the area involved, or with an instructor in a local training program. These individuals will not necessarily become co-authors should the case proceed to that stage, but their perspective can help to direct the author's efforts and to avoid unnecessary labor. If no such individual is readily available, consider writing a letter to the editor of the journal to which you want to submit. You could also contact one of the individuals listed as a consultant or editorial board member on the journal's title page.

The physician caring for the subject of the case report must be informed that his or her patient's case is being considered for publication. In some cases, the patient's physician should be a co-author. But this is not usually the case unless that physician initiated or participated in the study that is being described in the report. Instances have occurred in which two or more separate groups of individuals have unknowingly prepared manuscripts reporting the same case. These situations occur when a case has attracted a lot of attention or involved a large number of consultants.

Planning the Paper and Assignment of Roles and Authorship

Once you have become something of an expert on the subject of the report, begin planning the "nuts and bolts" of the paper. Outline the content of each of the structural elements of the case report (described in subsequent sections of the chapter). If photographs, artist's drawings, or statistical analyses will be required, they must be no less professional than the rest of the paper.

Most case reports have two to four authors, each of whom plays a different role in assembling the components of the final product. Who is and is not to be listed as an author should be agreed upon as early in the process as possible in order to avoid later conflict and antagonism. To be an author, each person must play a vital role, not necessarily in the care of the patient but in making the case report happen. Authors are those who are instrumental in library research, writing, editing, and preparation of tables or illustrations. It is helpful to draw up a rough schedule at this stage. The participants should agree to meet regularly until the paper is finished.

Further Investigation of the Case

Case studies are based primarily on the value of carefully designed scientific investigation carried out on a particular patient once the uniqueness or other value of that patient's illness has been recognized. In such instances, all the steps described thus far consist of preparation for additional data collection based on what has been learned to that point. Most case reports do not contain this step of further investigation. But in those that do, it must be thoroughly thought out and designed before any more data are collected. Simply ordering all the tests one can think of on a patient with an unusual condition will waste resources, subject the patient to needless risk, and be unlikely to produce the new knowledge required for a worthwhile case study. The collaboration of an expert with experience in investigating similar cases is vital to the success of this type of case report. Data collected prospectively in the in-depth study of a single patient must be handled like data collected in other types of clinical research, as described elsewhere in this book.

Preparation of the First Draft

Writing the first draft is the most difficult step for first-time authors and for many experienced scientific writers as well. You can get "unstuck" by simply striving to get *something* down on paper—to get the process rolling and to provide something on which to build. One effective approach is to first gather all your data and notes, assembled during background reading and meetings among the paper's authors. Then make a one-page outline of the paper, including major components and points to be covered. Next, sit down and work your way through the pile of notes, making a crude narrative that follows the outline. At this stage, pay no attention to grammar or punctuation—simply try to get it all down. This sloppy, too long, usually confusing document constitutes a first draft. The draft serves as the real foundation on which the final manuscript will be constructed.

There are many other good ways to write a paper. Someone who has never written a comprehensive term paper or formal essay in high school or college might well enlist the help of an individual with more experience, even if they were not involved in the case being reported. There are excellent books on basic scientific writing that can also be helpful to first-time and experienced authors alike.

Preparation of Tables and Illustrations

Most case reports require means other than tests to convey important aspects of the case and to clarify their instructional value. This is not to say that a table must be assembled, or x-rays photographed, just to "flesh out" the report. Tables and illustrations can be difficult to prepare correctly, and including them is more expensive for the journal, so each one must communicate information vital to the case that cannot be conveyed more effectively in another way. Tables and figures are not peripheral details to be taken care of as the final version is readied but are primary, central features of the paper. Along with the abstract, they will be the first parts of the paper to be looked at by reviewers, the editor, and the eventual reader.

Consultation and Discussion

After a first, complete, working draft has been put together, it is a good idea to have an experienced individual not connected with the project examine the entire draft. This may not be required if one of the authors has extensive experience both with the subject matter and with manuscript preparation, but it can help to add perspective and guide revision, thus making the manuscript better. Having the paper "pre-reviewed" locally, before submission to a journal and while it can still be revised, can improve its chances for acceptance in the hands of the journal's editor and reviewers. Such a pre-reviewer should be thanked with an acknowledgment, usually placed just above the references in the manuscript.

Manuscript Revision

Every good manuscript goes through several revisions before it is finally submitted for publication. How many times this will have to be done to produce the clearest, most concise final product varies with the complexity of the project, the experience of the authors, and the degree to which they agree on revisions. A good paper is not ready for submission the minute its parts have been assembled for the first time. Manuscripts sent to an editor in this condition have little chance for acceptance.

Preparation and Submission of Final Draft

Prospective authors must read carefully the "instructions for manuscript preparation" section of a recent issue of the journal to which the paper will be sent. Then they must follow these instructions to the letter. Following detailed submission instructions may seem a tiresome chore in the euphoria that comes with completion of a project, but it is no less important than the other stages of manuscript preparation.

Each author should receive a copy of the final manuscript as it is to be submitted for publication. In addition to ensuring that he or she agrees with everything that is said in the paper, this will guarantee that each author's name and professional affiliations are shown correctly on the title page. Keep in mind that a published paper is a permanent, public record.

Structure of a Case Report

Like other forms of scientific writing, the case report should be organized so that its message is presented to the reader in the clearest, most logical fashion. Properly written case reports, therefore, are not just baskets carrying unconnected facts, like the telephone directory; they are instruments of persuasion. In keeping with this notion that an author needs to convince the reader of the validity of what is said, there is a logical arrangement for any scientific paper, including case reports:

1. Statement of problem or posing of question
2. Presentation of evidence
3. Explanation of the validity of the evidence presented
4. Implications of the evidence: initial conclusion or answers; statement of additional supporting evidence

5. Assessment of conflicting evidence
6. Final conclusion

Case reports are generally brief and need not have separate sections for each of these components. Most reports have the logical format of introduction, case summary, presentation of additional data (if appropriate), discussion, and references. Some journals also require a brief abstract preceding the introduction. However, the fundamental purpose of the paper is to communicate information, and some cases may lend themselves better to some variation on this plan. In all cases, however, the "critical argument" sequence outlined above should be considered and its elements addressed.

Most case reports will lend themselves best to the structure summarized in the next sections.

Introduction

The introduction announces to the reader what the paper is about and why it is important. It generally should not be more than a paragraph. If definitions or a description of the syndrome being presented are necessary for the reader's understanding of the case summary, then the introduction should provide these.

Case Summary

The case summary is the heart of the case report, and it must include enough data to convince a critical reader that the author's contention is correct. Only those aspects of the patient's illness, the event, or the procedure described that are crucially important for this purpose should be included. Inexperienced authors often have difficulty distinguishing the clinically relevant from the extraneous in this respect, so having the case reviewed by an expert can be helpful.

Although only elements important to the report should be provided, the case summary should still adhere to the traditional format for presenting a case:

1. Chief complaint
2. Current illness
3. Personal and family history
4. Occupational and environmental history
5. Physical examination findings
6. Initial laboratory findings
7. Initial x-ray findings
8. Working diagnosis
9. Hospital course
   a. Initial treatment
   b. Chronology of response to treatment; complications; new forms of treatment; later physical or laboratory findings
   c. Current status or outcome; revised diagnosis or problem list

In most cases, some of these components will not be needed, and others need be mentioned only briefly, but the sequence should be followed.

Tables and Illustrations

Tables and illustrations are really part of the case summary, unless the paper also contains a results section following the case summary that presents data from original research based on or developed from the patient's illness. Numerical data, such as long sequences of arterial blood gas values or other measurements, if included at all, should generally be provided in a table. An alternative is to display these data visually using a graph, particularly when a small number of functions (such as Po_2, Pco_2, and pH) are reported repeatedly to describe the course of the patient's condition. Most journals publish explicit instructions for the preparation of tables and figures in their instructions for authors, and these must be followed.

Radiographs and other images are often reproduced in case reports because of their important role in diagnosing and managing diseases of the chest. However, it is difficult to reproduce chest films in a manner that shows the desired features clearly to the reader of the final published product. If the chest x-ray was normal, or showed right upper lobe consolidation or a pneumothorax, this can simply be stated. If information vital to the case report is on film, consultation with both the radiologist and a medical photographer will ensure the best possible reproduction. Once the radiologist has pointed out exactly what and where the features are that should be illustrated, you should go over this with the photographer so that he or she can use developing and printing techniques that best show these features.

Discussion

A case report should teach, and the teaching is done in the discussion. The discussion amplifies the case summary by pointing out and explaining its unique or otherwise important aspects. The elements of "critical argument" listed at the beginning of this section should be included. Typically, a case report's discussion section accomplishes this in three or four paragraphs that contain the following:

- Initial, brief summarizing statement of the reason for reporting the case
- Concise description of the disease or condition illustrated, if this was not done earlier, including any important features not found in the case presented
- Brief discussion of additional evidence, alternative explanations, atypical or complicating features, or other factors that need to be mentioned
- Clear statement of the lesson(s) to be learned from the case

Although some journals accept lengthy literature reviews introduced by case reports, the majority insist on brevity. Virtually all published case reports have shorter discussion sections than originally submitted to the editor. Thus, your goal should be to make only the points that have to be made, do this with the fewest possible words, and eliminate everything else. A five-page manuscript is no less a contribution than one four times that length, and it will be received more appreciatively by the journal's editor.

References

The references at the end of the paper should consist of a small number of citations. They should serve two specific purposes. First, because lengthy descriptions of the disease, treatment, and so on cannot be included in a case report, you should cite one or two authoritative sources of more complete information. These could be recent review articles or chapters in authoritative textbooks. Second, the references should back up any specific or controversial points made in the report. Citations should be specific, providing the reader with the exact source for the information referred to, rather than, for example, to an entire book, and they should also be to reference sources that are readily available to the reader of the paper. Do not cite references found in other papers unless you have personally read them; cited articles do not always contain the information suggested by their titles, or data justifying the conclusions drawn by previous authors who cited them.

Common Mistakes in Case Report Writing

Table 16.3 summarizes 12 mistakes commonly made by authors of case reports, particularly those with little previous experience with such projects.

Tunnel Vision

Through no fault of their own, prospective authors of case reports may believe their observation to be unique and "reportable" because they and those around them have never heard of it before, when in fact it is a well-documented but infrequent phenomenon. Steps 2 and 3 in Table 16.2, review of the literature and discussion of the case with an "expert," will prevent expenditure of needless effort in developing the project further.

Another form of tunnel vision is to assume the rest of the world uses the same procedures and equipment as you do. Stating that the patient underwent "standard tests for collagen vascular disease" will confuse many readers (What tests? Which collagen vascular diseases?) and fails to accomplish the basic goal of all scientific writing, which is to communicate information accurately and completely.

Insufficient Documentation of Case

One of the most frequent reasons that editors reject case reports submitted for publication is an inadequate database. It is not enough that the author really, truly believes that the patient had acute respiratory distress syndrome (ARDS) secondary to Legionnaire's disease. This diagnosis must be rigorously proven to the editor and to the reader. The proof is established not only with the accepted definitions and criteria but also by careful exclusion of other possible diagnoses. Case reports often provide more extensive documentation than would ordinarily be obtained in clinical practice. If features of the case are atypical or do not follow the expected course for the condition being reported, these must be explained convincingly.

Insufficient Documentation of Intervention

The author's belief that treatment of condition A with intervention B resulted in outcome C may be the reason for submitting the paper to a journal. Whether the journal's editor accepts

Table 16.3

Common Mistakes Made by Authors of Case Reports

In Selecting the Case Itself:
1. Tunnel vision: Unfamiliarity with experience or practice outside of one's own geographic region
2. Insufficient documentation of the case: Inadequate data base to establish the diagnosis or feature being reported
3. Insufficient documentation of intervention or outcome: Failure to prove the value of a new device, technique, or therapy
4. Poor patient care: Documentation of results of bad clinical practice rather than spontaneous events
5. Erroneous premise: Mistaken physiology or inadvisable therapy that happened to be associated with a favorable outcome on this occasion

In Preparing the Manuscript:
6. Wrong journal: Inappropriate subject matter or format
7. Literary inexperience: Unfamiliarity with scientific, professional, or medical writing
8. Inadequate literature review: Failure to locate and cite important background material
9. Ineffective illustrations or tables: Poor selection and communication of visual or numerical data
10. Poor references: Inappropriate selection of documentation or sources of more extensive information
11. Technical mistakes: Failure to adhere to journal's published instructions for manuscript preparation; inadequate proofreading prior to submission
12. Non-revision: Failure to follow through with suggestions by reviewers and editor to resubmit revised manuscript

that reasoning for publication is likely to depend upon the means by which the author proves his or her case. If a patient with ARDS recovers after receiving large doses of corticosteroids, one is tempted to conclude that recovery is related to the drugs. However, the essence of the scientific method is that such associations can, and must, be established far more rigorously. Perhaps the best way to begin is to consult with an individual having relevant experience.

Poor Patient Care

Some complications or outcomes submitted to journals as case reports occur not as spontaneous events but as a result of bad clinical management. Unless the intention of the author is to emphasize this for teaching purposes, such a paper would not be accepted for publication. Doing so would appear to give the journal's approval of the patient care described.

Erroneous Premise

Case reports that are based on a faulty understanding of physiology are occasionally submitted for publication (and some even have published). Others document potentially dangerous interventions that happened to be followed by a favorable outcome. In such cases, the problem is usually inexperience on the part of the would-be author, failure to review the relevant literature, and lack of discussion and consultation with more experienced individuals.

Submission to the Wrong Journal

Medical journals are published for well-defined audiences. Each has its own requirements for the format, length, and subject matter of papers it publishes. Prospective authors must familiarize themselves with the journal to which they intend to submit their manuscript. They must carefully read the journal's instructions for authors and a list of the articles that journal publishes. If the author is unfamiliar with a particular journal, an appropriate question would be why he or she wishes to submit a paper to it. If you do not read the journal, very likely your peers do not read it either.

Literary Inexperience

Often, authors submitting a case report have never before attempted to write something for publication. Few health care practitioners have had formal training in scientific writing and manuscript preparation. They should not be dissuaded from trying, because a case report is the ideal first paper, but they will need to study the subject or to collaborate with someone with appropriate experience.

Inadequate Literature Review

To serve its purpose of contributing to the sum of our knowledge on a particular subject, the case report must place the condition or event described in appropriate context. This requires that the author become thoroughly familiar with present knowledge on the topic prior to beginning to write. Cited references should be recent, and many more sources should be read than cited. The author must be confident that others have not published similar reports in the journal or field involved. Although it is a minor literary effort in comparison to some other types of publication, the case report is nonetheless a great deal of work—at least as much as a college term paper. Reviewing the literature makes up much of this work, but without this part of the project, the whole cannot succeed.

Ineffective Illustrations or Tables

Illustrations and tables are crucial to the case report's effectiveness, as already discussed, and must be of professional quality. Photographs of X-rays should not show more than the feature of interest: an entire 14- by 17-inch chest film should not be reproduced if a stenotic area in the cervical trachea is being illustrated. The film should be photographed and printed so as to emphasize the desired feature, and arrows should be included if the point referred to is not obvious to the reader. Tables are better than inclusion within the text if a series of numerical values must be reported, although such data have to be trimmed to only those results that are crucial to the case. Even if 16 different parameters of the patient's pulmonary function were measured, these should be omitted unless the value of the case rests on them.

Poor References

An author provides references so that the reader can amplify and verify statements made in the paper. All cited sources must therefore be recent and accessible in frequently used books or journals. The original description of an illness or therapy might be an exception to this rule, but review articles and chapters in textbooks must not be.

Technical Mistakes

There is no excuse for submitting a manuscript that does not conform to the journal's published instructions for authors. This applies not only to the paper's length and format, but also to restrictions on tables and illustrations and to the citation of references. In their rush to get the final draft into the mail, authors often fail to proofread their manuscript carefully enough and send it to the journal's editor with typographical errors, punctuation mistakes, and misspelled words. Every reference must be double-checked against its original source (not the rough draft), and, if possible, someone not connected with the paper should proofread it for grammar and typing.

Failure to Revise the Manuscript After Editorial Review

Not one manuscript in 100 is accepted on its first submission to a peer-review journal without requests that the author make some revisions. However, many papers fail to reach publication because the modifications suggested by reviewers or editor are not followed up by the author. If the manuscript cannot be made acceptable for publication, it will be rejected; otherwise, it will come back to the author with a list of changes the editor considers important in order to make it acceptable. Occasionally these suggestions are unreasonable or even impossible (for example, when additional data are required and the patient is no longer available or the records are lost), but in most cases the author can make the changes within a few hours. Comments from reviewers and editors are intended to improve the paper and ensure that it does not mislead or contain erroneous information. If the project was worth pursuing in the first place, it is worth the effort to revise the manuscript and attempt to meet the criticisms and suggestions made for it.

Questions

True or False

1. A case report consists of a description of an individual illness or treatment, followed by a discussion of the unique features it demonstrates.
2. A previously unreported clinical feature of a known disease is reportable as a case study.
3. A new diagnostic test or other assessment is not an appropriate report topic even if it is illustrated by an individual case.
4. Unlike an original study, the case report does not require a literature review.
5. A logical arrangement of the case report is: (1) statement of problem, (2) presentation of evidence, (3) explanation of validity of evidence, (3) implications of evidence, (4) assessment of conflicting evidence, (5) conclusions.
6. One common mistake made by authors of case reports is tunnel vision, or unfamiliarity with medical practice outside of one's own geographic region.

CHAPTER 17

The Poster Presentation

I n Chapter 15, on writing the abstract, we discussed the fact that scientific presentations at most medical conventions are either lectures or poster presentations. Poster sessions allow direct communication with the author(s) in a more relaxed and informal atmosphere and more time for the audience to examine illustrations (I once attended a poster session where they served wine!). These factors help to ensure proper interpretations of the information presented. The author or authors benefit too, in that dialogue with other researchers with similar interests may stimulate new ideas.

There are two main formats for poster presentations. In the first, called an open session, posters relating to various topics are set up in a large exhibit hall. The author or authors stand next to these posters and answer questions as interested viewers come by at random over a period of two to three hours. A more formal format is the poster symposium. Posters of related subject matter are grouped in a specified area at a specific time. A moderator, chosen for his or her expertise in the particular subject, directs each session. A relatively small audience views posters for a short period before the session begins. Then, at the moderator's request, the author gives a short (one- to two-minute) oral presentation outlining the significance of the study. Following this, the audience can discuss the work with the author. Often, discussions are generated among the members of the audience under the guidance of the moderator. Compared with oral abstract presentations, poster presentations are less formal and less anxiety producing for the beginner, and may have more of the atmosphere of a social event.

Poster quality at scientific meetings is sometimes barely acceptable. This is due primarily to poor planning and inexperience. The following suggestions should help to improve the effectiveness of a poster presentation.

Layout

A bulletin board will be provided by the sponsor of the conference for mounting the poster with thumbtacks. The usable surface of this board is usually four feet high and six feet long, and it will be elevated about two to three feet from the ground. The information presented by the poster follows the same format as the abstract of an article. The poster format includes a

Figure 17.1

Example layout for a poster presentation.

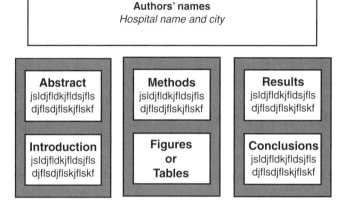

title (along with the names of the authors, institution, city, and state), introduction, methods, results, and conclusion (**Figure 17.1**).

The organization of information (eye movement) should flow naturally down columns or horizontally along rows. Material at the top and center of the poster will attract the most attention. Material in the lower left and right corners is less important, and these areas may be left blank to provide visual rest and to highlight the main points. Once the rough sketch is completed, it is helpful to redraw it full size on a blackboard. This will help to establish proportions and sizes of each section. Indicate text with horizontal lines, and draw in rough sketches of where the art will be.

Template

There was a time when authors made posters by hand, mounting pieces of typing paper on cardboard backing. I once even saw a well-known physician simply thumbtack handwritten notebook sheets to the poster board (I give him the benefit of the doubt and assume that his poster was lost in transit). Now, most authors create their posters in Microsoft® PowerPoint, then take the file to a printer (like Kinko's) and have the poster made into one large four- by six-foot sheet of thick, glossy paper. The poster is then rolled up, put into a cylindrical cardboard container, and transported as a carry-on at the airport.

Figure 17.2 shows the custom page layout settings I use in Microsoft PowerPoint. **Figure 17.3** (see pages 284–285) shows an actual poster created with this template that was presented at an international meeting.

Figure 17.2

Microsoft PowerPoint page setup dialog box illustrating the settings to use for a poster presentation slide template.

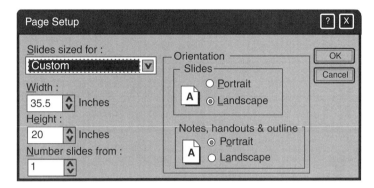

The single slide is saved as a .ppt file and used by a professional printer to create the poster.

Questions

True or False

1. Poster presentations allow direct communication with the author in an informal atmosphere and more time for the audience to examine illustrations.
2. Posters are usually not accepted in scientific meetings unless they are created by professional graphic artists.
3. Poster sections are similar to those of abstracts and papers: Title, Introduction, Methods, Results, and Conclusions.
4. You should strive for clarity and simplicity in your poster layout.

Figure 17.3

An actual poster created with a PowerPoint template.

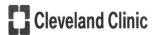

MID FREQUENCY VENTILATION:
Robert L. Chatburn, BS, RRT-NPS,
Cleveland Clinic,

Abstract

Studies support the use of small tidal volumes (6-8 mL/kg) during mechanical ventilation to reduce ventilator induced lung injury. The extreme of this philosophy is high frequency ventilation (HFV), which requires specialized ventilators. Conventional adult ventilation, even with low volumes, is applied with relatively low frequencies (<35/min). The purpose of this study was to develop a mathematical model that predicts a patient-dependent frequency that minimizes tidal volume while maximizing alveolar minute ventilation (AMV) during conventional pressure controlled continuous mandatory ventilation (PC-CMV). **METHODS**: We modified the Marini et al model of PC-CMV (J Appl Physiol 1989, 67:1081-92) to include variable dead space fraction (DSF). The new model allows input of patient data including height, compliance, resistance, DSF, inspiratory pressure (IP), PEEP, and duty cycle (%I) and outputs AMV, tidal volume, mean airway, and autoPEEP as functions of frequency. If IP is adjusted until peak AMV equals physiologically required AMV then optimum frequency and volume are those that produce peak AMV. The model simulated ARDS using resistance = 10 cm H$_2$O/L/s and compliance = 0.025 L/H$_2$O, DSF = 0.45, height = 170 cm. We varied model parameters to identify the effects of lung mechanics and DSF on output variables. **RESULTS**: At nominal ARDS parameters the optimum frequency was 45/min delivering 4.3 mL/kg with autoPEEP = 1 cm H$_2$O (see Figure 1). Changing resistance and compliance to double the time constant yielded optimum values at 28/min, 5.4 mL/kg. Increasing DSF to 0.60 yielded 46/min and 5.9 mL/kg. The lowest optimum tidal volume was always at %I = 50%; other values for %I yielded higher lower frequencies and higher tidal volumes. **CONCLUSON**: Measured lung mechanics and dead space can predict optimum settings with this model. PC-CMV optimized for minimum tidal volume and maximum alveolar ventilation results in lower tidal volumes and higher ventilatory frequencies than conventionally used but below that requiring specialized ventilators.

Introduction

Lower tidal volumes are now the standard of care for Acute Lung Injury/Acute respiratory Distress Syndrome (ARDS). A reduction in tidal volume leads to an increase in respiratory frequency. However, a limit of approximately 35 cycles/min has typically been used because of concerns related to auto PEEP (aPEEP), gas exchange and hemodynamic compromise. As a consequence, minute ventilation is commonly limited to the product of a V$_T$ of 6-8 mL/kg and a ventilatory frequency of 35 cycles/min. Thus, in practice, the selection of an "optimum" combination of frequency and V$_T$ reduces to setting a standard tidal volume and adjusting the frequency to get an acceptable PaCO$_2$, which is a rather primitive heuristic. As a result, conventional ventilators are probably not used to their fullest capacity in serving the dual goals of providing gas exchange while promoting lung protection. Another approach to minimizing tidal volume is high frequency ventilation (HFV), which requires specialized ventilators. Even with HFV, clinicians seldom consider any formal approach to optimizing settings in terms of frequency and V$_T$ combinations.

The only studies describing an algorithm for finding an optimum combination of frequency and V$_T$ are based on Otis's model that minimizes the mechanical work for a spontaneous, unassisted breathing. The assumption that this criterion is sufficient to be optimum for mandatory breaths during mechanical ventilation is the foundation of Hamilton Medical's Adaptive Support Mode.

Our algorithm for finding an optimum combination of frequency and V$_T$ (Mid Frequency Ventilation, MFV) is based on the idea of maximizing alveolar ventilation. "Optimum" in this context is the combination of frequency and V$_T$ that provides adequate gas exchange at the lowest alveolar end-inspiratory and tidal stretch.

The purpose of this study was to develop a mathematical model that predicts a patient-dependent frequency that minimizes tidal volume while maximizing alveolar minute ventilation (AMV) during conventional pressure controlled continuous mandatory ventilation (PC-CMV).

Methods

We used a mathematical model to describe pressure controlled continuous mandatory ventilation of a passive, single compartment, lumped parameter model. This model expresses alveolar minute ventilation as a function of ventilator settings (mandatory breath frequency, f, and inspiratory pressure above PEEP, P_{set}) and patient derived parameters (resistance [inspiratory and expiratory], compliance, and dead space fraction, D):

$$\dot{V}_A = f \times \left[\left(P_{set} \times C \right) \left(1 - e^{-60D/fR_iC} \right) \left(1 - e^{-60(1-D)/fR_eC} \right) / \left(1 - e^{-60(1-D)/fR_eC} \times e^{-60D/fR_iC} \right) - V_D \right]$$

A plot of alveolar minute ventilation vs frequency shows a local maximum Figs. 1 and 2. The set inspiratory pressure is adjusted such that the peak of the curve corresponds to the patient's required alveolar ventilation. Then, the frequency and V$_T$ corresponding to the local maximum on the curve are defined as the optimum values.

We programmed an Excel spreadsheet to allow input of model parameters and automatic plotting of results (Figure 1). We set the parameters of the model to simulate ARDS:
- resistance = 10 cm H$_2$O·s·L^{-1}
- compliance = 0.025 L/H$_2$O
- V$_D$/V$_T$ = 0.45
- height = 170 cm

We varied model parameters to identify the effects of lung mechanics and dead space fraction on output variables.

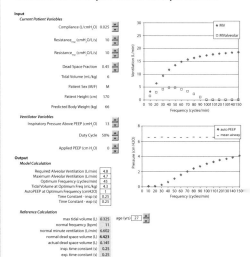

Figure 1. Spreadsheet implementation of MFV model

OPTIMUM SETTINGS FOR ARDS

FAARC, Eduardo Mireles-Cabodevila, MD

Cleveland, OH

Results

Figure 1 shows that for a simulated patient with ARDS, the optimum frequency was 45/min delivering 4.3 mL/kg with autoPEEP = 1 cm H_2O. Changing resistance and compliance to double the time constant yielded optimum values at 28/min, 5.4 mL/kg. Other manipulations of model parameters yielded results shown in Figure 2.

Some observations about the model performance include:
- Mean airway pressure = mean alveolar pressure only when $R_I = R_E$
- Optimum settings occur at 50% duty cycle when $R_I = R_E$
  - when $R_I < R_E$, optimum settings occur at duty cycle < 50%
  - when $R_I > R_E$, optimum settings occur at duty cycle > 50%
- Increasing V_D/V_T does not affect optimum frequency but increases optimum V_T

Conclusions

We have demonstrated, in a theoretical model, that increasing the ventilatory frequency above commonly used frequencies with pressure controlled ventilation at a constant duty cycle can potentially improve alveolar ventilation. Furthermore, we showed that we can achieve this with low tidal volumes and a constant mean airway pressure.

Interestingly, for many patients with relatively severe ARDS (ie, $R \leq 15$ cm $H_2O\cdot s\cdot L^{-1}$, $C \leq 35$ mL/cm H_2O, and $V_D/V_T \leq 0.5$) the model predicts that maximal alveolar ventilation can be obtained with tidal volumes less than 6 mL/kg at frequencies > 35 cycles/min.

Thus, PC-CMV optimized for maximum alveolar ventilation results in lower tidal volumes and higher ventilatory frequencies than conventionally used but below that requiring specialized high frequency ventilators.

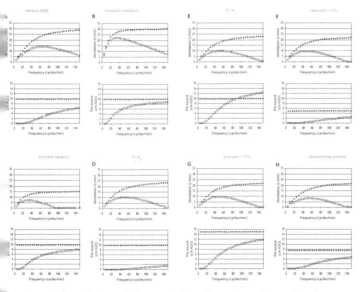

Figure 2. The effects of changes in lung mechanics and ventilator settings on the major outcome variables minute ventilation (closed diamonds), minute alveolar ventilation (open squares), mean airway pressure (closed triangles), and aPEEP (open circles). (**A**) nominal settings used for all experiments (inspiratory resistance = expiratory resistance = 10 cm $H_2O\cdot s\cdot L^{-1}$, compliance = 0.025 L·cm H_2O^{-1}, pressure limit 20 cm H_2O, PEEP = 0 cm H_2O, duty cycle = 50%). (**B**) the effect of increasing compliance to 0.075 L·cm H_2O^{-1}. (**C**) the effect of increasing resistance (with nominal compliance) to 20 cm $H_2O\cdot s\cdot L^{-1}$. (**D**) the effects of nominal compliance with inspiratory resistance of 20 cm $H_2O\cdot s\cdot L^{-1}$ and expiratory resistance of 5 cm $H_2O\cdot s\cdot L^{-1}$. (**E**) inspiratory resistance of 5 cm $H_2O\cdot s\cdot L^{-1}$ and expiratory resistance of 20 cm $H_2O\cdot s\cdot L^{-1}$. (**F**) duty cycle of 25%. (**G**) duty cycle of 75%. (**H**) pressure limit decreased to 15 cm H_2O.

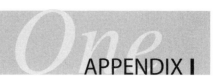

Basic Science Writing

Matthew "Matti" Mero, MA
Copy Editor, *Respiratory Care*

"I'm sorry to send you this long letter, but I haven't the time to write a short one."

Introduction

The sentiment of the quote above, in different forms, has been attributed to various authors. The point of it, I think, is that most first drafts are full of superfluous words and redundancy, and that, in almost all cases, good editing substantially shortens a document.

Editing is the process of re-scrutinizing your thinking by trying to reread your own writing from the perspective of the target audience. Many times I have finished writing a sentence or paragraph and said to myself, "Ah, well written! What a fine turn of phrase! Aren't I a good writer!" but later came back to it and said, "Dang! It's a nice turn of phrase but it's unclear, redundant, verbose, illogical, or poorly structured." To create good science writing, you must open your mind to the disgruntling possibility that your writing might not convey your science as clearly and simply as you first thought. It is difficult to see problems in material that you have read and edited repeatedly, especially if you liked it when you first wrote it.

You might ask, is it really worth the time to rigorously edit my science writing? After all:

- Does the writing really need to be so carefully crafted if the majority of the readers understand it well enough in its unedited form?
- Who has time to do nit-picky micro-editing?
- Editing is the job of editors, not writers.
- The important thing is to produce rigorous, thorough, and carefully reasoned science, not good-looking science, so if the science is good, what does it matter if the writing is not perfect?

Admittedly, not many people have the time or interest to do rigorous editing. You can decide to leave the editing to the editors. However, if you read this section I hope you will at least conclude that editors do not change text for arbitrary, capricious reasons, such as because the editor disagrees with the author's writing "voice." Instead, a good editor makes changes because there are opportunities to make the text clearer, shorter, easier to read, grammatically better, and/or more accurate.

Unless you are a writing genius, you will create merely text during your writing process; you create good writing during editing. Of science writing it is even fair to say, "Writing Is Editing!" Herein I will describe the tools to look at your writing with a rigorous editorial eye and help you avoid some common pitfalls. I hope to help you see the crucial difference between "clear to me" and "clear to my audience."

Your top four objectives should be:

• Clarity
• Completeness and full disclosure
• Concision
• Accuracy

Of those the most important is clarity because:

1. Clear writing reflects clear thinking, whereas unclear writing can make your thinking appear unclear, even if your research was well done, and thereby cast doubt on the validity of your findings. Whether a report is accepted for publication can depend on how well it is written, because the key decision-makers (the editor-in-chief and the peer reviewers) are busy, so if your writing is unclear they might not understand it on their first read and are thus more likely to reject it. If the writing is unclear, the reader may have difficulty knowing whether the writing's content is complete or accurate in the amount of time available to read it. If the reader has to read it twice to understand it, he or she is more likely to assume that the science is as shoddy as the writing.
2. Clarity is usually maximized by simplifying the language. Usually, the more you simplify, the more you clarify. However, "simplify" does not mean "dumb down;" it means using the right words in the right order, including all the necessary words, and excluding all the unnecessary words, to maximize readability.
3. "Concision" means saying it in the fewest possible words, which simplifies and thus clarifies.

Sometimes the objectives of completeness and concision seem to conflict. In attempting to ensure that the writing is complete, many authors inadvertently insert numerous superfluous words. But in attempting to make it concise, many authors fail to include words that the audience needs. My hope is to help you (1) identify superfluous words, (2) see when important words are missing, and (3) adopt a "tough love" mindset toward your writing, in which you will become more demanding about word choice and word order. Your scientific methods have to be rigorous, or your findings and conclusions will be rejected by your peers. I will show you how to apply that same demanding rigor to your writing.

There are two types of science writing. The first is material read primarily for pleasure and personal interest, such as newspaper articles about scientific things, publications such as *Science News* magazine, and the (wonderful!) science-for-the-well-educated-masses books from writers such as Jared Diamond. What I present here applies only to the other type, which is the professional scientific report. "Well written" means something very different for a professional scientific report than it does for a "read-for-pleasure" science article. Some of the things that make writing about science (and other read-for-pleasure writing) "well written" are exactly the things that can make a scientific report "poorly written."

Scientific reports are primarily read to obtain information as quickly as possible. Therefore, the objective is to make the writing as clear, simple, and concise as possible, and we do that by following some guidelines and rules that make science writing a relatively formal writing style. However, I think many authors have misconceptions about the formality of science writing, such as:

1. Use of the first-person voice, such as "I found that . . ." or "I think . . ." is somehow unacceptable. In fact, "I found that. . ." or "I think . . ." is often the best start to writing a clear, simple sentence that conveys the full meaning in the fewest words.
2. Scientific reports should be written in the passive voice, because the passive voice sounds more formal and erudite. Actually, the active voice is better for most sentences, but, as I'll explain, there are situations when the passive voice is better.
3. The formal style makes scientific reports inherently boring reading. That is simply false. Many authors, in misguided attempts to make their reports more interesting to read, use certain tactics of literary style commonly found in fiction and other for-pleasure reading, such as unusual turns of phrase and the "slender yellow fruit" strategy (which I'll explain later). But in science writing these literary tactics always make the writing redundant, wordy, less clear, and less precise than it should be. When writing a scientific report, remember that science is exciting. Don't try to make the writing interesting. Explain the science in the simplest, briefest (but complete) terms, and, if your science is good, your reader will say, "Now that's interesting."
4. When the paper has received the approval of the editor-in-chief and the peer reviewers, then the editing is done, with minor exceptions such as adding or deleting commas and catching "typos." In fact, the copy editor, who reads the paper after the peer reviewers, can make important contributions to the paper's clarity and concision. The editor-in-chief and the peer reviewers are primarily concerned with the accuracy and completeness of the science, and they read papers from an expert's perspective. The copy editor attempts to read the paper from the perspective of the journal's audience, many of whom do not know the subject matter nearly as well as the author, peer reviewers, or editor-in-chief. The copy editor's objective is to make the writing as clear and easy to read as possible, and in attempting to do that, many copy editors have rankled many authors. Authors hate copy editors who:
   • Make edits the author thinks are unnecessary.
   • Make edits that change the meaning from what the author intended.
   • Edit out the author's "voice."

All three of those certainly seem to constitute bad editing, but consider:

1. There are often editing reasons the author does not know about, and the copy editor does not have time to explain every edit.

2. The copy editor would not intentionally change the meaning, so the copy editor must not have understood the author's meaning. If the copy editor did not understand the passage, probably an important percentage of the audience won't understand it either. Therefore, the passage needed clarification. You might ask, why didn't the copy editor just ask the author what was meant? Actually, that is what the copy editor is doing. When the copy editor makes an edit, he or she is saying "Is this what you meant?" If the author's answer is "No, I meant this," no problem; the copy editor's changes should be taken as questions in the form of suggestions, which is the fastest, simplest way of asking.

3. "Voice" is the summation of a person's habits regarding sentence structure, syntax, and word choice, and certain sentence structures and syntaxes are clearer and easier to read than others. Also, in science writing, word choice is more constrained (by the need for accuracy and concision) than it is in for-pleasure writing. Thus, sometimes "voice" is in conflict with the objectives of clarity, completeness, concision, and accuracy/honesty.

Many authors have opined (or yelled) that the copyeditor should "lay off" because the meaning of a passage can be a "delicate thing, easily altered." I think science writing shouldn't be that way. The writing should be unambiguous and simple—not subtly nuanced code written only for those who know the "secret handshake." If there are subtle nuances to the subject matter, good writing can explain those nuances clearly, often in surprisingly few words. Rarely is science so complex that good writing cannot make plain the basic ideas.

I believe the editing principles I describe here can help you make science prose clearer, easier to read, and therefore more likely to be understood *on first read*, thereby maximizing the value to the readers (including reviewers and editors) and perhaps even optimizing the value of the research to the advancement of science, because everyone who reads it will quickly understand it.

The writing examples I give below are all from the field of respiratory medicine, but the principles apply to all professional science writing. I think the example passages illustrate that good editing can change science writing from "inscrutable jargon" to simple-yet-thorough explanation that most people can understand, while making it shorter!

Questions to Ask About Your Words

Are There Superfluous Words?

Identifying superfluous words can be difficult because they hide in common phrases that we tend to gloss over and in sentences that have a "nice ring" on first read. To rigorously scrutinize a sentence, try to set aside "pride of voice" in how you phrased it. If you concentrate on the content rather than the form of the sentence, you will probably find superfluous words. As I'll explain later, some sentences should be in the passive voice, *but passive-voice sentences are the most prone to superfluous words.* Changing a sentence to active voice usually helps to detect superfluous words, and when they are deleted (and the sentence thus shortened), you often see that the sentence should include additional information.

Example

Bacterial pathogens were believed to be the primary etiologic factor.

What's Wrong With That?

The sentence uses two-word terms ("bacterial pathogens" and "etiologic factor") when one-word terms ("bacteria" and "cause") are equally accurate.

Revised Version

We believe bacteria was the cause.

The revised version is so short, it is revealed as an "underachiever" that should include more information.

Improved Revised Version

We believe Pseudomonas aeruginosa and Haemophilus influenzae caused 27% of the deaths in Group A.

Did I Include Explanations That Are Not Necessary for My Audience?

Another category of superfluous words is remedial explanations.

Example

Inhaled β-agonists are also well tolerated, but are associated with decreased efficacy with chronic use. This development of tolerance (often referred to as tachyphylaxis) is not seen with muscarinic antagonists. The antimuscarinic drugs maintain their efficacy over the long term.

What's Wrong With That?

1. The parenthetical definition of "tachyphylaxis" is unnecessary for the intended audience. Assume that the audience is well versed in the relevant terminology.
2. "Chronic" is not a synonym for "long term."
3. The three original sentences can be summed into one sentence.

Revised Version

Inhaled β-agonist is also well tolerated but tachyphylaxis is common, unlike with muscarinic antagonists.

Did I Use the Right Word or Term?

The most common word-choice errors are:

- Wrong word by definition
- Unnecessary or incorrect use of long term
- Wrong form of the word (adjectival versus adverbial versus noun form)
- Wrong preposition

Wrong Word by Definition

Example

Heliox's thermal conductivity is much increased above that of air.

What's Wrong With That?

"Increased" is the wrong word by definition, because increase (or decrease) indicates a change in one thing, not a difference between two things. The correct word is "greater."

Revised Version

Heliox's thermal conductivity is much greater than that of air.

Example

Closed suctioning generates negative airway pressure and subsequently decreases lung volume.

What's Wrong With That?

"Subsequently" implies that one event occurred after another event, but not necessarily because of that other event. The point of the sentence is that the negative airway pressure caused the decrease in lung volume. Another technical point: by the laws of physics, pressure is never negative; it is either zero or positive. Only pressure *differences* can be negative. In this case, the correct term is "transrespiratory pressure," indicating the difference between the pressure at the airway opening and the body surface. This shows the difference in view points of an expert content reviewer (who should have caught this) and a copy editor (who may not have such detailed technical knowledge on this particular subject). However, in the context of this sentence, people generally understand that "airway pressure" is measured relative to atmospheric (i.e., body surface) pressure. So we will let it slide . . .

Revised Version

Closed suctioning generates negative airway pressure and consequently decreases lung volume.

Improved Revised Version

Closed suctioning generates negative airway pressure, which decreases lung volume.

Example

Table 2 illustrates the data.

What's Wrong With That?

"Illustrate" is incorrect; it means "describe via drawing" or "provide an example of." The table only shows the data; a figure would illustrate the data. In science writing, always use exactly the correct term; strive for precise use of language, for the same basic reason that you strive for precise measurements—because good science requires precision, not vague generalizations. Don't use pseudo-synonyms, such as "emulate" instead of "simulate," or "demonstrate" instead of "showed."

Revised Version

Table 2 shows the data.

Example

With steroids this fraction varies from less than 1% to 50%.

What's Wrong With That?

The word "varies" is incorrect because the point of the sentence is the range of values. Swapping the positions of the values makes the sentence a little easier to read.

Revised Version

With steroids the range is from 50% to less than 1%.

Unnecessary or Incorrect Long Term

Many authors use the longest terms rather than the most accurate or correct terms.

Example

The molecular and cellular pathogenetic mechanisms and etiologies of cystic fibrosis lung disease were studied with multiple methodologies.

Revised Version

We studied the causes of cystic fibrosis.

Example

This systematic regimen of bronchodilators brought much heightened mucociliary clearance.

Revised Version

The bronchodilator treatments significantly improved mucus clearance.

Example

At that point in time the therapeutic interventions were initiated.

Revised Version

At that point we began treatment.

Example

Our technique significantly improved mucociliary clearance.

What's Wrong With That?

Several factors affect mucus clearance (not just cilia), and we are not sure that the technique improved cilia function; it might have affected the other factors instead, so the correct word is "mucus," not "mucociliary." I think the author used "mucociliary" without carefully considering whether it was really the right term; instead, he used the longest, most erudite-sounding term he knew. Like some authors use "utilize" instead of using "use."

Revised Version

Our technique significantly improved mucus clearance.

Example

They are developing potent new chemical entities of biological origin.

What's Wrong With That?

It is superfluous to state that the research is on something potent; no one researches a drug that will not be potent. The term "chemical entities of biological origin" is vague and unnecessarily long. Be specific and concise.

Revised Version

They are developing organic molecules that may treat cystic fibrosis.

Scrutinize your terms. Did you use the correct term or just the longest, most erudite-sounding term? Using the simplest, shortest (but accurate) terms makes science writing easier to read and therefore more likely to be quickly understood. Don't try to demonstrate your technical vocabulary. Even with technical, recondite subjects, the correct term is often the simple, short, common term.

Wrong Form of the Word

One of the most common writing errors is misuse of adjectival and adverbial forms of words. I suspect that to many people the adjectival and adverbial forms sound more erudite because they are usually longer. Incorrect use of the plural form is another common error.

Example

The pathological findings showed that. . .

What's Wrong With That?

"Pathological" is the adjectival form of "pathology." The findings from the pathology lab are pathology findings, not pathological findings.

Revised Version

The pathology findings showed that . . .

Example

Her maximal FEV_1 was 1.4 L.

What's Wrong With That?

"Maximal" and "minimal" (adjectival forms of "maximum" and "minimum") are also commonly misused.

Revised Version

Her maximum FEV_1 was 1.4 L.

Incorrect use of plural-form words often occurs in sentences that have superfluous words.

Example

Hyperventilation results in rapid reductions in ICP.

What's Wrong With That?

"Reduction" should be singular, and there are superfluous words.

Revised Version

Hyperventilation results in rapid reduction in ICP.

Better Revised Version

Hyperventilation rapidly reduces ICP.

Example

Those patients are prone to infections, particularly pneumonias.

What's Wrong With That?

Incorrect use of plural "pneumonias."

Revised Version

Those patients are prone to infections, particularly pneumonia.

Example

The blood gas samples were ran through the analyzer.

What's Wrong With That?

Incorrect verb tense of the verb "run." The author has used the past tense rather than the past participle. Respiratory therapists seem to make this particular mistake very often.

Revised Version

The blood gas samples were run through the analyzer.

Wrong Preposition

Example

High inflation pressure increases the risk for barotraumas.

What's Wrong With That?

"For" is the wrong preposition.

Revised Version

High inflation pressure increases the risk of barotrauma.

Example

Plateau pressure was significantly lower with the treatment group for days 1, 3, and 7, by comparison with the control group.

What's Wrong With That?

1. There are two incorrect prepositions: "with" and "for."
2. The prepositional phrase "by comparison with" often signals suboptimal sentence organization and superfluous words. When you see the phrase "by comparison with," see if you can restructure the sentence to replace it with the word "than."

Revised Version

Plateau pressure was significantly lower in the control group than in the treatment group during days 1, 3, and 7.

Did I Use Acronyms and Technical Terms Correctly?

While writing, you can easily forget the words that an acronym stands for and, having forgotten, use the acronym incorrectly. As you reread your writing, say the words that the acronym letters represent and see if the sentence really makes sense.

Example

The MRI image (Fig. 1) indicated that . . .

What's Wrong With That?

MRI stands for "magnetic resonance imaging," so the word "image" is superfluous.

Revised Version

The MRI (Fig. 1) indicated that . . .

Example

The percent of droplets with an MMAD in the 1–5-mm size range increased.

What's Wrong With That?

MMAD stands for "mass median aerodynamic diameter," which is the median size of the droplets that form an aerosol. The median is the 50th percentile by definition, so the percentage of droplets with a given MMAD can never "increase." Thus, that use of MMAD is incorrect.

Revised Version

The percentage of 1–5 mm droplets increased.

Example

We conducted rapid-sequence intubation (RSI) and then instituted partial liquid ventilation (PLV).

What's Wrong With That?

It creates new acronyms. Compressing a multiple-word term into an acronym does not save an important amount of space on the printed page, and it offers no benefit to the reader, because (1) once the reader is familiar with the term he or she can read it very quickly, so the spelled-out term does not increase the reading time; (2) in the context of a report that includes various acronyms, many readers will repeatedly pause at a new acronym and think, "Uh, what does that one mean again?" As well, there is a risk of creating illogical and/or grammatically incorrect acronyms from terms that are not carefully thought out. For instance, "dry powder inhaler" (or DPI) is a standard term in respiratory medicine, but the person who originated the term apparently did not consider that the phrase "dry powder" is redundant, because there is no such thing as a "wet powder." Acronyms can make your report slightly shorter, but brevity is not the most important writing objective; brevity should be used as a tool to achieve readability and, thus, clarity. Brevity does not always improve readability, so don't create new acronyms.

Did I Use Terms Consistently?

Don't use a variety of synonyms for one thing. The term "slender yellow fruit strategy" comes from an apocryphal tale of an author who thought his writing was boring because he needed to mention a banana numerous times in his story and he decided to refer to the banana by as many other terms as he could think of, including "slender yellow fruit." In fiction and other for-pleasure reading, "slender yellow fruit strategy" is common and can "enliven" for-pleasure writing. But with science writing, remember that people will be reading your report not for the pleasure of reading, but to learn—as quickly as possible—your methods, results, and conclusions, and the reading is easier if you use one term to refer to one thing, consistently, throughout the report. Your writing will not be more interesting or in any way better by your demonstrating that you know all the colloquial terms experts use for a certain thing. Don't use multiple terms for one thing, unless you need to explain that you are using your term advisedly.

Example

The alveolar-arterial oxygen difference (which is often incorrectly called the alveolar-arterial oxygen gradient) was 12 mm Hg.

What's Wrong With That?

Nothing is wrong with it. That sentence is a good example of an author using the correct term but explaining that she knows that an incorrect term is widely used.

Example

Most practitioners consider an SvO_2 of 75% acceptable on venoarterial ECMO. In venovenous support the SvO_2 reflects the recirculation.

What's Wrong With That?

1. In the second sentence the author used "support" as a synonym for "ECMO." The reader might be able to surmise that that is what the author meant, but why challenge the reader to interpret various synonyms? Choose one term and stick with it. This will not make your writing boring. *The excitement is in the science, not the writing.*
2. "On" and "in" are incorrect prepositions.

Revised Version

Most practitioners consider an SvO_2 of 75% acceptable during venoarterial ECMO. During venovenous ECMO the SvO_2 reflects the recirculation.

Did I Create Unnecessary and/or Problematic Data Categories?

A common error is to unnecessarily group data into categories that don't help explain the data.

Example

We designated four therapies as "high-volume therapies": aerosol administration, oxygen therapy, bronchopulmonary hygiene, and incentive spirometry. We designated five therapies as "low-volume therapies": *suctioning, tracheostomy change, arterial-blood-gas sampling, and pulse oximetry. Figure 2 shows the 10-year trends in low-volume and high-volume therapies.*

What's Wrong With That?

There is no value (and some detriment) in separating the therapies into two groups.

Did I Include Error or Range Values for All Numbers?

Most numbers should include measurement-error values or range values.

Example

The estimated cost was $3,447.11 per new employee.

What's Wrong With That?

$3,447.11 is an exact number, not an estimate. Indicate the possible range of values.

Revised Version

The estimated cost was $3,400 $\pm$ $420 per new employee.

Is the Sentence Logically Organized?

To determine if a sentence is logically organized, the first question is, where in the sentence do you find out what the sentence is about? The earlier the better. Make the sentence easier to read by revealing early in the sentence what the sentence is about.

Example

Because of the arteriovenous fistula, a continuous heart murmur, and advanced age for a patient of Rendu-Osler-Weber syndrome, and in light of her family history, our initial diagnosis was revised.

What's Wrong With That?

You don't find out what the sentence is about until the end of the sentence. At the beginning of the sentence you encounter a list of factors (arteriovenous fistula, etc.) that you have to read through before you find out what those factors relate to. With that sentence structure you have to load each of the listed factors into your memory and then, at the end of the sentence, mentally connect them all to the thing that they influenced (the initial diagnosis).

Revised Version

We revised our initial diagnosis because we discovered an arteriovenous fistula and a continuous heart murmur, and because of her family history and advanced age (for a patient with Rendu-Osler-Weber syndrome).

Example

Data regarding ICU length of stay, ICU readmission, admission Acute Physiology and Chronic Health Evaluation (APACHE) III score, and the frequency of positive blood cultures are routinely collected in our medical ICU.

What's Wrong With That?

You don't find out what the sentence is about until the end of the sentence. Also, the phrase "length of" is superfluous; we can write simply "ICU stay."

Revised Version

In our medical ICU we routinely collect data on ICU stay, ICU readmission, admission Acute Physiology and Chronic Health Evaluation (APACHE) III score, and the frequency of positive blood cultures.

If the sentence is organized so that it reveals early what it is about, then the reader can pause and consider how each phrase of the sentence relates to what the sentence is about or advances the understanding of the subject.

Does the Sentence Use the Correct Voice?

Use the active voice for your first "stab" at a sentence. To keep your mind in the active voice, memorize a simple active-voice sentence such as "This is true and that is false," and try to boil down your thoughts to that simple, declarative style.

Passive-voice sentences typically have so many superfluous words, we're tempted to conclude that the passive voice causes superfluous words. But sometimes you should use the passive voice to reveal early in the sentence what the sentence is about. Compare these two sentence structures:

A affects B. (active voice)
B is affected by A. (passive voice)

In cases where you want to describe how only one thing affects only one other thing, use the active "A affects B" form, like this:

The timing of administration affects drug efficacy.

But to describe how several variables influence something, use the passive-voice form:

A is affected by B, C, and D.

Example

Changes in the patient's respiratory drive, secretion buildup in the tube, changes in the temperature and compliance of the ventilator circuit, and changes in the patient's disease state affect the peak pressure during volume-controlled ventilation.

What's Wrong With That?

You don't find out what the sentence is about until the end of the sentence. Also, the list of factors that affect the peak pressure isn't in the most logical order; the item "patient's disease state" belongs with "patient's respiratory drive."

Revised Version

During volume-controlled ventilation, the peak pressure is affected by the patient's disease state and respiratory drive, by secretion buildup in the tube, and by changes in the temperature and compliance of the ventilator circuit.

Example

As can be seen, when work load is incrementally increased, the cardiorespiratory system is called upon to deliver increasingly higher amounts of oxygen and to clear increasingly higher amounts of carbon dioxide.

What's Wrong With That?

It's in the passive voice, and for that sentence there is no need for the passive voice.

Revised Version

When work load increases, the cardiorespiratory system must deliver more oxygen and clear more carbon dioxide.

Example

The current sentence does provide an example of how the use of the passive voice can often lead to the inclusion of words that are not necessary.

Revised Version

Passive-voice sentences usually contain superfluous words.

Is the Sentence Too Long or Too Short?

Don't assume that a long sentence is a bad sentence, nor that there is some inherent virtue in a sentence being short. If a sentence is logically organized, it can be quite readable despite being long, and just because a sentence is short doesn't mean it's clear. It often makes sense to write one longer sentence rather than two or three shorter sentences. Don't try to make your sentences short; try to make them logically organized and therefore easily readable no matter how long they are. In attempting to keep sentences short, writers often cut one thought into two or more sentences. Computer programs that supposedly measure the reading-difficulty of a piece of text operate (partly) on the unfounded assumption that a longer sentence is more difficult to read. Actually, you can make a piece of text more difficult to read by "chopping up" into short sentences a logical chain of thought, such as a sequence of causes and effects. Chopping up into little sentences also causes superfluous words and redundancy.

Example

A consistent observation in many studies is that exercise under hyperoxic conditions reduces the minute ventilation at a given level of exercise. This results in a mild respiratory acidosis at any given level of exercise, compared to that which would be seen on room air.

What's Wrong With That?

1. It's two sentences that could be one clearer sentence.
2. The term "hyperoxic conditions" is not explained; later in the report the author explained that he simply meant "while the subject is inhaling supplemental oxygen." *Don't create or use terms without explaining them.*
3. Superfluous words. Once we see that the sentence is about what happens when an exercising subject inhales supplemental oxygen, we need to know that the comparison is with room air. Clarifying one thing often obviates explaining another thing.

Revised Version

Many studies have found that, during exercise, supplemental oxygen reduces minute ventilation at a given level of exercise and causes mild respiratory acidosis.

Example

Symptom triggers such as environmental allergens, changes in weather, and exposure to cold air are all predictors of positive airway hyperresponsiveness. Family history of asthma is also a significant predictor. The relative risk with these parameters is low as well, ranging from 1.6 to 1.9.

What's Wrong With That?

1. It's three sentences that could be one clearer sentence.
2. The word "positive" is superfluous.
3. Incorrect use of the word "parameters," which should be reserved for its mathematical meaning in science writing.

Revised Version

Airway hyperresponsiveness predictors include family history of asthma and symptom triggers, such as environmental allergens, changes in weather, and exposure to cold air, but the relative risk from those variables is low (1.6–1.9).

Example

The study was a retrospective chart review of 632 patients with an overall failure rate of planned extubations of 4.9%.

What's Wrong With That?

The two parts of the sentence are related but should be separated into two sentences.

Revised Version

The study was a retrospective chart review of 632 patients. The overall failure rate of planned extubations was 4.9%.

Does the Beginning of the Sentence Have an Obvious Logical Connection to the Previous Sentence?

A sentence is probably suboptimally organized if it doesn't "explain itself" in the first five words. Will the reader stop and think, "Wait a minute; how does this sentence relate to the previous sentence or to the heading of this section?" Sometimes you need to point back to a previous sentence or section to clarify the logical connection between what you said previously and what you're about to say. Such point-back phrases are not redundant if they improve readability. The general structure of this type of sentence is:

1. Pointer to (i.e., reminder of) information or concept you previously discussed
2. Indication of what the current sentence is about
3. New information, new concept, or advancement of earlier concept

Example

In considering the causes of exercise impairment in chronic obstructive pulmonary disease, oxygen supplementation can conceivably improve performance in a number of different ways. Pulmonary vasoconstriction and dysrhythmias secondary to hypoxemia plus right heart dysfunction may be reduced to provide better cardiovascular function.

What's Wrong With That?

The logical connection between the sentences is not apparent until the end of the second sentence. The sentences can be merged into one clearer sentence.

Revised Version

Now that we know how chronic obstructive pulmonary disease causes exercise impairment, we see that oxygen supplementation should improve exercise performance by relieving hypoxemia and thereby relieving pulmonary vasoconstriction, dysrhythmia, and right-heart dysfunction.

The beginning of the revised sentence now points back to previous information in the report, which makes clear the relationship of the current sentence to the whole report.

You may have difficulty deciding when to include a point-back phrase; the decision is one of numerous decisions about what items do and do not need explanation. If you write simply and clearly, and make your sentences structurally logical (i.e., so that each sentence reveals early what it is about), few sentences will need pointers to previous information, but watch out for sentences that don't "explain themselves" in the first few words.

Does the Sentence Say Something That Really Needs to Be Said?

If you rigorously scrutinize a sentence, eliminate superfluous words, and put the words in logical order, you'll sometimes find that the point of the sentence is too obvious to merit mention.

Example

The findings are self-explanatory, but a few observations may be in order to orient the reader.

What's Wrong With That?

The sentence is self-contradictory, indicating that the findings need no explanation (which is incorrect, because no findings are self-explanatory), and then indicating that some explanation might be useful. Delete the whole sentence.

Example

The effects of inhaled corticosteroids in asthma relate to the basic pathophysiology of this disease and the known pharmacologic effects of this class of drugs.

What's Wrong With That?

The beneficial effects of any drug for any condition relate to the pathophysiology of the disease and pharmacology of the drug, so the sentence states something that is not worth stating. Delete the whole sentence.

Example

Ventilatory modes and techniques have been variously utilized in specific circumstances to accomplish therapeutic success.

What's Wrong With That?

The sentence indicates only that ventilatory modes and techniques have been used to treat patients, which is so obvious it's not worth saying. Delete the whole sentence.

Is It Redundant?

While writing it often seems worthwhile to rephrase something for emphasis or to give the reader multiple perspectives on an idea, but such restatements are usually superfluous.

Do Not Restate for Emphasis

Example

Early recognition of ventilator auto-triggering is important to avoid adverse outcomes that can result directly from excessive hyperventilation or indirectly from clinician attempts to pharmacologically suppress respiratory drive. This point is extremely important, because failure to recognize auto-triggering caused by a bronchopulmonary fistula could lead to inappropriate escalation of sedatives and/or neuromuscular blockers, because the patient might be assumed to be breathing spontaneously.

What's Wrong With That?

1. The passage is redundant and has superfluous words. For emphasis, use italics or a phrase such as "It is extremely important to . . . ."
2. It's two sentences that could be one better sentence.

Revised Version

Early recognition of bronchopulmonary-fistula-related auto-triggering is extremely important, because auto-triggering can cause excessive hyperventilation and inappropriate escalation of sedatives and/or neuromuscular blockers (if the patient is incorrectly believed to be breathing spontaneously).

Scrutinize Commonly Used Phrases for Redundancy

Example

The patient's past history was unremarkable.

What's Wrong With That?

History is, by definition, of the past, so "past history" is redundant (and funny when you consider the possibility of the patient's "present history" or "future history"). Yes, the term "past history" is so widely used that it is nearly a "term of art," but many such terms are clichés that are used thoughtlessly, and many of them suffer some illogic.

Revised Version

Her history was unremarkable.

Example

ARDS can best be defined as an acute pathophysiological state resulting from a multitude of complex cellular and biochemical events that represent sequelae of either severe pulmonary injury or nonpulmonary insults.

What's Wrong With That?

1. The phrase "acute pathophysiological state" is redundant because "ARDS" means "acute respiratory distress syndrome."
2. The phrases "pathophysiological state" and "represent sequelae of" are pompous longhand for "condition" and "are caused by."
3. The word "multitude" is hyperbolic.

Revised Version

ARDS results from a series of cellular and biochemical events caused by severe pulmonary or nonpulmonary injury.

Example

The nebulizer delivery system used to deliver aerosolized medication can have a significant effect on the amount and quality of aerosol delivered to the patient.

What's Wrong With That?

The sentence is redundant and it explains things that don't need to be explained to the audience for whom it is written. It is not necessary to inform the reader that a nebulizer system delivers aerosolized medication to the patient.

Revised Version

There are significant differences in the amount and quality of aerosol delivered by various nebulizer systems.

Example

Inhaled nitric oxide acts as a selective pulmonary vasodilator in children with congenital heart disease, and the increased saturation values signify a selective lowering of pulmonary vasoconstriction.

What's Wrong With That?

If inhaled nitric oxide is a pulmonary vasodilator then it is redundant to state that it lowers pulmonary vasoconstriction. Notice also that the sentence's structure suggests that inhaled nitric oxide causes pulmonary vasodilation in children with congenital heart disease but not necessarily in other patients; in fact, it causes pulmonary vasodilation in any human.

Revised Version

Inhaled nitric oxide causes selective pulmonary vasodilation, which increases saturation and thus benefits children who have congenital heart disease.

Did I Phrase It Tentatively?

Avoid making conclusions without adequate evidence. However, many facts and conclusions are noncontroversial, and there is no sense in phrasing things with terms that suggest you *don't* know something that you *do* know. Such unnecessarily tentative phrasing causes superfluous words and wastes the reader's time and mental energy. If you know that something is true, state that it is true, not that it might be true or that it is still under debate.

Example

Airway pressure-release ventilation may lower airway pressure while providing adequate oxygenation, so the incidence of ventilator-induced lung damage may also be decreased.

What's Wrong With That?

Later in the report the author describes convincing research that airway pressure-release ventilation definitely lowers airway pressure and decreases the incidence of ventilator-induced lung damage.

Revised Version

APRV provides adequate oxygenation with lower airway pressure and thus helps avoid ventilator-induced lung damage.

Example

It has been shown by several well-done studies from expert researchers that the addition of a holding chamber significantly improves delivery of aerosol.

What's Wrong With That?

If several credible studies came to the same noncontroversial conclusion, you can eliminate tentative phrasing. Also, what does "it" refer to?

Revised Version

Addition of a holding chamber significantly improves aerosol delivery.

Is the Syntax Convoluted, Peculiar, or in a Literary Style?

Many authors make misguided attempts to "spice up" their prose by using unusual and unexpected phrasings and syntax—a writing tactic often used in for-pleasure writing. In scientific reports, such literary tactics:

- Tend to focus the reader on the form rather than the content of the sentence
- Are more likely to be confusing on first read and thus make the reading take longer and/or make your message more difficult to understand
- Decrease the chance of your report being accepted for publication

In science writing, word choice and word arrangement should be as simple and concise as possible, because the objective is to convey the meaning as quickly as possible—not to try to entertain the reader with interesting turns of phrase. Remember: the reader is presumably trying to "keep up with the scientific literature," so the simpler you write it, the faster and easier the reader can read it.

Example

At present, the current findings do reveal that the most substantive advantage among a super-majority of the sickest patients was rendered by the albuterol Ventolin, surprisingly not the anti-arrhythmic beta-adrenoreceptor-blocking sotalol hydrochloride.

What's Wrong With That?

1. The syntax is peculiar.
2. Several terms ("substantive advantage," "supermajority," and "sickest") are vague. Use specific terms and values whenever possible. Do not use approximate synonyms, such as "substantive advantage" instead of "significant improvement."
3. The methods section should have already indicated that Ventolin is a type of albuterol and that sotalol hydrochloride is a type of anti-arrhythmic beta-adrenoreceptor-blocker. Thoroughly describe drugs, devices, techniques, and your terms in the methods section, and thereafter consistently use one term for each thing. For drugs, use the generic name, not the brand name.
4. Superfluous words.

Revised Version

Among the patients who had "severe" obstruction (as measured with our obstruction rating system), 89% significantly improved with albuterol, whereas, to our surprise, sotalol hydrochloride significantly improved only 20% of the severe-obstruction patients.

Example

Vis-à-vis the nominal dose difference, the customary difference range is 11- to 12-fold between metered-dose inhalers and nebulizers, in favor of the nebulizer.

What's Wrong With That?

I think the writer was concentrating on creating an interesting turn of phrase, not on communicating the meaning in the simplest possible way. Also, the phrase "in favor of" suggests that there is an advantage to delivering a larger dose, but in this case the opposite is true; most of the larger dose from a nebulizer is lost to the ambient air.

Revised Version

The nominal dose from a nebulizer is 11–12 times larger than that from an MDI.

Are There Confusing Word Strings?

Another common problem in science writing is strings of words in which it is hard to tell which word modifies which.

Example

The left side malignancy female patient 6 month mortality was 24%.

What's Wrong With That?

The phrase "left-side malignancy female patient 6 month mortality" is a confusing word string. To eliminate confusing word strings: (1) restructure the sentence so that it reveals as soon as possible what the sentence is about, (2) insert the appropriate articles, pronouns, prepositions, and/or participles to separate (and thus clarify) the words, and (3) hyphenate adjectival multiple-word phrases to help the reader comprehend your meaning.

Revised Version

Mortality among the female patients who had left-side malignancy was 24% at 6 months.

Do Any of the Words Contradict Each Other?

Self-contradictory phrases and sentences are common in science writing.

Example

The drug effect lasted up to an hour or more.

What's Wrong With That?

The phrase "up to an hour" contradicts the phrase "or more." The effect lasted for either (1) less than an hour or (2) more than an hour; it can't be both. Use specific names and values.

Revised Version

Salmeterol's effect lasted 54 $\pm$ 23 min.

Example

As much as a 20–50% increase can ensue.

What's Wrong With That?

The phrase "as much as" conflicts with the phrase "20–50%." Does it mean that the increase is at least 20%? If the objective is to indicate the range of possible increase, the phrase "as much as" should be deleted. If the objective is to indicate the maximum possible increase, only one value should be included.

Revised Version

The increase can be as much as 50%.
or
The increase will be 20–50%.

Example

The mean value was approximately 0.033 mL.

What's Wrong With That?

The word "approximately" seems to contradict the value 0.033 mL, which is a fairly precise amount. There is no indication of how approximate the value is. Instead of vague words such as "approximately," be as specific as possible and give a standard deviation value whenever possible.

Revised Version

The mean ± standard deviation was 0.033 ± 0.14 mL.
   The revised version reveals that the standard deviation was large, relative to the mean value.

Did I Lay Out the Information in Chronological Order?

Describe things (e.g., previous research or sequences of cause and effect) in chronological order unless there is a compelling reason not to. That is, after you reveal what the paragraph is about, list things in chronological, cause-and-effect sequence.

Example

Cystic fibrosis lung disease leads to chronic respiratory insufficiency. This is because inflammatory processes are activated by mucus hypersecretion, since the mucociliary escalator cannot adequately mobilize the supranormal amounts of mucus, and the stagnant mucus tends to become infected.

What's Wrong With That?

It's illogically organized. The sequence of causes and effects should be in chronological order.

Revised Version

Cystic fibrosis causes mucus hypersecretion and the mucociliary escalator cannot adequately mobilize the supranormal amounts of mucus, so mucus stagnates in the small airways. The stagnant mucus tends to become infected, which leads to inflammation, which leads to deposition of fibrin in the airway walls. That further decreases the efficiency of the mucociliary escalator, exacerbating the problem. The chronic clogging, inflammation, and hardening of the airways leads to respiratory insufficiency.

The revised passage is longer, but easier to understand on first read, and it "fills in the blanks" of the sequence of causes and effects.

Did I State the Topic and Then Stay on Topic?

While reading our own writing, we tend to overlook missing concepts and missing logic-steps. *The logical connections between the sentences are obvious to the author, so the author can easily overlook that a paragraph fails to state the topic and then discuss it in a logical sequence.* If the topic is not clear at the beginning of the paragraph, the sentences can feel like an annoying tour through the miscellaneous.

Example

We report a case in which a laryngeal mask airway endotracheal tube was used because tracheal intubation was difficult. Subsequently left-lung atelectasis developed, but the wire coil that gives the tube support (and was thought to identify the entire tube) ended 2 cm above the main carina. At bronchoscopy the tube was in the bronchus intermedius. Even in retrospect the true end of the tube could not be seen radiographically.

What's Wrong With That?

The topic of the paragraph is not clear at first. The first sentence suggests that the topic might be that the laryngeal mask airway is useful for difficult intubations. The beginning of the second sentence seems to change the subject; it hints that the topic might actually be atelectasis related to using that type of tube, but then the sentence raises the issue of the wire coil in the tube. The third sentence seems to slightly change the subject again. In the fourth sentence we see that the passage is primarily about the tube's radiographic invisibility, but it's not clear how important are the other topics mentioned.

Revised Version

We report a case in which the distal 3 cm of a laryngeal mask airway endotracheal tube was radiographically invisible. The radiopaque wire coil built into the tube was mistakenly believed to mark the end of the tube, so the radiograph made it appear that the end of the tube was 2 cm above the main carina. This type of tube extends 3 cm beyond the end of the wire coil, and the final 3 cm of the tube can be difficult or impossible to see on a radiograph. Bronchoscopy revealed that the end of the tube was in the bronchus intermedius. In this case, even in retrospect, the true end of the tube could not be seen on the radiograph.

In the revised passage the first sentence reveals the topic, and the subsequent sentences stay on topic and logically lay out and connect the information. Reveal what the paragraph is about at the beginning of the paragraph, and try to make each sentence follow logically from the previous sentence.

Did I Put the Information in the Right Format (Text, Table, or Figure)?

How do you decide whether information belongs in text, a table, or a figure? Tables and figures provide a "mental break" from long blocks of text, and such mental breaks tend to make the reading experience more engaging, so some would say that more tables and figures make a report more readable. And, to some extent, readability can feel like clarity. But you should ask of table or figure, will it really better illustrate the information or clarify my point? Conversely, are you struggling to write a textual description of something that could be more easily summarized in a table or figure?

Example

Refer to **Table I.1**.

Table I.1

Risk Factors for Pediatric Acute Respiratory Distress Syndrome

- Sepsis
- Gastric aspiration
- Pulmonary contusion
- Burns
- Toxic gas or smoke inhalation
- Multiple urgent transfusions

What's Wrong With That?

There is not enough information in it to warrant the table format. Write the information into a sentence.

Revised Version

The risk of pediatric acute respiratory distress syndrome is higher if the patient has any of the following: sepsis, gastric aspiration, pulmonary contusion, burns, toxic gas or smoke inhalation, or multiple urgent transfusions.

However, if you think the reader might benefit from a mental break at that point in the text, or, for instance, that the reader might want a quick-reference list of those reasons, keep the table, but consider adding more information to it, as in **Table I.2**.

Table I.2

Risk Factors for Pediatric Acute Respiratory Distress Syndrome

Risk Factor	Percent Who Develop ARDS
Sepsis	30
Gastric aspiration	15
Pulmonary contusion	40
Burns	55
Toxic gas or smoke inhalation	60
Multiple urgent transfusions	45

Example

Smith et al. conducted a randomized, double-blind, placebo-controlled trial of nitric oxide for hypoxic respiratory failure. They considered ECMO rate, mortality rate . . . . Jones et al. conducted a randomized, placebo-controlled, double-blind, dose-response study of nitric oxide for hypoxic respiratory failure. The outcome variables were . . . . Henry et al. conducted a retrospective, matched cohort study of nitric oxide for hypoxic respiratory failure. They found that . . . ; etc.

What's Wrong With That?

Describing previous reports in text form usually requires a lot more words than if the information is organized into a table. A table allows quick and easy comparison of the reports. List the studies in chronological order. Use terms consistently, even if the studies you are describing used different terms for one thing.

Revised Version

See **Table I.3**.

Table I.3

Studies of Inhaled Nitric Oxide for Hypoxic Respiratory Failure

First Author	Year	Design	Control	*n*	Nitric Oxide Concentration (ppm)	Measured Variables	Findings
Smith[31]	1996	Randomized, double-blind	Placebo	248	5, 20	ECMO rate, mortality rate, Pao_2, $P_{(A-a)O_2}$	Significantly lower ECMO rate and CLD rate. Significantly lower $P_{(A-a)O_2}$ at 1 h. No difference in mortality rate.
Jones[32]	1998	Retrospective	None	155	5, 20, 80	ECMO rate, cost	50% less need for ECMO. Significantly less expensive than ECMO on per-hour basis.
Henry[33]	2000	Retrospective, matched cohort	Normal therapy	50	6, 20	Pao_2, ECMO rate, hospital cost	Significantly better sustained Pao_2. Significantly lower ECMO rate, CLD rate, and hospital cost.
Mero[34] (present study)	2003	Randomized, placebo-controlled, double-blind, dose-response	Placebo	103	5, 10	Pao_2, ECMO rate, hospital cost	No difference in sustained Pao_2. Significantly lower ECMO rate and CLD rate. Nonsignificantly lower hospital cost.

Example

Look at **Figure I.1**.

Figure I.1

An unnecessary figure.

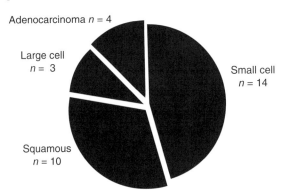

What's Wrong With That?

The figure is not warranted, because it does not contain enough information. Nor does the figure make the data easier to comprehend. A table is not warranted either. Write the data into a sentence.

Revised Version

The cases included 14 small cell, 10 squamous cell, 3 large cell, and 4 adenocarcinoma.

Is There Redundancy Among the Sentences?

Eliminate redundancy.

Example

Though oxygen is the most frequently administered gas in respiratory care, the utilization of other specialty gases has become common practice in many neonatal and pediatric intensive care settings and emergency departments across the United States. This paper is a review of the literature and evidence of four such specialty gases: heliox, nitric oxide, hypoxic or sub-ambient gas, and carbon dioxide. Heliox (helium-oxygen mixture) has been used since the 1930s in the management of patients with upper airway obstruction from a variety of different etiologies. Nitric oxide, a relatively new gas when compared to heliox, was discovered in the early 1980s but has been a prolific area of study for the last two decades. Nitric oxide has proven to be a selective pulmonary vasodilator when delivered by inhalation. This has led to many investigative studies with patients with cardiopulmonary disorders that have defects or diseases that enhance or promote pulmonary vasoconstriction. The use of hypoxic gas therapy or carbon dioxide is usually reserved for infants with a specific congenital heart defect: hypoplastic left heart syndrome. The role of both these gases are to equilibrate the pulmonary vascular and systemic vascular resistance. A balance between pulmonary and systemic vascular resistance assures adequate oxygenation and tissue perfusion. Hypoxic gas therapy assists with achieving this pulmonary-to-systemic balance by maintaining an oxygen saturation (pulse oximeter) in the low 70s that increases pulmonary vascular resistance and leads to decrease in pulmonary blood flow. Carbon dioxide therapy achieves a slightly higher $PaCO_2$, in the range of 45–50 mm Hg, and a subsequent increase in pulmonary vascular resistance and a decrease in pulmonary blood flow.

What's Wrong With That?

On first read you might not see any glaring problems, but applying the editing principles described above can make it easier to read and about 40% shorter.

Revised Version

Though oxygen is the most frequently administered gas in respiratory care, other specialty gases are also commonly used in neonatal and pediatric intensive care and emergency *departments in the United States, including heliox (helium-oxygen mixture), nitric oxide, hypoxic gas (i.e., < 21% oxygen), and carbon dioxide. Heliox is less dense than air or nitrogen, so it causes less inhalation resistance and turbulence, thus decreasing the airway pressure and work of breathing, which alleviates the affects of airway obstruction. Inhaled nitric oxide is valuable because it can dilate pulmonary vasculature without causing systemic vasodilation. Hypoxic gas and carbon dioxide help manage hypoplastic left heart syndrome, a congenital heart defect that decreases oxygenation and tissue perfusion in neonates. Hypoxic gas lowers blood oxygen saturation (to around 70%), whereas carbon dioxide raises $PaCO_2$ (to 45–50 mm Hg), either of which increase pulmonary vascular resistance and decrease pulmonary blood flow, which equilibrates pulmonary and systemic vascular resistance and thus improves oxygenation.*

Is the Information in the Right Part of the Report?

The "Introduction, Methods, Results, Discussion, Conclusions" outline helps prevent placing text in the wrong part of the report, but such misplacement nevertheless happens. For example, many authors discuss some of the background information (e.g., previous reports on the subject) in the introduction section and the rest of it in the discussion section. One illogical but widely accepted science-writing convention is that the review of previous research goes in the discussion section. Logically, it should go in the introduction section, so the reader begins with the background and context of your methods and results, but this is one of those science-writing conventions that there is little hope of changing. Whether you put it in the introduction or the discussion, organize your review of previous research into one coherent, chronologically ordered section.

Example

Discussion
Airway hyperresponsiveness is common in asthma patients. Bronchoprovocation to assess airway hyperresponsiveness might be useful for diagnosing asthma, when the patient's history is suggestive but spirometry values are normal. The best use of bronchoprovocation is contro-versial because airway hyperresponsiveness is characteristic of but not specific to asthma.

What's Wrong With That?

All that information belongs in the introduction section, not in the discussion section. Don't reiterate material from the introduction in the discussion section.

Is There Redundancy Between Parts of the Report?

Don't reiterate passages, values, facts, or conclusions from one section of the report in another section. The most common version of this mistake is restating information from the results section in the discussion section.

Example

Discussion
We found significant differences in 2 of the 5 outcome variables.

What's Wrong With That?

The results section already stated those results. Only restate results as necessary to discuss your interpretation of the results.

Revised Version

We believe the 2 outcome variables that showed significant differences were more important clinically than the 3 that did not.

Also, don't restate data from a table or figure in the text, except as necessary to explain your current point.

Example

Table 3 shows that 39% of the patients showed statistically significant improvement and 61% did not.

What's Wrong With That?

Some sentences may need to mention data that appears in a table or graph (e.g., "We were surprised that 81% of the patients had sepsis."), but, generally, the point of creating a table or graph is to eliminate sentences that merely list data, as opposed to discussing the meaning of the data.

Revised Version

Though only 39% of the patients showed statistically significant improvement (see Table 3), many of the patients' improvement was nearly statistically significant.

Does the Abstract Follow These Rules?

- The abstract must not contain anything that does not also appear in the body of the report.
- The abstract must summarize the main points from the body of the paper. Do not include "teaser" statements such as "This paper will discuss . . . ." Instead, reveal the main points with statements such as "Our data indicate that . . . ."
- The abstract must not make off-topic or merely peripherally related generalizations.
- The abstract must not be merely introductory remarks.
- The abstract must not suggest conclusions that are not clearly supported by the evidence in the body of the report.

Glossary

This is a "teaching" glossary. It contains many terms and explanations that do not appear in the text.

Accuracy   The degree to which a measured value reflects the true value; sometimes expressed as the difference between true and measured values as a percentage of the true value. *See* Error.

Algorithm   A well-defined set of rules that when routinely applied lead to a solution of a particular problem (often expressed as a flowchart).

Alpha (α) level   The maximum tolerable probability of making a Type I error. *See* Significance level.

Analysis of variance (ANOVA)   An inferential statistical test used to test the significance of differences between three or more mean values.

Bell curve   The characteristic shape of the normal and t distributions; having the shape of a vertical cross-section of a bell.

Benchmarking   A procedure for identifying best practices among a group of similar organizations.

Beta (β) level   The probability of making a Type II error.

Bias   Deviation of results or inferences from the truth, or processes leading to such deviation; the difference between the mean value of a set of measurements and the true value.

Ascertainment bias   Arises when a higher exposure to a risk factor causes a higher probability of detecting the event of interest.

Detection bias   The tendency to look more carefully for an outcome in one of two groups being compared.

Publication bias   Occurs when the publication of research depends on the direction of the study results and whether they are statistically significant.

Recall bias   Occurs when patients who experience an adverse outcome have a different likelihood of recalling an exposure than the patients who do not have an adverse outcome, independent of the true extent of exposure.

Selection bias   May occur whenever a treatment is chosen by the individual involved. A classic example of this problem occurred in the Lanarkshire milk supplementation experiment of the 1920s. In this trial, 10,000 children were given free milk and a similar number received none. The groups were formed by random allocation. Unfortunately, well-intentioned teachers decided that the poorest children should be given priority for free milk rather than sticking strictly to the original groups. The consequence was that the effects of milk supplementation were indistinguishable from the effects of poverty. Another example of selection bias is *volunteerism*, where the study entrant selects him- or herself.

Blind (*or* Blinded *or* Masked)   The participant in a study is unaware of whether patients have been assigned to the experimental or control group. Anyone associated with the study (e.g., patients, researchers, data analysts, writers) may be blinded. To avoid confusion, the term *masked* is preferred in studies in which vision loss of patients is an outcome of interest. If both the researcher and the patient are unaware of the assigned treatment, the study is *double blinded.* If only one of the two is blinded, the study is *single blinded.* Blind assessment first began in the late eighteenth century as a tool for fraud detection mounted by elite mainstream scientists and physicians to challenge the suspected delusions or charlatanism of unconventional medicine. Some of the first experiments were carried out to evaluate mesmerism and were literally conducted with blindfolds. They took place in France at the house of Benjamin Franklin, the American minister plenipotentiary, who was head of a commission of inquiry appointed by King Louis XVI.

Calibration   The adjustment of the output of a measuring device to match the value of a known input. A common example in respiratory care is the calibration of an oxygen analyzer by exposing the sensor to pure oxygen and adjusting the readout to display 100%.

Calibration verification   Measuring a known (assumed true) value with a calibrated device and noting the difference between the measured and true value. If the difference is below some predetermined threshold, the device is judged accurate enough for use. If not, it is recalibrated.

Causation   The process whereby a given event, called a cause, *invariably* precedes a certain other event, called the effect.

Clinical trial   Planned experiment involving participants, usually patients, to determine the most appropriate therapy by comparing one therapeutic approach with another, usually standard care.

Cohort study   A type of prospective study in which the same group of subjects is followed over a period of years, and data are periodically recorded.

Confounding factor (*or* variable)   A factor that distorts the true relationship among the study outcome variables because it is also related to the outcome variables. Confounding variables are often unequally distributed among the groups being compared. Randomized studies are less likely to have their results distorted by confounding factors than are non-randomized studies.

Continuous variable   A variable that can theoretically take any value and in practice can take a large number of values with small differences among them.

Control   Any operation that is designed to limit any of the conceivable sources of error (confounding factors) in a study. Experimental control refers to the manipulation of conditions under which the observations are made. Statistical control involves the treatment of data to remove the effects of confounding factors.

Control group   Subjects who are as closely as possible equivalent to an experimental group and exposed to all the conditions of the study except the experimental treatment. In many studies, the control group receives either the standard of care or no treatment at all.

Cost analysis   If two strategies are analyzed but only costs are compared, this comparison would address only the resource-use half of the decision (the other half being the expected outcomes) and is termed a cost analysis.

Cost-benefit analysis   A form of decision analysis in which both the costs and the expected outcomes (benefits) are measured on the same continuous scale (either both as costs or both as dimensionless numbers) and compared as a ratio (either as cost/benefit or as benefit/cost). This relationship allows the comparison of two or more courses of action (e.g., new therapies or purchases of equipment).

Cost-effectiveness analysis   An economic analysis in which the expected outcomes are expressed in natural units. Some examples would include cost per life saved or cost per unit of blood pressure lowered.

Cost-minimization analysis   An economic analysis conducted in situations in which the expected outcomes of two or more alternative courses of action are identical, so the only issue is their relative costs.

Cost-utility analysis   A type of cost-effectiveness analysis in which the expected outcomes are expressed in terms of life-years adjusted by peoples' preferences. Typically, one considers the incremental cost per incremental gain in quality-adjusted life-years (QALYs).

Crossover design   The same individual is included in both treatment and control conditions or in multiple treatment conditions in the same study; the individual acts as his or her own control. Random allocation is used to determine the order in which the treatments are received. The simplest design involves two groups of subjects. One group receives each of two treatments, A and B, in the order AB, while the other group receives them in the reverse order, BA. Because the treatment comparison is within one subject rather than between subjects, fewer subjects may be required to achieve a given statistical power. Carryover effects (conditions from one experiment that effect a subsequent experiment) may be a problem. An attempt to minimize this problem is to include a washout period between the two treatments (the period required for a treatment to cease to act once it has been discontinued).

Crossover effects   Residual effects of the treatment received on the first occasion that remain present into the second occasion.

Decision analysis   A systematic approach to decision making under conditions of uncertainty. It involves identifying all practical alternatives and estimating the probabilities of potential outcomes associated with each alternative, assigning value weights to each outcome, and on the basis of probabilities and values, arriving at a quantitative estimate of the relative merit of the alternatives.

Deductive reasoning   Reasoning that proceeds from a general law to a conclusion that is specific to a particular situation. Reasoning from general to particular.

Degrees of freedom   An elusive concept that occurs throughout statistics. Essentially, it means the number of independent units in a sample used to calculate a statistic. Another way of thinking about it is 1 minus the number of sample values that can be determined from knowledge of the other values. For example, if the mean value of 3 numbers is 4 with $x_1 = 3$ and $x_2 = 4$, then x_3 must equal 5. One of the three sample values can be determined by knowledge of the other two, so the "degrees of freedom" is $n - 1 = 2$.

Delphi technique   A questionnaire strategy in which a panel of experts complete consecutive questionnaires generated on the basis of the answers to the previous questionnaires; designed to achieve a consensus among the panel of experts.

Dependent variables   The variables the investigator measures in response to the causal (treatment or independent) variable; outcome variables.

Dichotomous variable   A variable that can take one of two values, such as yes or no, dead or alive, 1 or 0, etc.

Drift   The gradual changing of an instrument's accuracy during use due to uncontrollable electrical, chemical, or physical factors.

Effectiveness study   A study designed to answer a question of the type: " Does the treatment work in clinical practice settings with unselected patients, typical care providers, and usual procedures?"

Effect size   The difference in outcomes between the intervention and the control groups divided by some measure of variability, usually the standard deviation.

Efficacy study   A study designed to answer a question of the type: "Does the treatment work in a tertiary care setting with carefully selected patients under tightly controlled conditions?"

Endpoint   Endpoints are events or outcomes that lead to completion or termination of a study or follow-up of an individual (e.g., death or major morbidity).

Error   The difference between measured and true values, sometimes expressed as a percentage of the true value; bias plus imprecision.

Experimental variable   The variable(s) manipulated by the researcher; the independent variable(s).

Exposure   A condition patients come in contact with (either a potentially harmful agent or a potentially beneficial one) that may affect their health.

False negative   In a treatment study, treatment is considered ineffective when it actually is effective. In a diagnosis study, the patient has the target condition, but the test suggests the patient does not.

False positive   In a treatment study, treatment is considered effective when it actually is not effective. In a diagnosis study, the patient does not have the target condition, but the test suggests the patient does.

Generalizability   The ability to apply results from a sample to a population. For example, results from a study of bronchodilators on a group of asthmatics may be generalizable to all asthmatics in the world if the sample had the same characteristics as the world population of asthmatics and in the same proportion (e.g., age, gender, severity of illness, socioeconomic status).

Gold standard   A method having established or widely accepted accuracy, providing a standard to which measurements can be compared (e.g., for calibration).

Halo effect   The tendency to overrate a subject's performance on some task because of the observer's perception of the subject doing well during a prior evaluation.

Hawthorne effect   A term used for the effect that might be produced in an experiment simply from the awareness by the subjects that they are participating in some sort of scientific research (due to the novelty of the situation of being treated in a special way). The psychological reaction to the study conditions can be mistaken for the effect of the experimental variable(s). It was first described in some classic experiments at the Hawthorne plant of the Western Electric Company in Chicago during the late 1920s and early 1930s.

Hello-goodbye effect   A phenomenon first described in psychological research that may arise whenever a subject is assessed on two occasions, with some intervention between the visits. Before an investigation, a person may present himself in as bad a light as possible, thereby hoping to qualify for treatment, and impressing staff with the seriousness of his problems. At the end of the study, the person may want to please the staff with his or her improvement, and so may minimize any problems. This minimization may lead to the false conclusion that some improvement exists when none has actually occurred, or to magnify the beneficial effects that did occur.

Hidden time effects   Effects that arise in data sets that may simply be a result of collecting the observations over a period of time.

Historical controls   A group of patients treated in the past with a standard therapy, used as the control group for evaluating new treatment on current patients. Although this study design is used frequently in medical investigations, it is not recommended because possible biases (due to other factors that may have changed over time) can never be eliminated.

Hypothesis   A statement of relationship among variables that is assumed true until data are obtained that prove it wrong. The *null hypothesis* is usually a statement of no difference or no association between groups (the observed difference in values of a statistic are due to chance alone). The *alternate hypothesis* is the opposite of the null and usually states that there is a difference or that the difference is in a particular direction (one group statistic is larger or smaller than another).

Imprecision   The extent to which repeated measurements of the same quantity vary from one another; usually characterized by the variance or the standard deviation as an estimate of the random error of measurements.

Incidence   The number of new cases of disease occurring during a specified period of time; expressed as a percentage of the number of people at risk.

Inclusion criteria   Criteria used to define the population who will be eligible for a study.

Independent variables   Explanatory or predictor variables that may be associated with a particular outcome.

Induction   A process of reasoning that proceeds from specific facts in a particular situation to general propositions or laws. Reasoning from particular to general.

Inference   A judgment based on other information rather than on direct observation. Statistical inference is the process by which one is able to make generalizations from the data.

Informed consent   The situation where a competent person, in possession of all the relevant facts, has agreed to participate in a research study.

Intention-to-treat principle (*or* analysis)   A procedure in which all patients randomly assigned to a treatment are analyzed together as representing that treatment, whether or not they completed or even received it. This method is intended to prevent bias due to using compliance with treatment (a factor often related to outcome) to determine the groups for comparison. It maintains the power of randomization.

Interaction effect   The effect of two or more independent variables acting in combination rather than independently of one another; the effect of one factor is not consistent over all levels of another individual factor in a two-factor (two-way) analysis of variance (ANOVA).

Interval level Measurement scale that has the following properties: (1) the values are distinguishable; (2) they are ordered; (3) the intervals between the points on the scale are equal; and (4) the zero point is not absolute; it does not represent the absence of the quantity being measured. An example is temperature on the Celsius or Fahrenheit scales.

Inverse rule of 3s A rough rule of thumb that says if an event occurs on average once every n days, we need to observe $3n$ days to be 95% confident of observing at least one event. For example, if the event occurs once every 10 days, we need to observe $3 \times 10 = 30$ days for at least one event to occur.

Likert-type scale A scale, typically with three to nine possible values, that includes extremes of attitudes or feelings (such as strongly agree, agree, undecided, disagree, strongly disagree). A number is attached to each possible response, and the sum of these ratings is used as the composite score. Likert-type scales are used to obtain ratings from study participants. A commonly used Likert-type scale is the Apgar score used to evaluate the status of newborn infants.

Linearity The degree to which variation in the output of an instrument follows input variation.

Literature review A summary of earlier published work on a topic of interest, containing a critical review of what is known.

Longitudinal study Study that requires obtaining repeated measures over time.

Meta-analysis A quantitative procedure for combining the results of several studies into a pooled estimate of the independent variable on the dependent variable.

N of 1 clinical trial A special case of a crossover design for determining the efficacy of a treatment for a specific patient. The patient is repeatedly given a treatment and placebo, or different treatments, in successive time periods.

Negative results Research findings that suggest the null hypothesis be accepted; nonsignificant results.

Nominal variable Variable that takes on distinct, mutually exclusive categorical values (e.g., male or female, yes or no). The values have no particular order and the intervals between the values are meaningless. Numbers associated with the categories have no quantitative value and are used only as labels.

Nonparametric test A class of statistical test that is not based on the estimation of a parameter for the underlying population, usually does not assume a particular sampling distribution, and can be used with nominal or ordinal data.

Observational study Study providing questions about overt behaviors or events and answers using human observers to record the behaviors or events over a period of time. The researcher has little or no control over the behaviors or events.

Occam's (or Ockam's) razor Also known as the parsimony principle, popularized by William Occam, a fourteenth-century philosopher. The principle states that unverified assumptions should be kept to the bare minimum and the hypothesis with the fewest assumptions is preferred. Michael Faraday warned against the tendency of the mind "to rest on an assumption" and when it appears to fit in with other knowledge to forget that it has not been proved.

Ordinal variable A variable having the following properties: (1) mutually exclusive; (2) ordered but the intervals between the values are not equidistant; (3) there is no meaningful zero point.

Outlier An observation that appears to deviate markedly from the other members of the sample. Extreme values may reflect some abnormality in the measurement process.

Parameter A numerical characteristic of a population (e.g., the population mean) or a mathematical model (e.g., the probability of success in binomial distribution).

Percentile The point in a cumulative percentage plot below which the percentage of cases indicated by the given percentile falls. For example, an IQ of 100 represents the 50th percentile of intelligence scores; 50% of people have IQ scores below 100. In a normal distribution, the mean represents the 50th percentile.

Phase I drug study Studies that investigate a drug's physiological effect or ensure that the drug is not toxic; often conducted with normal volunteers.

Phase II drug study Initial studies on patients that provide preliminary evidence of possible drug effectiveness.

Phase III drug study Randomized control trials designed to definitively establish the magnitude of drug effects.

Phase IV (or post-marketing surveillance) drug study Studies conducted after the effectiveness of a drug has been established and the drug marketed, typically to establish the frequency of unusual toxic effects.

Pilot study A study carried out before a research design is completely formulated. The purposes of a pilot study are to assist in (1) the definition of the problem; (2) the development of the hypotheses; (3) the estimation of sample sizes; and (4) the establishment of priorities for further research.

Placebo (From the Latin "I will please.") A treatment designed to appear exactly like a comparison treatment, but which has no active component or effect. It is used to control for psychological bias (*see* Hawthorne effect) by matching the experimental and control groups in terms of equivalent exposure to the treatment administration. In studies of surgical procedures, the placebo treatment is called a sham surgery (e.g., opening the abdomen but not removing the appendix).

Play-the-winner rule A procedure sometimes considered in clinical trials in which the response to treatment can be classified as positive (a success) or negative (a failure). One of two treatments is selected at random and used on the first patient. If the response is positive, the same treatment is used on the next patient; if the response is negative, the other treatment is used on the next patient. The goal is to minimize the number of patients assigned to the inferior treatment.

Power The probability of rejecting the null hypothesis when it is false; correctly identifying an effect when it is there. Power $= 1 - \alpha$. When comparing tests of the same hypothesis, the one with the highest power is preferred. Power is also the basis for estimating the sample size needed to detect an effect of a particular magnitude (effect size).

Precision The degree to which repeated measurements of the same quantity agree with one another. Often quantified in terms of the variance or standard deviation as an estimate of the random error of measurements. *See* Imprecision.

Prevalence A measure of the number of people in a population who have a particular disease at a particular time. Point prevalence is the number of cases at a particular moment divided by the number in the population at that moment. Period prevalence is the number of cases during a specified period divided by the number in the population at the midpoint of the period.

Prospective study A type of research design, also known as a longitudinal study, in which the collection of data proceeds forward in time (as opposed to a retrospective study). A cohort study is a type of prospective study in which the same group of subjects is followed over a period of years and data are periodically recorded.

p **value** The probability that the observed results or results more extreme would occur if the null hypothesis were true and the experiment were repeated many times.

Quality-adjusted life-year (QALY) A unit of measurement for survival that accounts for the effects of suboptimal health status and the resulting limitations in quality of life. For example, if a patient lives for 10 years and her quality of life (measured on some scale) is decreased by 50% because of chronic lung disease, her survival would be equivalent to five quality-adjusted life-years.

Random Governed by chance such that the occurrence of previous events is of no value in predicting future events. For example, the long-term probability of observing "heads" on the toss of a coin is 0.5, but the actual outcome of the next toss cannot be determined based on the number of heads in previous tosses. The "gambler's fallacy" occurs when, for example, a gambler observes 10 heads in a row and then bets heavily that the next toss will not be heads because the probability of 11 heads in a row is very low. In fact, 11 heads in a row is rare, but that fact is irrelevant; each toss is independent of the last with probability of heads on a given toss remaining at 0.50.

Randomization A technique in experimental research to equalize the composition of the various groups under study so that they are as similar as possible on all pertinent characteristics (including confounding factors). Subjects are allocated to the different study groups according to the laws of chance (e.g., by flipping a coin, drawing ballots, or using a table of random numbers).

Ranking The process of sorting a set of values into either ascending or descending order.

Ratio level Measurement scale that has the following properties: (1) the values are distinguishable; (2) they are ordered; (3) the intervals between the points on the scale are equal; and (4) the zero point is absolute; it represents the absence of the quantity being measured. Examples are height, weight, and temperature measured on the Kelvin scale.

Regression to the mean The phenomenon first noted by Sir Francis Galton (one of the originators of statistics): "each peculiarity in man is shared by his kinsmen, but on the average to a less degree" [Popenoe PB, Johnson RH. (1918). *Applied Eugenics* (p. 138). New York: The Macmillan Company]. For example, tall parents tend to produce offspring who are tall but on average are shorter than their parents. The term is used now to describe how a measurement that appears extreme on its first measurement will tend to be closer to the average value for a later measurement. For example, in a screening program for hypertension, only persons with high blood pressure are asked to return for a second measure. But on average, the second measure will be less than the first.

Repeatability The closeness of repeated measurements of the same quantity by the same observer under the same conditions and using the same equipment over relatively short time intervals; precision.

Reproducibility   The closeness of repeated measurements of the same quantity by different observers under different conditions and different equipment over a relatively long time.

Retrospective study   The type of design in which the dependent variable is observed first and the data are traced back and related to possible relevant independent variables that are hypothesized as being associated with the dependent variable; considered to be a non-experimental design.

Rosenthal effect   The phenomenon where the expectations of the researchers in a study influence the outcome. For example, an observer who believes that a particular treatment is effective may underreport observations inconsistent with this belief.

Sampling   The process of selecting a fraction of a population for inclusion in a study.

Area sampling   A probability sample in which the primary sampling units are households used in large-scale studies conducted by the government. On a smaller scale, beds in a hospital could serve as a sampling unit.

Cluster sampling   Used in large-scale descriptive studies involving target populations with geographically dispersed sampling units. The cluster, or primary sampling unit, might represent a hospital or a block within a neighborhood. The elementary sampling unit on which measurements are made might be the patients in the hospital or the residents of the block. Commonly used in epidemiological studies.

Convenience sampling   Subjects are selected because they are easy to identify and happen to be available for participation in the study at a certain time.

Purposive sampling   A sample in which the sampling units are deliberately (non-randomly) selected according to certain criteria that are known to be important and are considered to be representative of the population.

Quota sampling   Similar to a convenience sample, but the use of controls prevents overloading the sample with subjects having certain characteristics. The controls are established by determining the distribution of the sampling units according to those variables deemed to be important.

Random (probability) sampling   A method whereby each sampling unit in the target population has the same, known probability (greater than zero) of being selected in the sample. Neither the sampler nor the sampling unit has any conscious influence over the inclusion in the sample; selection is by chance.

Sequential sampling   The sampling units are taken into the study sequentially, and the number to be included in the study is not fixed in advance.

Stratified random sampling   The target population is subdivided into homogeneous subpopulations. Then, a random sample or a systematic sample is selected from each subpopulation.

Systematic sampling   After a random start, every nth unit (name on a list, patient in a bed, house on a block) is selected in the order in which the units are arranged.

Sampling unit   The individual members of a target population (e.g., humans, animals, plants, inanimate objects).

Science   Organized curiosity.

Significance level   The level of probability at which the null hypothesis will be rejected. A result is statistically significant (by definition) if the null hypothesis is rejected. That is, the probability of the observed result (the p value) is below an arbitrary threshold (conventionally set as 0.05). The significance level is the threshold value for p. Remember that a small p value may be the result of a large sample size, so that even small differences or slight correlations are detected. Thus, the observed results may be statistically significant but clinically unimportant.

Statistic A numerical characteristic of a sample, such as the sample mean and standard deviation.

Theory A general statement of apparent relationships or underlying principles of certain observed phenomena, which has been verified to some degree by testing specific hypotheses.

Type I error The error of rejecting the null hypothesis when it is true. For example, if the significance level of a test is set at $\alpha = 0.05$, and the p value for a statistical test turns out to be $p = 0.01$, then reject the null hypothesis. The probability of this rejection being in error is 0.01.

Type II error The error of accepting the null hypothesis when it is false. For example, if the significance level of a test is set at $\alpha = 0.05$, and the p value for a statistical test turns out to be $p = 0.25$, then accept the null hypothesis. To calculate the probability of being in error, β, you need the power of the test (often calculated by statistics programs along with p). For example, if the power was 0.80, then $\beta = 1 - \text{power} = 1 - 0.8 = 0.20$.

Validity A criterion for evaluating the quality of a method for measuring variables (often applied to humanistic measurements such as patient satisfaction; surveys and psychological tests are often referred to as "measuring instruments").

Construct validity The extent to which an instrument is consistent with and reflects the theory underlying it.

Content validity The extent to which an instrument adequately encompasses the pertinent range of subject matter.

Face validity The extent to which an instrument appears as a logical measure of what it is supposed to measure.

Predictive validity The extent to which an instrument is correlated with an objective criterion measure (e.g., job satisfaction with job turnover). This is the most important assessment of validity.

Visual analog scale A measurement technique designed to obtain data; requires respondents to select a point on a linear scale to indicate the intensity of their feelings or opinions.

Peer Review Checklists

The following checklists are examples of what have been used by reviewers for *Respiratory Care*. No = criterion not met; ? = not certain that criterion has been met and reviewers' comments will explain; and NA = not applicable.

Original Study Checklist

No	?	NA	**Introduction**
			1. Is the background information adequate to introduce the research problem?
			2. Are the references adequate?
			3. Are specific study objectives or hypotheses stated?
			4. Is the writing in this section clear and concise?
No	**?**	**NA**	**Methods**
			5. Are there outcome variables described for each study objective or hypothesis?
			6. Are there appropriate descriptions of how calculated values were determined?
			7. Are outcome variables that do not relate to the objectives or hypotheses avoided?
			8. Are the measurement procedures appropriate for the study objectives or hypotheses?
			9. Is there enough detail to judge validity and for readers to replicate the study?
			10. Is there adequate description of calculated values?
			11. Were appropriate statistical methods chosen for this study design?
			12. Are the tables, figures, and captions adequate?
			13. Is the writing in this section clear and concise?

No	?	NA	**Results**
			14. Are there complete data for each procedure or test described in the Methods section?
			15. Do the data, or descriptions of the data, appear to be valid?
			16. Are data that do not relate to the study objectives or hypotheses avoided?
			17. Are the tables, figures, and captions adequate?
			18. Does the text avoid presenting the same data as the tables or illustrations?
			19. Is the writing in this section clear and concise?
No	**?**	**NA**	**Discussion and Conclusion**
			20. Is there an explanation of how the results address the problem statement or hypotheses?
			21. Are theoretical and practical aspects of the results discussed?
			22. Do you agree with the interpretation of the results discussed?
			23. Is there a comparison of this study with previously published studies?
			24. Are the references adequate?
			25. Is there a discussion of the limitations of the study?
			26. Is there a section that clearly states the author's conclusions?
			27. Is the writing in this section clear and concise?
No	**?**	**NA**	**Miscellaneous**
			28. Does the paper's title reflect the paper's content?
			29. Is the abstract informative: briefly outlining hypotheses, methods, results, and conclusions?
			30. Is there a Product Sources listing?

Device/Method Evaluation Checklist

Yes	No	?	NA	**Introduction**
				1. Is the background information adequate to introduce device/method?
				2. Are the references adequate?
				3. Is it stated whether this is a descriptive study, accuracy study, or agreement study?
				4. Is the writing in this section clear and concise?
Yes	**No**	**?**	**NA**	**Device/Method Description**
				5. Is there enough detail to explain device/method if unfamiliar to readers?
				6. If device: is it explained that it is a new product, commercially available, or prototype?

Yes	No	?	NA	**Evaluation Methods**
				7. Are there appropriate descriptions of how calculated values were determined?
				8. Are the measurement procedures appropriate for the study objectives or hypotheses?
				9. Is there enough detail to judge validity and for readers to replicate the study?
				10. Is there adequate description of calculated values?
				11. Were appropriate statistical methods used? See *Resp Care* 1996;*41:* 1092–1099.
				12. Are the tables, figures, and captions adequate?
				13. Is the writing in this section clear and concise?
Yes	**No**	**?**	**NA**	**Evaluation Results**
				14. Are there complete data for each procedure or test described in the Methods section?
				15. Are there cost data if appropriate?
				16. Do the data, or descriptions of the data, appear to be valid?
				17. Are data that do not relate to the study objectives or hypotheses avoided?
				18. Are the tables, figures, and captions adequate?
				19. Does the text avoid presenting the same data as the tables or illustrations?
				20. Is the writing in this section clear and concise?
Yes	**No**	**?**	**NA**	**Discussion and Conclusion**
				21. Is there an explanation of how the results address the study purpose?
				22. Are theoretical and practical aspects of the results discussed?
				23. Do you agree with the interpretation of the results?
				24. Is there a comparison of this study with previously published studies?
				25. Are the references adequate?
				26. Is there a discussion of the limitations of the study?
				27. Is there a section that clearly states the author's conclusions?
				28. Is the writing in this section clear and concise?
Yes	**No**	**?**	**NA**	**Miscellaneous**
				29. Does the paper's title reflect the paper's content?
				30. Is the abstract informative: briefly outlining hypotheses, methods, results, and conclusions?
				31. Is there a Product Sources listing?

Case Study Checklist

Yes	No	?	NA	**Introduction**
				1. Is the background information adequate to introduce the case study?
				2. Does the diagnosis satisfy accepted criteria?
				3. Are data supplied to confirm the diagnosis?
				4. Does the report provide an adequate description of the patient's presentation and condition?
				5. Is the writing in this section clear and concise?
Yes	**No**	**?**	**NA**	**Case Summary**
				6. Is the case summary complete?
				7. Does the treatment make good theoretical and physiological sense?
				8. Is the treatment safe?
				9. If the treatment is new, is it needed (i.e., are current methods inadequate)?
				10. If the treatment is new, is it an improvement?
				11. Is the treatment cost effective?
				12. Is the writing in this section clear and concise?
Yes	**No**	**?**	**NA**	**Discussion**
				13. Is the significance of the case clear?
				14. Is the case uncommon or of exceptional teaching value?
				15. Is the writing in this section clear and concise?
Yes	**No**	**?**	**NA**	**Illustrations**
				16. Do the illustrations add value to the case report?
				17. Are the illustrations clear and well labeled?
Yes	**No**	**?**	**NA**	**Miscellaneous**
				18. Does the paper's title reflect the paper's content?
				19. Is the abstract informative: briefly outlining introduction, case summary, and discussion?

Answers

Chapter 1: Why Study Research?

Definitions

- *Basic research:* Seeks new knowledge rather than attempting to solve an immediate problem.
- *Applied research:* Seeks to identify relationships among facts to solve an immediate problem.
- *Quality assurance:* Delivery of optimal patient care with available resources and consistent with achievable goals.

True or False

1. True
2. True

Multiple Choice

1. a

Chapter 2: Ethics and Research

Definitions

- *IRB*: Institutional Review Board; panel of experts who evaluate and approve research protocols involving humans.
- *Informed consent:* The voluntary permission given by a person allowing him- or herself to be included in a research study after being informed of the study's purpose, method of treatment, risks, and benefits.

True or False

1. True
2. False

Multiple Choice

1. d
2. f
3. b

Chapter 3: Outcomes Research

Definitions

- *Disease management:* The systematic, population-based approach to identify patients at risk, intervene with specific programs, and measure outcomes.
- *Continuous quality improvement:* A cycle of activities focused on identifying problems or opportunities, creating and implementing plans, and using outcomes analysis to redefine problems and opportunities.
- *Outcomes research:* The scientific study of the results of diverse therapies used for particular diseases, conditions, or illnesses.
- *Evidence-based medicine:* An approach to practice and teaching that integrates pathophysiological rationale, caregiver experience, and patient preferences with valid and current clinical research evidence.
- *Benchmarking:* A continuous process of measuring products, services, and practice against one's toughest competitors.

True or False

1. False
2. True
3. False
4. True
5. True

Multiple Choice

1. b
2. c
3. a
4. b
5. d

Chapter 4: The Scientific Method

Definitions

- *Hypothesis:* A short statement that describes your belief or supposition about a specific aspect of a research problem.
- *Rejection criteria:* A set of criteria set up before the experiment and used to test the hypothesis.

True or False

1. False
2. True

Multiple Choice

1. d
2. e

Chapter 5: Developing the Study Idea

Definitions

- *Inductive reasoning:* Reasoning from specific observations to general theories.
- *Deductive reasoning:* Reasoning from general theories to specific observations.
- *Operational definitions:* Terms based on specific operations, observations, or measurements used in the experiment.
- *Feasibility analysis:* Judging the overall practicality and worth of a proposed research project.

True or False

1. True
2. True
3. False

Multiple Choice

1. a
2. f
3. c
4. d

Chapter 6: Reviewing the Literature

True or False

1. False
2. False
3. True
4. True
5. False

Multiple Choice

1. a
2. c
3. e
4. b
5. d

Chapter 7: Designing the Experiment

Definitions

- *Assessable population:* The collection of cases available to the investigator as defined by the study criteria.
- *Target population:* The entire collection of cases to which research results are intended to be generalized.
- *Sample:* A subset of the population.
- *Variable:* An entity that can take on different values.
- *Independent variable:* The manipulated variable; the treatment.
- *Dependent variable:* The measured variable; the outcome of the treatment.
- *Nuisance or confounding variable:* Extraneous (usually uncontrollable) variable that can affect the dependent variable.
- *Placebo:* A treatment designed to appear exactly like a comparison treatment, but which has no active component.
- *Hawthorne effect:* Psychosomatic effects caused by a subject's awareness of being in a study.

True or False

1. False
2. True
3. True
4. False
5. True
6. True
7. False
8. True

Multiple Choice

1. a
2. e
3. b
4. c
5. d

Chapter 8: Steps to Implementation

True or False

1. True
2. False
3. True
4. False

5. True
6. False
7. False
8. True

Chapter 9: Making Measurements

Definitions

- *Systematic errors:* Errors that occur in a predictable manner and cause measurements to consistently under- or overestimate the true value.
- *Random errors:* Errors that occur in an unpredictable manner due to uncontrollable factors.
- *Accuracy:* The maximum difference between a measured value and the true value, often expressed as a percentage of the true value.
- *Precision:* The degree of consistency among repeated measurements of the same variable.
- *Resolution:* The smallest incremental quantity measurable.
- *Calibration:* The process of adjusting the output of a device to match a known input, thus minimizing the systematic error.
- *Calibration verification:* The process of measuring a known value with a calibrated device and making a judgment of whether or not the error is acceptable.

True or False

1. False
2. True
3. False
4. False

5. True
6. True
7. True

Multiple Choice

1. b	**4.** a	**7.** c
2. d	**5.** f	**8.** d
3. b	**6.** b	**9.** e

Chapter 10: Basic Statistical Concepts

Definitions

- *Qualitative variable:* A categorical variable not placed on a number scale.
- *Quantitative variable:* A variable measured using a scale of numbers.
- *Discrete variable:* A variable with gaps or interruptions, such as a variable measured with whole numbers.
- *Confidence interval:* The range of values believed to contain the true parameter value.
- *Error interval:* The range of values expected to contain a given proportion of all future individual measurements at a given confidence level.
- *Null hypothesis:* States that no difference or no association exists.
- *Alternate hypothesis:* States that there is a difference or association.
- p *value:* The probability that the observed results or results more extreme would occur if the null hypothesis were true and the experiment were repeated many times.
- *Alpha (level of significance):* The predetermined level of probability at which the null hypothesis will be rejected.
- *Type I error:* The error of rejecting the null hypothesis when it is false.
- *Type II error:* The error of accepting the null hypothesis when it is false.
- *Power (statistical):* The probability of rejecting the null hypothesis when it is false.

True or False

1. False	**6.** True
2. True	**7.** False
3. False	**8.** True
4. True	**9.** False
5. True	**10.** True

Multiple Choice

1. a	**11.** a	**21.** c
2. d	**12.** b	**22.** b
3. c	**13.** c	**23.** d
4. b	**14.** d	**24.** b
5. a	**15.** e	**25.** c
6. b	**16.** b	**26.** a
7. c	**17.** a	**27.** c
8. b	**18.** b	**28.** b
9. a	**19.** a	**29.** devils, demons, death,
10. c	**20.** c	and damnation

Chapter 11: Statistical Methods for Nominal Measures

Definitions

- *Contingency table:* A table used to display counts or frequencies of two or more nominal variables.
- *Proportion:* The number of objects of a particular type divided by the total number of objects in the group.
- *Percentage:* The proportion multiplied by 100%.
- *Ratio:* The number of objects with a given characteristic in a group divided by the number of objects in the group without the characteristic.
- *Odds:* The probability of an event occurring divided by the probability of the event not occurring.
- *Rate:* The quantity of something occurring per unit of time.
- *Sensitivity:* The ability of a diagnostic test to correctly identify patients with the condition of interest.
- *Specificity:* The ability of a diagnostic test to correctly identify patients who do not have the condition of interest.
- *Positive predictive ability:* The probability that the condition of interest is present when the diagnostic test is positive.
- *Negative predictive ability:* The probability that the condition of interest is absent when the diagnostic test is negative.
- *Receiver operating characteristic (ROC) curve:* A plot of the true positive rate against the false positive rate for a diagnostic test over a range of possible cutoff values.

True or False

1. True
2. False
3. True

Multiple Choice

1. a
2. c
3. d
4. b

Chapter 12: Statistical Methods for Ordinal Measures

Multiple Choice

1. a
2. b
3. c

4. d
5. e

Chapter 13: Statistical Methods for Continuous Measures

Multiple Choice

1. a	**5.** a	**9.** a
2. d	**6.** b	**10.** d
3. b	**7.** c	**11.** b
4. c	**8.** c	**12.** c

Chapter 14: The Paper

True or False

1. True	**5.** True
2. False	**6.** False
3. True	**7.** False
4. True	

Chapter 15: The Abstract

True or False

1. True
2. True
3. False
4. False
5. False

Chapter 16: The Case Report

True or False

1. True	**4.** False
2. True	**5.** True
3. False	**6.** True

Chapter 17: The Poster Presentation

True or False

1. True
2. False
3. True
4. True

Model Paper

W hat follows is an actual manuscript in the form it was submitted to *Respiratory Care* for review and possible publication. Appendix VI shows the comments of the peer reviewers and the authors' responses. The paper was subsequently published in *Respiratory Care* 2009;54(4):495–499.*

A Comparison of Respiratory Care Workload and Staffing Patterns Using Two Different Nebulizer Devices

Edward Hoisington, RRT[1]
Rob Chatburn, RRT-NPS, FAARC[2]
James K. Stoller, MD, MS, FAARC[3]

[1] Supervisor, Section of Respiratory Therapy, Respiratory Institute, Cleveland Clinic
[2] Research Manager, Section of Respiratory Therapy, Respiratory Institute, Cleveland Clinic
[3] Jean Wall Bennett Professor of Medicine; Executive Director, Leadership Development; Head, Cleveland Clinic Respiratory Therapy, Respiratory Institute, Cleveland Clinic, Cleveland, OH

Pertinent relationships with any organization with a direct financial interest in the subject of the manuscript:

• Hoisington: none

• Chatburn: member Scientific Advisory Board, Cardinal Health

• Stoller: none

*This paper is reprinted courtesy of *Respiratory Care* and the American Association for Respiratory Care.

Correspondence:

James K. Stoller, MD, MS

Respiratory Institute (A90)

Cleveland Clinic Foundation

9500 Euclid Avenue

Cleveland, Ohio 44195

Telephone: (216) 444-1960

Fax: (216) 445-8160

E-mail: stollej@ccf.org

ABSTRACT

Aerosol therapy using small volume nebulizers (SVN) accounts for a large proportion of the respiratory care workload. Treatment time is mostly nebulization time, which is highly variable depending on SVN design. Our study purpose was to compare the effect of reducing nebulization time on workload distribution. **HYPOTHESIS:** Time saved on aerosol workload can be used to increase time spent on optional value-added respiratory therapy patient care activities. **METHODS:** Workload distribution on the day shift was compared on a post-operative floor for two consecutive 30-day periods. SVNs delivered bronchodilators (3 mL unit dose). SNVs used for control period—Vixone (nebulization time averaged 9 minutes); for intervention period—Salter 8960 Nebutech HDN (nebulization time limited to 3 minutes). Daily volumes were recorded for 21 possible procedures assigned standard times. Procedure volumes were compared using the Student's t-test. Procedure times were compared with Mann Whitney

Rank Sum test. Values of $p \leq 0.05$ were considered significant. **RESULTS:** Daily procedure volumes were similar in both periods (33.8 [baseline] vs. 33.3 [intervention], $p = 0.679$) as was the daily volume of SVN treatments (11.9 [baseline] vs. 11.8 [intervention], $p = 0.806$). The daily time required was higher in the baseline than in the intervention period (4.7 hours [baseline] vs. 3.6 hours [intervention], $p < 0.001$). The daily time available to deliver optional value-added respiratory therapies was higher for the intervention than control period (0.75 hours vs. 0.50 hours, $p < 0.039$). We projected a reduction of 1.8 full-time equivalents (net yearly savings of $66,491). **CONCLUSIONS:** SVN workload can be substantially reduced without adverse events by reducing nebulization time. Workload savings were converted into value-added patient care activities. Concurrent SVN therapy was eliminated. Appropriate selection of technology and retraining can play a large role in coping with the national labor shortage.

INTRODUCTION

The administration of aerosol therapy using small-volume nebulizers (SVNs) accounts for a large proportion of the inpatient respiratory therapy workload in large healthcare organizations. For example, at the Cleveland Clinic, time spent delivering SVN treatments accounts for approximately 40% of the clinical workload outside of the intensive care units.

The time necessary to administer a SVN treatment depends mainly on the aerosol output rate and the volume of the medication being administered.[1] Thus, modification of the nebulizer equipment to deliver drug more rapidly could have an important effect on the workload requirements to administer SVN therapy. The purpose of this study was to compare the workload requirement using a common SVN with a newer nebulizer that can deliver a standard dose of bronchodilator medication in less time.[2] The specific hypothesis examined is that the time saved on aerosol workload could be used to increase the time available to spend on other valued RT patient care activities.

METHODS

The study was approved by the Cleveland Clinic Institutional Review Board. Respiratory care workload and staffing were compared during two intervals: a baseline period in which a standard nebulizer (VixOne Westmed, Tucson, Arizona) was used, and an intervention period during which a rapid nebulizing device (Salter 8960 Nebutech HDN, Salter Labs, Arvin, California) was used. The compared intervals were 30 consecutive 8-hour day shifts between March 14, 2007, and April 13, 2007 (baseline period) and between April 14, 2007, and May 13, 2007 (intervention period). All nebulizer therapies were administered by a single group of 8 respiratory therapists on a single post-operative thoracic surgical patients ward. Nebulized treatments were typically administered three times daily under a physician order, usually endorsing a respiratory care plan that was generated using a respiratory therapy consult service to optimize allocation of treatments.[3–4] All patients ordered to receive SVN treatments were considered for inclusion in the study, with exclusion only of those unable to tolerate the SVN.

The primary outcome variable, workload requirement (minutes), was calculated based on the standard times for each type of patient care activity (Table 1) and the number of activities performed during one 8-hour shift. Standard times were derived from previous time and motion studies performed at the Cleveland Clinic. For

purposes of analysis, workload was divided into 3 groups: workload associated with
SVN treatments, workload for all other physician-ordered treatments, and workload
for desired but less time-sensitive procedures (e.g., desaturation studies, Respiratory
Therapy Consult Service assessments[4]).

Table 1

**Standard Times for Scheduled Patient Care Activities Used for
Making Assignments**

Procedure	Standard Time			
	(hr)	**(min)**	**Type**	**Description**
SVN	0.150	9	ordered	Aerosol by small volume nebulizer
MDI	0.100	6	ordered	Aerosol by metered dose inhaler
BPH	0.167	10	ordered	Broncho-pulmonary hygiene (airway clearance techniques)
PEP	0.167	10	ordered	Positive expiratory pressure therapy for airway clearance
Incentive Spirometry	0.083	5	ordered	
Tracheal Suctioning	0.133	8	ordered	
Naso-tracheal Suctioning	0.133	8	ordered	
Desaturation Study	0.333	20	**optional**	Titration of oxygen therapy by pulse oximetry during ambulation for home O_2 evaluation of need
Noninvasive Vent	0.500	30	ordered	Noninvasive mechanical ventilation
Antibiotic Aerosol	0.250	15	ordered	
ABG sticks	0.250	15	ordered	Arterial puncture for blood sample

Procedure	Standard Time			
	(hr)	(min)	Type	Description
IPPB	0.150	9	ordered	Intermittent positive pressure breathing
Bedside Spirometry	0.133	8	ordered	Bedside PFT for OR clearance
O_2/Pulse Ox intermittent	0.067	4	ordered	Titrating resting Fio_2 requirement using pulse oximetry
Tracheostomy tube changes	0.333	20	ordered	Changing tracheostomy tube per departmental guidelines
Sputum induct	0.250	15	ordered	
Tracheostomy care	0.250	15	ordered	Q-shift tracheostomy care
Rounds	0.500	30	**optional**	Attending physician-led patient rounds
Assessments	0.250	15	**optional**	Assessment of respiratory status change
Patient education	0.250	15	**optional**	Review of written patient education handouts with patients/caregivers

The standard time needed to administer a SVN treatment using the VixOne nebulizer was counted as 9 minutes. Based on design characteristics of the Nebutech nebulizer, full drug delivery occurs within approximately 2.5 minutes (based on our own observations), though as a conservative estimate, treatment time with this device was considered to be 3 minutes.

To confirm and extend the observations from the baseline and intervention periods, a third measurement period 6 months later (July 23, 2007, to September 28, 2007) was considered (called the follow-up period) during which workload volume (number of procedures SVN vs. other) was measured on 2 randomly sampled days per week over a 10-week period on all wards of the Cleveland Clinic Hospital. For this follow-up period, the SVN workload was calculated as the product of the volume of nebulizer treatments and the standard time per treatment (as above). The "other" workload was calculated as the product of the volume of "other" procedures and the aggregate "standard" time for "other" procedures. This aggregate standard time was estimated as the combined time for other procedures from the baseline and intervention periods divided by the combined volume for other procedures in the same periods (thus yielding an average time per other procedure). Then, using the workload volume data from this follow-up period, the effect of a 3-minute vs. a 9-minute standard time for nebulizer treatment was evaluated with regard to overall workload time and staffing requirements.

The mean numbers of total daily procedures and SVN treatments in the baseline and intervention periods were compared using the Student's *t*-test. Total daily procedure times in the baseline and intervention periods were compared using the Mann Whitney Rank Sum test. Proportions were compared with Chi-Square test. Values of $p \leq 0.05$ were considered statistically significant for all comparisons.

RESULTS

Actual durations of nebulizer treatments were timed during all periods, allowing calculation of a compliance rate of the 3-minute benchmark for the Salter 8960 Nebutech HDN treatments. Eighty-two percent of nebulized therapies with the Salter device were administered in fewer than 3 minutes whereas 18% of such treatments exceeded 3 minutes. We did not measure compliance to the 9-minute standard because in practice, the therapist may take as long as they think necessary to complete the treatment.

Table 2 shows the total procedures and times during the baseline and intervention periods. The daily procedures administered were similar in the baseline and intervention periods (33.8 [baseline] vs. 33.3 [intervention], $p = 0.679$) as was the mean daily total number of SVN treatments (11.9 [baseline] vs. 11.8 [intervention period], $p = 0.806$). However, the daily time required for RT therapies was higher in the baseline than in the intervention period (4.7 hours [baseline] vs. 3.6 hours [intervention], $p < 0.001$) due to the reduction in SVN treatment time. Also, the percent of the total respiratory therapy workload allocated to administering SVN treatments was significantly lower in the intervention than in the baseline period (16% vs. 38%, $p < 0.001$), as was the median total daily time necessary to administer SVN (1.8 hours vs. 0.6 hours, $p < 0.001$). Importantly, these time-savings were achieved with no stacking of SVN treatments observed in the intervention period.

Table 2

Data Summary for the Baseline and Intervention Periods

	Period 1			*Period 2*		
	Procedures	**Time**	**Percent of Time**	**Procedures**	**Time**	**Percent of Time**
SVN	358	54	39	353	18	17
Other ordered procedures	624	72	52	592	68	64
Optional procedures	32	13	9	54	20	19
Total	**1014**	**139**		**999**	**106**	

As shown in Table 2, the total time (for the period) available to administer "optional" or less time-sensitive respiratory therapy procedures (e.g., ambulatory desaturation measurements, patient assessments, tracheostomy care) was significantly higher in the intervention period than in the baseline period. Our main hypothesis was that the daily time saved on aerosol workload could be used to increase the time available to spend on the optional activities. This hypothesis was confirmed by the observation that the median daily time devoted to optional procedures was higher in the intervention period than the control period (0.50 hours [intervention] vs. 0.75 hours, $p < 0.039$).

No adverse events associated with nebulizer administration were observed in either baseline or intervention periods. Also, in talking with patients using the Nebutech device who had previously used conventional nebulizers, the respiratory therapists had the impression that the patients preferred the shorter treatment time. However, no formal survey instrument was administered in this study.

To further assess the impact of a shorter nebulizer administration time on global staffing and on the cost of respiratory therapy treatments, data from the follow-up period were analyzed (Table 3). The reduction of nebulization time from 9 minutes at baseline to 3 minutes using the newer device allowed a reduction in total respiratory staff required to administer ordered respiratory therapy treatments by 1.8 full-time equivalents. Assuming an average hourly salary of $21.00/hr (not counting fringe benefits) this reduction of full-time equivalents translates into a saving associated with using the faster nebulizer of $78,839.00. This savings would accrue against net increased cost for the newer nebulizer of $12,348 (4,900 nebulizers/year at $3.18/ nebulizer for the Nebutech device vs. $0.66/nebulizer for the VixOne device), suggesting a projected net yearly savings of $66,491 in using the Nebutech device.

Table 3

Data from Follow-Up Period Showing Potential Labor Savings If Standard 9-Minute Treatment Time Replaced by Hypothetical 3-Minute Treatment Time

	Standard 9-Minutes/Treatment					Reduced 3-Minutes/Treatment			
	Work (minutes)			Assign-ments		*Work minutes)*			Assign-ments
Area	Aerosol	Other	Total	(target = 300)	Area	Aerosol	Other	Total	(target = 300)
G70	18	27	45		G70	6	27	33	
G71	5	16	20		G71	2	16	17	
G81	51	79	130		G81	17	79	96	
G90	28	54	82	277	G90	9	54	63	
G91	42	50	93		G91	14	50	64	274
G110	220	283	503	596	G110	73	283	356	
G111	132	132	264		G111	44	132	176	
H50	11	51	62	326	H50	4	51	55	
H51	31	42	73		H51	10	42	52	
H60	15	46	62		H60	5	46	51	334
H61	8	14	22		H61	3	14	17	
H63	5	30	35		H63	2	30	32	
H70	10	51	61		H70	3	51	55	
H71	8	61	69	322	H71	3	61	64	
H80	66	68	134		H80	22	68	90	257
H81	69	78	147	281	H81	23	78	101	
P	0	0	0		P	0	0	0	
M50	3	6	9		M50	1	6	7	
M53	21	35	55		M53	7	35	42	
M60	24	32	55		M60	8	32	40	
M63	5	8	13		M63	2	8	9	
M71	29	16	45		M71	10	16	26	
M80	24	36	61		M80	8	36	44	
M81	1	3	4	242	M81	0	3	3	272
Total	**825**	**1218**	**2043**		**Total**	**275**	**1218**	**1493**	
	Grand Total		2043			*Grand Total*		1493	
	Required Staff		6.8			*Required Staff*		5.0	
						Potential Staff Savings		**1.8**	

DISCUSSION

The major finding of this study is that use of a device which more rapidly delivers aerosol treatments confers benefits of: reduced total time needed to administer aerosol therapies, a smaller percentage of the total time for RT therapies that was required for administering aerosol treatments, an expanded opportunity to administer other valued respiratory treatments to patients, and a reduction in necessary full-time equivalents for RTs to complete workload assignments. Furthermore, the time savings associated with more rapid nebulization offset the added expense of the newer nebulizer device, such that an annual savings of $66,491 was projected. These benefits were appreciated with no excess adverse effects of nebulized therapies and with no stacking of treatments.

Importantly, assumptions underlying our analysis warrant discussion. First, our assumption of benefit associated with using the rapid nebulizer device depends on the degree to which RTs' time would be allocated to other unmet RT needs. Also, a more detailed financial analysis of the new device would require calculating additional technical revenue related to incremental RT activities (because of greater available time) against the additional cost of the device. Because this analysis was beyond the scope of the current study, arguments in favor of the new device must be articulated in terms of enhanced efficiency and better allocation of RT services rather than in pure cost savings. However, in other settings, a reduction in workload may translate to a reduced need to hire vacant positions and thus a true cost savings.

Also, several limitations of this study warrant discussion. First, nebulization times related only to single bronchodilator treatments (e.g., albuterol alone), so that times related to neither combined drug nebulized treatments (e.g., albuterol and ipratropium) nor to nebulized antibiotic treatments were measured in this study. Based on historical data, such "complex" nebulized treatments comprise about 45% of the total nebulizer treatments. If we had extended our procedure to these complex treatments, the benefits of rapid nebulization would have been even greater.

Another limitation is that our study was conducted in only a single center, so that the generalizability of our conclusions about the workload distribution impact of more rapid nebulization can be questioned until validated by extending the study to other centers. Also, our study lacked any formal assessment of the clinical efficacy of more rapid nebulization or of patients' preferences regarding more rapid nebulization treatments. Informal queries in this study suggested patients' preferences for the shorter nebulization times, though we are also anecdotally aware that patients may also prefer their usual treatments. More formal assessment of patients' subjective experience of the Nebutech device is needed.

In summary, the current study suggests that use of devices to more rapidly deliver nebulized medications confers benefits related to enhanced RT workload distribution and potential financial savings. Our study invites further assessment to test the generalizability of these conclusions and to broaden assessment of administering nebulized treatments more rapidly (e.g., regarding patient preferences, use of combined nebulizer medications, associated clinical outcomes).

REFERENCES

1. Chatburn RL, McPeck M. A new system for understanding nebulizer performance. *Resp Care* 2007;52(8):1037–1050.

2. Hess D, Fisher D, Williams P, Pooler S, Kacmarek RM. Medication nebulizer performance. Effects of diluent volume, nebulizer flow, and nebulization brand. *Chest* 1996; 110(2):498–505.

3. Stoller JK, Mascha EJ, Kester L, Haney D. Randomized controlled trial of physician-directed versus respiratory therapy consult service-directed respiratory care to adult non-ICU inpatients. *Am J Respir Crit Care Med.* 1998 Oct;158(4):1068–1075.

4. Stoller JK, Haney D, Burkhart J, et al. Physician-ordered respiratory care vs. physician-ordered use of a respiratory therapy consult service: early experience at the Cleveland Clinic Foundation. *Resp Care* 1993;38(11):1143–1154.

Response to Reviewers

T his is the actual text of the authors' response to the reviewers' comments on the manuscript in Appendix V. The response is written to the journal editor—who serves as judge and jury—deciding if the reviewers' comments were fair, if the authors' responses were appropriate, and ultimately, if the paper should be published. Note that each comment of each reviewer is stated (for the convenience of the senior journal editor) along with the response to the comment.

Reviewer #1

1. In the methods section on the Nebutech treatment duration of 2.5 minutes, it is stated this is "based on our own observation." You need to clarify if this is the observation and capture of actual treatment times in the patient care setting or if this was an observation in a lab setting. There should be adequate information for others to duplicate your methods if desired.

   a. We modified the Methods to describe how treatment times were measured to check compliance with the protocol and to validate our bench observations of shorter treatment times. The Results section was modified to show the actual mean treatment time for a random sample of data.

2. In the results section, you indicated "we did not measure compliance to the 9-minute standard because in practice, the therapist may take as long as they think necessary to complete the treatment." Seems you should indicate that this was an existing time standard validated over the past XX years, and therefore previously validated. The existing statement can lead the reader to assume "as long as necessary" could be 2 minutes or 20 minutes . . . this is not a major issue, but a suggestion.

   a. We modified the Results as suggested.

3. Regarding the determination of the savings of 1.8 FTEs, it is important to ensure the reader understands how this was derived. Table 3 was confusing, as I was not able to see how you came up with total work minutes decreasing from 2043 to 1493 would result in a 1.8 FTE reduction. If you use the 30 day SVN count in Table 2, there are 353 treatments. Provided each treatment saves 6 minutes, which accounts for 2118 direct variable minutes saved each

month, or 436 hours per year. 436 hours per year is about 0.25 FTE. I sense I am not following the authors' logic in determination of FTE savings, and others may not as well. Considering the importance of understanding this metric, a clarification is needed.

a. Although the Methods section offered an explanation about how Table V.3 was created, we added text to the Results section to explain how to read the table: "In this table, each row represents the aerosol and other workload (in minutes) for a particular hospital ward. As described in the Methods, aerosol workload was calculated as the product of average aerosol volume (from the follow-up period) and either 9 or 3 minutes standard treatment time. The other workload was the product of average other volume and an average time for other procedures of 8.3 minutes. Then, workload for several wards was summed to provide a hypothetical assignment with a target of 300 minutes (e.g., 277 minutes for G70 through G90). Each assignment is assigned a color on the table for clarity. Note that assignments for wards G91 and G110 total 596 minutes and would be shared by two therapists. The required staff (e.g., 6.8) is simply the sum of ward total workloads divided by the ideal assignment workload of 300 minutes."

Reviewer #2

1. Page 5 para 3: The authors cite 9 minutes and 3 minutes as the administration times for the two study SVNs. Unfortunately, no methods are described for how the authors actually measured this time and the completeness of nebulization.

   a. We modified the Methods to describe how treatment times were measured to check compliance with the protocol and to validate our bench observations of shorter treatment times. The Results section was modified to show the actual mean treatment time for a random sample of data.

2. Page 6 para 3: Under results, the authors state that compliance for the alternative SVN was not measured. This is a curious omission. This information would have been very helpful.

   a. The results were modified as suggested by Reviewer #1 to state: "We did not measure compliance to the 9-minute standard because we had previously validated it with time-motion studies."

3. Page 5 para 1: The authors should explain what bronchodilators are administered three times daily. In their previous publications (references 3 and 4), they mention short acting agents such as albuterol and ipratropium. It would be surprising if they were still administering those agents, rather than longer acting agents, on a regular three times a day basis.

   a. We modified the text to read: "Nebulized treatments (3 mL unit doses of either albuterol or levalbuterol) were typically administered three times daily under a physician's order . . ."

4. Page 7 para 1: Please clarify what is meant by "stacking of treatments." Please state clearly whether therapists routinely treat one patient at a time or have multiple treatments being administered to different patients simultaneously.

   a. We modified the text as follows: "Therapists do not routinely administer multiple treatments to different patients simultaneously (i.e., stacking) but this practice has been described as occurring during times of heavy workload."

5. Discussion: The authors should acknowledge that for hospitalized patients, there are other methods to administer bronchodilators. For instance, long-acting agents can be administered by DPIs, which would save substantially more time than using SVNs and would provide longer lasting effect. There have been studies in this area which have clearly demonstrated clinically relevant benefits and cost savings.

   a. We have added this statement to the Discussion: "We acknowledge that there are other methods of delivering inhaled drugs with short treatment times, such as dry powder inhalers. However, the intent of this study was to evaluate a means of decreasing treatment times that did not involve changing physicians' ordering practice or therapists' skill set."

Reviewer #3

1. Abstract: Under Methods: "SNVs used . . ." I think you mean SVNs.
   a. Thanks for pointing out this typographical error. We have fixed it.
2. Under conclusion I am concerned with statement ". . . reduced without adverse events . . ." Since effectiveness of shorter nebulized treatments was not measured, it should be noted.
   a. The reviewer's point is fairly taken. In response, we have added this statement as a further limitation of the study: ". . . while we did not observe any adverse effects during the intervention period, the study was not designed to specifically examine the effects of a shorter treatment time."
3. Methods: Based on designed characteristics of the Nebutech nebulizer, full drug delivery occurs within approximately 2.5 minutes. Based on manufacturer's features of the Nebutech HDN 8960 nebulizer: "Nebulizes 3 cc within 7 minutes or less." It may be helpful to other clinicians who may want to implement the findings of this study to know what the average volume of medication used was for the treatments in this study. (i.e., 2cc or 2.5cc would obviously take less time to nebulize).
   a. To address the reviewer's point, we added this sentence to the Methods: "Nebulized treatments (3 mL unit doses of either albuterol or levalbuterol) were typically administered three times daily under a physician order . . ."

Index